Language Development, Differences, and Disorders

Language Development, Differences, and Disorders

A Perspective for General and Special Education Teachers and Classroom-Based Speech–Language Pathologists

Kathleen R. Fahey
and
D. Kim Reid

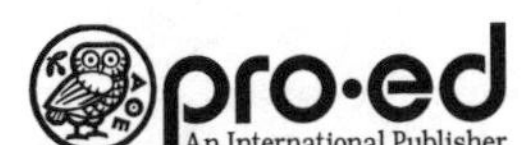

8700 Shoal Creek Boulevard
Austin, Texas 78757-6897
800/897-3202 Fax 800/397-7633
Order online at http://www.proedinc.com

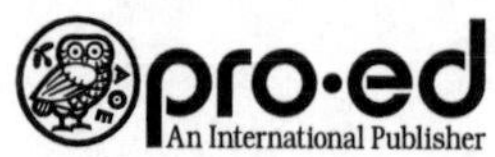

8700 Shoal Creek Boulevard
Austin, Texas 78757-6897
800/897-3202 Fax 800/397-7633
Order online at http://www.proedinc.com

Library of Congress Cataloging-in-Publication Data

Fahey, Kathleen R.
Language development, difference, and disorders : a perspective for general and special education teachers and classroom-based SLPs / Kathleen R. Fahey, D. Kim Reid.
p. cm.
Includes bibliographical references and index.
ISBN 0-89079-822-2 (hardcover)
1. Children—Language. 2. Language acquisition. 3. Language disorders in children. 4. Speech therapy for children. 5. Language arts—Remedial teaching. I. Reid, D. Kim. II. Title.
LB1139.L3F35 2000
418—dc21 99-27839
CIP

This book is designed in Goudy and Avant Garde.

Printed in the United States of America

2 3 4 5 6 7 8 9 10 03 02

To Daniel—my love and soul mate.
To John—a book for a big man. Love, Mom

Contents

Chapter 3

The Development of Oral Language 79

Kathleen R. Fahey

Chapter 4

The Development of Written Language 135

Maud Kuykendall and Kathleen R. Fahey

Part II

Language Differences

Chapter 5

Language Acquisition and Usage: Multicultural and Multilinguistic Perspectives 177

J. M. Lagrander and D. Kim Reid

Chapter 6

Ebonics and Hispanic, Asian, and Native American Dialects of English 219

D. Kim Reid

Part III

Language Disorders

Part IV

Classroom-Based Language Interventions

Preface

This book is for general education teachers, special education teachers, and speech–language pathologists (SLPs), who are increasingly being asked to collaborate with each other in providing educational opportunity and support to students with language differences and language disorders. Teachers of bilingual education and English as a Second Language (ESL) will also find the text of interest. In addition, the book is suited for use as a textbook for students in teacher education, special education, bilingual or ESL education, and speech–language pathology programs, at both the undergraduate and graduate levels.

The book is designed to allow easy access to topics that apply to individual student concerns, such as Asian and Latino culture and language, or specific language problems of students, such as those related to hearing impairment or cognitive abilities. As a textbook, it includes a wide breadth of information about language development, language difference, and language disorders, which serves as a foundation for the intervention chapters that deal with classroom-based strategies for improving oral and written language problems.

The central purpose of the book is to integrate information about language into a source that educators can use to make collaborative decisions for the benefit of children in their classrooms. Terminology is defined and an effort made to keep jargon to a minimum. In doing so, the use of language to talk about language is both clear and precise. Tables and figures are used liberally and illustrations punctuate the end of each chapter, both to entertain the reader and to take advantage of the power of figurative language to make our meanings richer.

The educational philosophy conveyed throughout the book is decidedly constructive and sociocultural. That is, the belief that students and teachers engage in supportive interactions that facilitate continued growth in language, thinking, reasoning, and problem solving underpins each chapter. This perspective pervades the discussions about language development, cultural and linguistic variations, language problems, the need for collaboration, and classroom-based assessment and intervention considerations. Students with language differences or disorders are *not* viewed as having deficiencies that are inherent within themselves. Rather, context contributes to difficulties and can be manipulated to ameliorate them. Students are viewed as capable learners who need the support and guidance of educationists (i.e., various professionals concerned with schooling) to maximize their interactions with others. Although language disorders are discussed in terms of the labels often associated with them, this is only so that we, as collaborators, can effectively dialogue about the characteristics that require our attention in assessment and intervention planning. In addition, each student and the student's parents are considered as active and collaborative members of the educational team.

The book is organized into four sections: Part I, Language Development; Part II, Language Differences; Part III, Language Disorders; and Part IV, Classroom-Based Language Interventions. Part I, Language Development, sets the tone for the necessary dialogue among general education teachers and the many others that support students with language differences and disorders, including special education teachers, SLPs, school psychologists, audiologists, and other specialists. It presents a comprehensive summary of the developmental changes in discourse, oral language systems, and written language from preschool through high school. Part I also presents a challenge to all teachers and specialists regarding the nature of the interactions in classrooms among teachers and students. Chapter 1 describes the particular discourse registers that are commonly used in school and distinguishes them from family and social discourse that children learn at home. Discussions of the patterns of school discourse include a critical review of the traditional Initiate–Respond–Evaluate (IRE) model of instruction and an argument for change to dialogic instruction that engages students in participatory interactions with teachers and peers. Chapter 2 focuses on the development of discourse, conversations, and explanations as students advance through school. The focus of Chapter 3 is on the development of the systems of oral language (i.e., articulation–phonology, morphology, syntax, semantics, pragmatics, and metalinguistics), and Chapter 4 presents the development of written language. These four chapters provide an in-depth background of the normal acquisition of language.

In Part II, two chapters focus on the language differences that teachers and specialists are likely to encounter in today's schools. In Chapter 5, language is discussed in the context of race, class, and gender. This discussion frames such differences in relation to the dominant culture and power structures (white, Eurocentric, male) that characterize U.S. society and concludes with the educational implications of such language differences. Chapter 6 includes a detailed description of several dialects of English, including Ebonics, Hispanic, Asian, and Native American influences on English. The commonalities of language dialects are presented and each is described noting historical information about the origin of people using the dialect today. The specific phonological, morphological, syntactic, and prosodic features are contrasted with Standard American English (SAE). Examples show the features of each dialect. Readers are reminded that all languages are rule governed and equally functional and that each has value and status within the culture of its users. It is the sociopolitical environment associated with education and affluence that favors SAE. Students learn SAE through immersion in natural contexts, but also require specific information about the differences and similarities between it and their languages and dialects.

Language and speech problems are the focus of Part III. Chapter 7 presents eight conditions that often include problems with the development of the oral language systems. The conditions are language and learning disabilities, central auditory processing disorders, attention-deficit/hyperactivity disorder, mental retardation, traumatic brain injury, pervasive developmental disorder and autism, fetal exposure to substance abuse, and maltreatment. Each of the conditions is described and a short case example is included to help readers see how the characteristics of problems appear in individual children. Chapter 8 is modeled after Chapter 7, providing descriptions and case examples of students with problems in speech and language associated with hearing loss and deafness, visual impairment and blindness, motor speech problems such as dysarthria and developmental apraxia of speech, cleft lip and palate, and speech production problems (i.e., articulation–phonology, stuttering, voice).

Part IV focuses on classroom-based collaboration, assessment, and interventions for students with language (oral or written), learning, or speech problems. Chapter 9 discusses the important role of collaborative relationships between general and special education teachers, SLPs, parents, and students, and presents several models of collaboration. This chapter establishes the strong commitment educationists must have in collaboration if classroom-based assessment and intervention practices are to benefit students. In Chapter 10, a description of the principles of teaching and learning within an integrated and holistic approach sets the parameters for using classroom-based assessment and intervention strategies for students with language and learning impairments. Chapter 11 discusses ways that such principles are used for assessment and intervention of students with hearing, vision, and speech problems. The discussion of classroom-based assessment and intervention for students with written language problems in Chapter 12 highlights many strategies that teachers, specialists, and parents should use to facilitate students' development of reading and writing. All of the chapters related to assessment and intervention focus on student participation, functional assessment of successes and problems that directly impact classroom learning, and interventions that develop metacognitive strategies and enable students to be successful in contextual oral and written language activities.

Acknowledgments

First, we thank Don Hammill, president and founder of PRO-ED, and James Patton, executive editor for books, for listening to our ideas for this book and supporting and guiding us throughout its development. We are privileged to have the opportunity to work with these fine professionals.

The thorough reviews, excellent suggestions, and editorial comments made by Katharine Butler and Charlann Simon greatly assisted us in the organization, content, and presentation of the information. We are very appreciative of the work each put into their reviews.

We are grateful to Ginny Helwick, Maud Kuykendall, Jay Lagrander, and Molly McCarthy Leamon, our four colleagues—all at least part-time teachers in the public schools—who co-authored chapters with us. These women worked collaboratively with each of us to provide information and insight to Chapters 4, 5, 9, and 12. They not only made scholarly contributions to the content, but kept us focused on what is relevant and useful for classroom teaching and learning.

Probably the most important intellectual influence in any professors' lives is the discussions they engage in with their students. Our students (and colleagues) in speech–language pathology and special education at the University of Northern Colorado certainly deserve our appreciation. They asked good questions, challenged our thinking, and read and critiqued drafts of several chapters while they were taking our courses. Their feedback and fond support for this project were very helpful.

Next, we need to thank our angels—the people who gave of their time and talents to assist us with the important details inherent in a document this size. Gen Guinan was invaluable in her help with computer and diskette incompatibilities, formatting documents and references, and a hundred other little things—always with a calming smile and a word of encouragement. Norma Alkire was wonderful for her cheerful assistance with printing, formatting, and the seemingly endless typing of references. Anyone who makes you tea when you arrive at their home for the fourth time on the same night is definitely an angel! Lorea Blum assisted with light editing and the construction of the table of contents. She made what for us would have been a formidable task both simple and pleasant. We are also grateful for the substantial efforts of Daniel Fahey, who designed and produced the tables and figures, and to

Thomas Balchak, who created the wonderfully pertinent illustrations for each chapter.

Our love and gratitude for their patience, encouragement, and help go to the members of our families. My husband, Dan, continuously showed his pride and enthusiasm for this endeavor. My stepchildren, Anna and Molly, were quiet and considerate when I needed to work, even during their school vacations. My parents and brothers encouraged and supported me, and my nieces and nephew allowed me to experience their language development, strengths and challenges. I am sure Kim would want me to say a word of thanks to her parents and her peripatetic son, traveling companion, and friend, John Reid-Hresko. John was very helpful in the last days of struggling to meet deadlines. He even snowproofed the boots for Lithuania!

We are also grateful for the opportunities we have had to teach and learn from students with language differences and problems and the practitioners who serve them. They are the reason for our work and for our initial choice of disciplines, which continue to be a source of discovery, pleasure, and, not least of all, our livelihoods. We hope that the information in the book we have written will lead all of us, together, to become better learners and teachers.

KRF

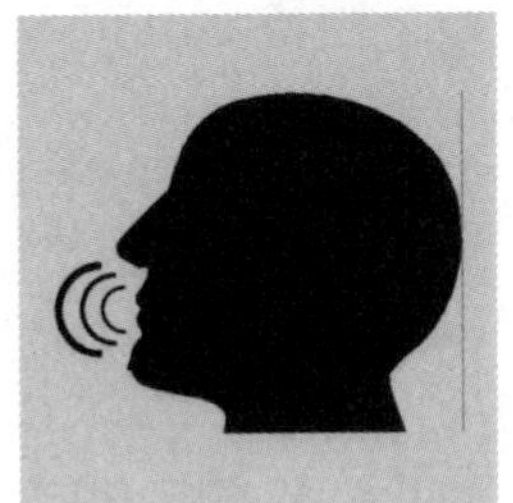

Part I

Language Development

Discourse in Classrooms

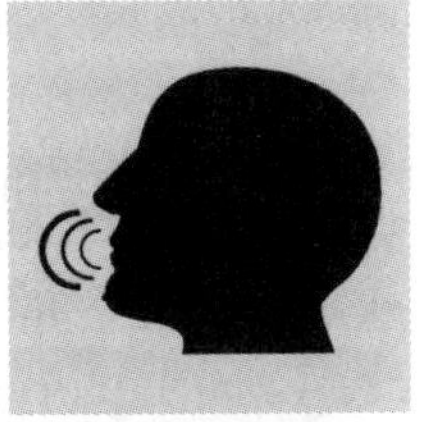

Chapter 1

D. Kim Reid

One of the most significant insights in education in recent decades is that teaching and learning are largely linguistic processes: *language is both the content of and the context for instruction*. In her landmark book on classroom discourse (i.e., units of language that are two sentences or larger), Cazden (1988) noted that mastering the content of the curriculum means mastering language—learning how to read; write; use mathematical symbols; express the concepts of social studies, science, and literature; and so forth. However, language is not only about content. It is also the means for creating the learning context. A substantial portion of students' school days are spent using language to interact with teachers and other students as well as the designated curriculum. The way particular teachers and the specific students in their classrooms use language defines the classroom environment—who can talk, about what topics, when, to whom, and under what circumstances. The language of schooling is both unique and demanding. It is substantially different from the language that is used in any other life situation—at home, on the playground, or even on the way to and from school.

Is it any wonder, then, that students' learning difficulties in school are usually associated with language functioning? Language is implicated in every special education category. Whether or not the defining problem is language disability per se, the co-occurrence of disability and language problems is strikingly high. In addition, students from groups that are not in the mainstream (i.e., the white middle and upper middle classes) of our society, especially those whose language differs in some important way from classroom requirements for language usage (e.g., language or dialect differences), are often overrepresented in special education and/or are continuously low in achievement throughout their school years, despite the fact that there is little evidence that they are actually disabled (Individuals With Disabilities Act [IDEA], 1990; IDEA Reauthorization, 1997). Because learning (and teaching too!) is a linguistic process in a specific cultural setting, language is an important predictor of school success.

Because it is not possible to understand how the mind works without understanding the culture in which it develops (Bruner, 1996), educationists (i.e., various professionals concerned with schooling) have begun a concerted effort to learn about learning and development in context, in the real world of classrooms. However, as common sense indicates, students react differently to any specific classroom environment: People are not mechanistically determined by their culture. It is as if at birth we become participants in an ongoing play (Bruner, 1990). The plot, known by the other actors, is already in progress and what the others with whom we interact say both constrains what we can say and how we can act and leads us toward an already established set of expectations. In the play of life, however, there is no script, our lines are not prescribed: we have agency and can negotiate our parts in interaction with the others. Consequently, it is the *interface* or *interaction* between individual people and their culture (the ongoing play) that enables us humans to define ourselves and to develop community.

Consequently, the emphasis in this book is on this interface or interaction. It is the perspective that will guide the study of how students engage in meaning making, especially how they use language to accomplish that task. It is useful for teachers of general or special education and for the speech–language pathologists (SLPs) who work in schools to understand how student characteristics, curricular demands, and classroom environments interact. It is important to distinguish between language differences and language disorders and to learn how to ameliorate their effects. In this text, instructional and assessment approaches are both social and holistic, but at the same time do not ignore the important subcomponents of oral and written language. The recognition of the importance of interface or interaction, two terms used interchangeably in this book, also heightens concerns for establishing classroom and professional communities and for working collaboratively within them. Finally, by acknowledging the relations between schools and the larger society and by examining the role language actually plays in classrooms, both teachers and SLPs can become more deliberate about the linguistic environments they create and, hence, become more effective practitioners.

The Politics of Language and Schooling

Wilhelm (1994) described the classroom as "the scene of a daily process of significant social negotiation in which teachers and students construct and reproduce a nation's 'preferred' knowledge, that is, those attitudes, norms, and information that legitimate existing relationships and power domains" (p. 223). Schools, then, serve as the major socializing institution of the society. As a consequence, whatever is right or wrong about our society as a whole is also right or wrong within classrooms, in the interactions between teachers and students (see Poplin, 1992).

Given our national history, it is not surprising that students with special needs and those with language differences—both groups by definition outside the norm—have typically been marginalized and isolated in schools (for in-depth treatments of this topic, see Darder, 1991; Lazerson, 1983; Macedo, 1994). The Eurocentric curriculum, for example, heroizes Christopher Columbus, Manifest Destiny, and corporate efficiency even in the poorest inner-city or reservation school without regard to the effects such conquerors, policies, and successes have had on the material existence of the children learning those lessons and their families. As a result of our desire to create an American culture, we have created schools that try to make all students conform to the culture we have inherited from our Western European ancestors. The educational system is configured to take a diverse group of students and make them fit into the one curriculum, reflecting the one dominant culture deemed by those in power to be "American" and, therefore, appropriate. The results have not always been satisfactory for our nation. For example, large numbers of students from nonmainstream families are limited in the contributions they are able to make to our society by their limited school success. By paying attention to the ways we use (and abuse) language in classrooms and by working collaboratively and pooling our collective intellectual resources, we can deliberately and systematically work to become more accepting of difference, as our democratic ideals prescribe, and to create more inclusive and more equitable opportunities for those who need them. Language and the access to knowledge it allows are undeniably political tools (Friere, 1998).[1] So, it behooves us as a nation to understand how language serves the functions of politicizing schools and how in specific contexts it operates to support or impede the learning and achievement of individual students. Consequently, this book is about what we refer to as *normal* language development and language *differences* as well as language *disorders*. Our focus is on how they affect learning and teaching.

The Three Languages of Classrooms

Cazden (1988) pointed out that when students enter school, they must learn three new and different discourses that exist simultaneously in the classroom:

[1]On January 8, 1998, for example, the Canadian government formally apologized to its Native American and Eskimo citizens for years of harmful political treatment. The government specifically mentioned the destructive nature of having sent the children of these marginalized groups to boarding schools in an effort to eradicate their languages.

the language of the curriculum, the language of control, and the language of personal identity. These different discourses are often confusing and difficult for students with language differences or language learning disabilities, largely because school personnel seldom make them explicit to students. Instead, students arrive in schools and teachers immerse them in the language of the classroom and expect them to figure out the rules. Consequently, there is a curriculum that must be mastered—that of knowing how to use these three classroom languages—that is hidden from the students; it is never discussed. Although the form of educational discourse always fits pedagogical functions, students, especially young students just entering school, seldom understand what pedagogical functions are. Instead, they often feel hurt or discouraged when disciplined for talking out or violating other unspoken rules of classroom interactional behavior.

The Language of Curriculum

Many students entering school have difficulty with the language of the curriculum. Some may not have had the kinds of preschool experiences that introduced them to the vocabulary of schooling. Words like *word*, *alphabet*, and *page* may be unfamiliar, because the children have not been read to at home. Others will not have practiced answering the types of questions that teachers ask, questions about what color things are or how many items are in a picture. Still others will speak dialects teachers find unacceptable or perhaps a different language altogether. A few will have slowed development because of hearing loss or blindness or brain injury. Some will have such limited experience with the world that they will not understand many of the concepts addressed. These groups of children will appear to be not as smart as their peers who have been read to and taught by their parents, who speak Standard American English (SAE), who have enjoyed an intact sensory system, and who have been provided a more typical range of early childhood experiences. Students with such difficulties will likely be vulnerable to failure throughout their school years (Bashir & Scavuzzo, 1992). Because so much of the curriculum is presented in language, both verbally and in writing, students with language differences and disabilities have very few other resources to rely on to help them learn.

The Language of Control

The language of control determines who talks when and under what circumstances. Cazden (1988) reported a study by the Scottish linguist Stubbs

Table 1.1
Functions of Teachers' Control Talk and Examples of Each

1. Attracting attention: Hey, you guys, wait a minute! Just listen.
2. Controlling the amount of talking: Anything else you could say about that?
3. Checking understanding: A happy what? I didn't understand you.
4. Summarizing: What I'm trying to say is that . . .
5. Defining: Can somebody tell me what that means?
6. Editing: That's getting closer.
7. Correcting: The word you wanted is *affected,* not *effected.*
8. Specifying a topic: That's a whole different ball game.

Note. Adapted from *Classroom Discourse: The Language of Teaching and Learning* (p.160), by C. B. Cazden, 1988, Portsmouth, NH: Heinemann.

who found eight different types of talk that teachers use to control the flow of activities in classrooms. They are listed in Table 1.1. These eight categories indicate that teachers orchestrate who talks, what students attend to, how long they speak, whether a given topic is sustained, and the way students think about the content. Nearly all of this orchestration is fast-paced and verbal and serves as an instructional scaffold (i.e., an instructional support that enables students to do what they could not do without help). Because control, like curriculum, is largely verbal, students with language differences and disabilities get little help to assist them in understanding what they are supposed to do, how they are supposed to think, and when they should speak. Much of the curriculum is, therefore, once again hidden from them. In addition, classroom teachers typically exercise control in a manner that maintains both distance and power—expectations of a system designed to prepare students to take their place in the larger, industrial society (although it should be noted that U.S. society is increasingly less industrial and more service oriented every year).

The Language of Personal Identity

Finally, in the classroom, students must use language to create personal identities. Cazden (1988) noted that sharing time (or show-and-tell) is important in that regard because it may be the only time for students (a) to create their own texts, that is, to decide for themselves what they will talk about and how they will talk about it; (b) to talk for an extended time; and (c) to share personal experiences. Yet, those students who need the most practice in sharing often get the least (Michaels, 1990), because teachers frequently become frustrated with the stories of students with language differences and disabilities.

Unfortunately, educationists know little about how students use language to construct personal identities, especially within classrooms. Cazden (1988) remarked that the approach to studying classroom discourse has been "colonial" in nature. Researchers have studied what is relevant to educators and other service providers, rather than looking at classroom discourse from the point of view of the students who are engaged in it.

In sum, it is clear that students with language differences and language learning disabilities have difficulties with all three languages of the classroom. Gaining access to knowledge, then, is difficult and early problems tend to be sustained and compounded as the students progress through school. Perhaps by focusing on these language problems, recognizing their importance, and working collaboratively to help students and their teachers overcome them, educationists will be able to create a different kind of learning environment, one that does not underserve students from low-status or special needs groups.

The Nature of Educational Discourse

In addition to the three languages of schooling that exist simultaneously within every classroom, there are particular *registers*, or ways of using language that differ across situations, that students are expected to use in classrooms. Within the school day, these discourse registers may vary with the particular student to whom a teacher is talking or according to the topic of study. There are differences within the language of curriculum, for example, that prescribe how students learn to talk about literature, science, and mathematics. When students read literature, they must be concerned with settings, plots, imagery, and so forth. When discussing science, they need language to propose theories; to explore their merits by asking questions and evaluating and refuting others' propositions; and, finally, to formulate and elaborate an accepted theory (Gallas, 1995). Mathematics, on the other hand, requires the manipulation of an entirely different symbol system—numerical language—as well as discussions of sets, equivalence, relationships, and so forth (Bushman, 1995). Teachers instruct students in the nuances of such discourses and hold students accountable for using them. In short, in classrooms, educators privilege the use of certain registers, as well as ways of structuring discourse, and these become the mark of the "educated" person.

The Scientific Concepts Register

Prior to entering school, most European American, middle class and upper middle class children are introduced to one of the most basic and perhaps most pervasive instructional discourse registers, the scientific concepts register, which is based on scientific concepts but not limited to science content. Their parents engage them in games and other verbal interactions that match the "hidden curriculum" typically expressed in the language used by teachers (Heath, 1983). At school entrance, most very rapidly learn to replace language that refers to experiential events with descriptions that evoke categories of specific sensory data. The following interchange, reported by Wertsch (1991, pp. 113–115), comes from a show-and-tell session in an upper middle class Chicago kindergarten.[2] T refers to the teacher, C1 to the child Danny, C2 to a different child, and so forth.

1. T:	Danny (C1), please come up here with what you have. (*C1, with a piece of lava in his hand, approaches* T.)
2. C2:	I love (*unintelligible*).
3. T:	Marissa, we're waiting for you.
4. C3:	(*Addressed to* C1) Where did you get it?
5. C1:	From my mom. My mom went to the volcano and got it.
6. T:	And you know what? You were with her.
7. C1:	No, I wasn't.
8. T:	Yes. You may have forgotten. I think you were just a little guy and you were sleeping. Mommy just told the story in the office that you were sleeping the day you went to Mt. Vesuvius to get this lava rock. Isn't that something that . . . Is there anything you want to tell about it?
9. C1:	I've had it ever since I was . . . I've always . . .
10. T:	(*In a low voice to another child*) Careful.
11. C1:	I've always been, um, taking care of it.

[2]From *Voices of the Mind: A Sociocultural Approach to Mediated Action* (pp. 113–115), by J.V. Wertsch, 1991, Cambridge, MA: Harvard University Press. Copyright 1991 by Harvard University Press. Reprinted with permission.

12. T:	Uh hum.
13. C1:	It's never fallen down and broken.
14. T:	Uh hum. Okay. Is it rough or smooth?
15. C1:	Real rough and it's . . . and it's . . . and it's sharp.
16. T:	Okay. Why don't you go around and let the children touch it. Okay? (*C1 takes it around the group, which is sitting on the floor*) Is it heavy or light?
17. C1:	It's heavy.
18. T:	It's heavy.
19. C1:	A little bit heavy.
20. T:	In fact, maybe they could touch it and hold it for a minute to see how heavy it is.
21. C4:	I didn't get a chance to hold it.
22. T:	And what do you have Lauren (C5)? You've got a . . .
23. C5:	Heather's holding this book.
24. T:	And what do you want us to find out in this?
25. C5:	There's something really neat.
26. T:	Yes?
27. C5:	(*Several children talking while C5 shows T something in the book*) . . . by your heart.
28. T:	By your heart?
29. C5:	Uh hum.
30. T:	Okay. You found something (*unintelligible*) heart. This one? Is that the picture you're interested in?
31. C4:	I'll hold.
32. C5:	Yeah.
33. T:	What does "heart" start with?

34. C5:	"H."
35. T:	"H." Okay. There she found in her dictionary a picture of the heart. And a picture of the veins and artery that lead to the heart. Okay. Did you find anything about volcanoes in here?
36. C5:	Uh. No.
37. T:	I'll bet there is under the sound for the letter "V." It's very possible. Let's see. Oh, look at this boys and girls . . . There is a volcano. It says, "an opening in the surface of the earth through which lava, gasses, and ashes are forced out. One of the most" . . . Danny . . . "one of the most active volcanoes in Hawaii." Isn't that something? Now, I wonder, should we look up lava?
38. SEVERAL CHILDREN:	Yeah, yeah, yeah.
39. T:	Okay. We want lava. Yes?
40. T:	Okay. Wow. Wait till you hear what this says. It's something to do with (*unintelligible*). It says, "Lava is melted rock that comes out of a volcano when it erupts. It is rock formed by lava that has cooled and hardened. [*sic*] So that must have been hot lava that, that came out of the volcano. Once it cooled off, it got hard and, and now it's rock.
41. C1:	And it's . . . Know what? And it's still . . . it's still . . . Look . . . Shows from where it got . . . from where it was burned.

In discussing this example, Wertsch (1991) pointed out that the way the teacher talks is very different from the way Danny talks (see also Cazden, 1988). Danny begins focusing on his experiences with the rock (see especially lines 9, 11, and 13), but very shortly the teacher begins shaping his presentation, asking him whether the rock is rough or smooth (line 14) and heavy or light (line 16). She is not only instructing him in the oppositional contrasts of rough–smooth and heavy–light, she is teaching him to describe the rock using categories that are decontextualized (i.e., they can be used to describe any rocks, not only the one Danny has)—a discourse built on scientific concepts. When the teacher suggests they look up *volcano* and *lava* in the dictionary, she moves one step further away from Danny's original experiential framework to talk about language in terms of a purely linguistic context: She is defining words in terms of other words, rather than concrete objects.

This ability to approach school assignments in terms of categories and word meanings, rather than personal experiences and objects, is crucial to school success. In the following transcript from a first-grade classroom, also taken from Wertsch (1991, p. 133), the teacher is focusing on helping the students make decisions by generating a superordinate term.

1. T: Okay. Let's turn over . . . This is fun. There's one picture in every row that does *not* belong. Which one doesn't belong in the first one? John, what doesn't belong?
2. C: Key.
3. T: Key. Put an X in the key. Why doesn't the key belong Mickey?
4. C: Umm . . . They can't open doors.
5. T: Oh . . . That's not a good answer. Why doesn't the key belong with the banana?
6. C: Because the key isn't a fruit.
7. T: Well, a ham isn't a fruit. What are all those things? Things you can . . .
8. C: Eat.
9. T: Eat. Things you can eat. You can eat a ham. You can eat a tomato. You can eat a banana. Can you eat a key?
10. C: No.

Wertsch (1991) explained that this ability to think about a problem in linguistic terms is a distinction in the behavior of schooled and unschooled persons. This distinction was first noted in 1976, in Luria's reports of his very influential study with Russian peasants. The peasants who had not attended school viewed the items they were asked to categorize as objects. A 39-year-old woman, for example, stated that there was no way to eliminate any item in a group of pictures that included a hammer, saw, hatchet, and log. When told that another person had said that the log did not belong, the woman replied that the other person must have had a lot of firewood! Schooled participants, on the other hand, assumed that what they were being asked to categorize were not the objects themselves, but rather the decontextualized word meanings represented by the pictures, that is, the superordinate terms. These transcripts of school discourse are only two examples of how instructional registers privilege scientific over everyday concepts and how much of classroom discourse is basically text referencing other texts—a far cry from the experiential education advocated by Dewey (1938/1963, 1944) and others who tried to find instructional means to link everyday and scientific concepts.

Furthermore, as mentioned earlier and as Wertsch (1991) also noted, there is a clear power differential in these types of discourse structures. Teachers direct the exchanges through the language of control: overt directives (e.g., lines 1 and 20 in the first transcription and lines 1 and 3 in the second) and questions (to which, when they are content oriented, he or she often knows the answer) that function as directives (e.g., lines 16 and 37 in the first transcription and lines 5 and 9 in the second). What the teacher wants is to regulate students' mental processing. Show-and-tell is an instructional vehicle that allows students to learn what scientific concepts are, to recognize that the scientific concepts register is privileged in school, and to adopt the new form of language usage that the teachers so carefully scaffold.

For normally developing, middle and upper middle class children, the transition from talking about everyday to scientific concepts is generally quite easy. Although students maintain the ability to use both, they recognize that the scientific concepts register is preferred in school. For others, however, adopting the scientific concepts register may be more difficult. For example, in 1972 Labov recognized that forcing some culturally different children to conform to a narrow range of linguistic and cognitive behaviors denied them the opportunity to demonstrate their actual competence. He specifically noted that it would be unlikely for the cognitive skills of many African American students to become evident when school situations differed markedly from the cultural experiences they had in their homes and communities. Heath (1982) found similar problems for the poor and working classes, Philips (1982) for Native Americans, McCullum (1989) for Hispanic Americans, and Au (1980) and Tharp and Gallimore (1988) for Hawaiian Americans. In short, the transition is likely to be difficult for any students not already immersed in a Eurocentric curriculum in their homes.

It is not, however, the mismatch between home and school language behaviors per se that causes the difficulties. It is because of the ways such differences are treated in schools (Mehan, 1984; Young, 1983) that many students from outside the white, middle class mainstream often fail in school or wind up in classes for students with special needs. As educationists, we assume that our responsibility is to teach all students, which suggests that we need to seek ways to help students cross linguistic borders. However, although language is an instructional enabler used by teachers and specialists to shape mental processing, the language of instruction and its impact have been largely ignored in most textbooks and courses about teaching methods (Reid, 1998). Consequently, how teachers use or react to language and the judgments they make about students in the process, because they are seldom thought through, may often have unintended, negative effects (Edwards, 1989; Gee, 1989b, 1990; Hymes & Cazden, 1980; Poplin, 1992, 1993; Reid & Button, 1995). One well-researched example of the kinds of problems that can arise is described in detail next.

Reteaching Narrative Structure

Michaels and Collins (Michaels, 1981, 1985, 1987, 1990; Collins & Michaels, 1986; Michaels & Collins, 1984) have described one type of problem that classroom teachers unknowingly create. They analyzed teacher–student exchanges related to the shaping of narratives during sharing time (i.e., show-and-tell), rather than varieties of classroom languages (as did Cazden, 1988) or registers (as did Wertsch, 1991). Michaels and Collins demonstrated that teachers unconsciously scaffold students into using narrative structures (at first orally and later in writing) that conform to a very specific, SAE form. Through this use of the language of control, they unknowingly do more than determine who can talk when. They also unintentionally play a causal role in the development of what may later come to be *labeled* as language or learning disorders. Michaels (1990) referred to this widespread phenomenon as the "dismantling" of narrative, because the stories the teachers tried to reshape were structured in ways the children had learned at home. Correcting such narratives, therefore, meant that the children needed to set aside their already learned narrative forms.

Related to the idea that teachers can sometimes do harm by not thinking sufficiently carefully about their language expectations and language teachings in the classroom is that many teachers think of sharing time as *noninstructional*, as a time when students talk about their experiences or describe objects they have brought from home. Michaels, like Wertsch, however, found that teachers mold the behaviors of their students during these sessions. They use language-of-control techniques such as prompting (e.g., teaching students to be lexically explicit by saying, "Tell us what that is called"), offering clarifying questions and comments (e.g., "How does it work?"), and discouraging them from assuming shared background (e.g., "Describe it for us")—note that they are simultaneously teaching students aspects of the scientific concepts register. These interventions are designed to shape the children's narratives into a form that teachers think is acceptable for school.

However, as noted, the children already know about narratives. Even very young children are familiar with narratives, because they are fundamental to all human cultures. The way they learn to frame their narratives reflects the traditions of meaning-making through talk that they learned in their families and communities. Whereas European American students tend to frame their descriptions in a given time and place and relate them in an account that has a beginning, a middle, and an ending (called a *topic-centered* narrative; see

Table 1.2

Topic-Centered Narrative by a White, Middle Class, 5-Year-Old Girl

This story was told as the girl turned book pages, pretending to be reading. It was a story about her recent birthday party.

How the Friends Got Unfriend

Once upon a time there was three boys 'n three girls

They were named Betty Lou, Pallis, and Parshin, were the girls

And Micheal, Jason, and Aaron were the boys

They were friends

The boys would play Transformers

And the girls would play Cabbage Patches

But then one day they got into a fight on who would be which team

It was a very bad fight

They were punching

And they were pulling

And they were ?banging

Then all of a sudden the sky turned dark

The rain began to fall

There was lightning going on

And they were not friends

Then um the mothers came shooting out 'n saying

"What are you punching for?

You are going to be punished for a whole year"

The end.

Note. From "Literacy, Discourse, and Linguistics: Introduction," by J. P. Gee (1989), *Journal of Education,* Boston University School of Education, *171*(1), pp. 14–15. Copyright 1989 by Trustees of Boston University and the author. Reprinted with permission.

Table 1.2), African American students (especially females) juxtapose several anecdotes thematically. Their *topic-associating* discourse is longer and shifts in time, place, and key characters (see Table 1.3). Michaels (1990) reported that teachers see it as "'rambling,' 'unplanned,' 'skipping from one thing to the next,' and as 'having no point'" (p. 311). Even though most classroom teachers have great difficulty with this structure—in part, at least, because it is a structure very few even know about—carefully detailed analyses (see Gee, 1989b) indicate that African American students often use literary devices (syntactic parallelism, repetition, word play, structural symmetry) that these same teachers admire in literary texts. Furthermore, African American adults rate these topic-associated stories very highly. Michaels argued, then, that in examining

> occurrences of narrative discourse and its transformation in school, we can see the ways that home and school worlds connect, mingle, or conflict. We can also see, over time, how certain forms of discourse, certain ways of making and displaying meaning, often nonnarrative in nature, come to be privileged, promoted, and "taken" into children's talk and writing. (p. 306)

Teachers often experience great difficulty interacting appropriately with students whose narrative forms differ from those that schools currently privilege; their attempts to teach (to correct) often interrupt or even cut off the student's story. A Catch-22 situation follows. Because teachers find it difficult to engage and collaborate with students whose discourse structures are unfamiliar (and undervalued), the students who need to be initiated into the descriptive, prose narratives that teachers are looking for seldom have an opportunity to learn how to use them. Such students are given fewer turns to talk and are interrupted so often that they seldom finish a story and, consequently, come to feel discouraged. As a result, we educationists sometimes create negative situations that perpetuate racism and classism in our schools (Hidalgo, McDowell, & Siddle, 1993; Mehan, 1992; Minami & Kennedy, 1991; Shapiro & Purpel, 1993). If we were more circumspect about our use of language in classrooms, we might easily teach students to use the language of schooling by having sharing time in which "home stories" are acceptable and appreciated, and other times, perhaps later in the school year, when "school stories," whose structure would be explicitly taught, would be required.

Formal Instructional Language in Advanced Grades

Expectations for language usage during show-and-tell exist partway between everyday language and the formal language of schooling privileged in more

(*text continues on page 20*)

Table 1.3

Topic-Associated Narrative of a 7-Year-Old African American Girl

This story was told as part of a sharing time session at school. Segments of text with a single intonational contour that indicates closure are marked with "//." Segments of text that seem to indicate that there is more to come end on a separate line with no symbol to mark them. The symbol "." indicates a break in timing. A measurable pause is marked by ". . . ". The symbol ":" is used to mark vowel elongation.

Puppy

L:a:st

last

yesterday

when

uh

m' my father

in the morning

an' he

there was a ho:ok

on the top o' the stairway

an' my father was pickin' me up

an' I got stuck on the hook

up there

an' I hadn't had breakfast

he wouldn't take me down =

until I finished a:ll my breakfast =

cause I didn't like the oatmeal either //

an' then my puppy came

he was asleep

an' he was—he was

he tried to get up

(continues)

Table 1.3 *Continued.*

an' he ripped my pa:nts
an' he dropped the oatmeal 'all over hi:m

an'
an' my father came
an' he said "did you eat all the oatmeal"
he said "where's the bo:wl" //
he said "I think the do
I said
"I think the dog . . . took it" //
"well
I think I'll have t' make another can" //

an' so I didn't leave till seven
an' I took the bus
an'
my puppy
he always be following . me
he said
uh
my father said
um
"he—you can't go //

an' he followed me all the way to the bus stop
an' I hadda go all the way back
by that time it was seven thirty //
an' then he kept followin' me back and forth =
an' I hadda keep comin' back //

(*continues*)

Table 1.3 *Continued.*

an' he always be followin' me =
when I go anywhere
he wants to go to the store
an' only he could not go t' pla:ces
whe:re
we could go
like
to:
like
t' the stores
he could go =
but he have t' be chained up

an' we took him to the emer:gency
an' see what was wro:ng with him
an' he got a sho:t
an' then he was cry:in'
an' . . . la
last yesterda:y
an'
now
they put him asleep
an'
he's still in 'e ho:spital
an' the doctor said that he hasta
he got a shot because he:
he was
he was ne:rvous
about my home that I had

(continues)

Table 1.3 *Continued.*

an' he
an' he could still stay but
he thought he wasn't gonna be a
he thought he wasn't gonna be able =
t' let him go: //

Note. From "The Narrativization of Experience in the Oral Style," by J. P. Gee, 1985, *Journal of Education,* Boston University School of Education, *167*(1), pp. 32–34. Copyright 1985 by Trustees of Boston University and the author. Reprinted with permission.

advanced grades. Wertsch (1991) pointed out that, unlike the teacher's expectations for sharing time, in formal instructional language students may not talk of events and experiences that occur outside of the classroom or of which the speaker has special, personal knowledge. This practice of excluding personal experience has the effect of grounding instructional discussions in knowledge shared by the members of the class, usually presented through texts (primarily textbooks). While teachers invite decontextualized background knowledge, they simultaneously cut off or ignore expressions of personal voice. As an example, see line 14 in the first example of classroom discourse. The following transcripts from Leamon's (1997, p. 79) study of the use of personal voice among students with special needs enrolled in a general education classroom also indicate how teachers simply cut off personal comments in favor of those that are textual, shared, and content-oriented.

T: That's Acapulco.

S: Looks like the Bahamas.

T: Yeah, it looks great doesn't it?

S: Ms. J, that looks like a hotel we stayed in.

T: Does it? (*Teacher moves on to the next picture.*)

Very soon thereafter, I [Leamon] observed a similar interaction.

T: That's Guadalajara and this is Acapulco right there.

S1: Yes.

S2: I'm going to go there in June with my uncle.

T: (*Cuts them off.*) So think how you can present this information.

Leamon noted that there were no differences in the way that the teacher treated students in general and special education. The teacher maintained a content orientation shared by all members of the class through their textbook regardless of the student's ability level, sometimes acknowledging and sometimes not the students' expression of their personal knowledge, but never encouraging it. The point was to focus on the decontextualized text: language carefully grounded in other language.

This textual nature of school discourse increases as students advance in grades. Teachers generally talk more to students but scaffold less. Classroom discourse tends toward large- or small-group interactions that require both highly developed pragmatic skills (e.g., learning how to disagree) and knowledge of the registers related to discussions of science experiments, current events, and literary analyses. Simultaneously, contextual supports (e.g., pictures in texts, graphic organizers, films, hands-on experiences) are dramatically reduced as students advance in grades. Students develop both oral and written products (e.g., reports, speeches, short stories) independently, usually using text (particularly written texts—books, the Internet, etc.) as the basis for their work.

Furthermore, the actual curriculum—as opposed to the official or intended curriculum—"consists in the meanings enacted or realized by a particular teacher and class" (Barnes, cited in Cazden, 1988, p. 2), mostly through linguistic interactions. Consequently, the linguistic environment varies from hour to hour and from teacher to teacher as students move from one subject to another. In addition, teachers make only some aspects of curriculum explicit. They make assumptions that students have already learned how to write a paragraph, for example, forgetting that the demands implicit in their assignments often call for paragraphs that are organized more complexly than many students can handle. These untaught expectations, as already noted, are considered the "hidden curriculum." But, there is also an "underground curriculum," often related to the establishment of personal identity, that occurs between and among students and is not sanctioned by the teacher. Furthermore, instruction tends to become more traditional as students reach junior high and high school. Teachers do a lot of "presenting" and infrequently allow students to engage in student–student interchanges. As the transcripts we have examined indicate, most talk, even at the elementary level, goes on between the teacher and each student one at a time. Because the language of schooling is so closely related to the development of discourse in school-aged students, we have noted many more of its characteristics in Chapter 2.

Summary

The language of schooling not only is quite different from everyday language, but is also the mark of those who are considered "educated." When they enter school, students are required to use language to think about and describe objects in ways that are specific to classrooms and to structure narratives in accordance with expectations for speakers of SAE. As they move through the grades, they learn that it is less and less acceptable to bring into the classroom their personal voice or home discourse if it differs from SAE. These characteristics of school discourse complicate learning for many students with language differences and disorders. Consequently, as educationists, we need to give these issues more critical appraisal.

Patterns of Classroom Discourse

As Cazden (1988) pointed out, one of the difficulties with the kinds of research analyzing the nature of school discourse is that the focus has been on what teachers do and what teachers intend or assume to be happening. Very little attention has been paid to the language of personal identity. Consequently, we know more about management and content than we do about the effects that such classroom discourse structures have on students' learning and motivation for learning. Some of the most recent work has begun to examine student responses.[3]

The IRE Model

The most traditional and still the most common classroom participation structure (illustrated in all of the transcripts previously examined) is the IRE model (Mehan, 1979). This structure consists of a question–answer sequence in which the teacher *Initiates* a question that is followed first by a student's *Response* and then by the teacher's carefully calibrated *Evaluation* of that

[3]Much of this and the next section is drawn from Reid (1998).

response. This pattern continues with another question, usually to a different student; the response; and yet another teacher evaluation—and so on. Teachers using the IRE model of classroom discourse, particularly at the elementary and middle school levels, most frequently ask what Heath (1982) described as "known-information" questions, those that ask students to name objects, to identify the features of things, or to describe things out of context. Most known-information questions are interrogative in form, but pragmatically directive. Although middle class parents teach their daughters and sons how to answer such questions, Heath found that low-income parents do not. Low-income parents typically use statements or imperatives, rather than questions. And when they do use questions, they often ask for comparisons or analogies. Information-seeking questions are rare. Low-income students are, therefore, put at a disadvantage in school. So are students with language differences: They use their poorest language when the classroom participation structure is tightly circumscribed (Ruiz, 1995). Likewise, students with special needs find this type of classroom interaction stressful because of its fast-paced, one-right-answer requirement for precision (students are expected to answer in the few specific words the teacher anticipates [Reid, Kurkjian, & Carruthers, 1994]) and its competitive character.

The model creates an environment in which peer–peer interactions are limited. Even when the IRE structure is used to scaffold discussions, these discussions are necessarily limited to interactions in which each student addresses the teacher. Contrast this participation structure with instructional conversations in which students talk to each other pretty much at will or with the participation structure known as *revoicing*.

Revoicing

O'Connor and Michaels (1993) illustrated the advantages of revoicing by describing a classroom lesson on ratios. Students had been asked to keep track of the proportions of sugar and lemon juice they used to make lemonade and to enter their values onto a graph. A problem arose when one student, Paula, forgot how many spoonfuls of lemon juice she used with 2 spoonfuls of sugar. The discussion was about how she should handle this situation.

The students were deciding whether it was permissible for Paula to substitute an average of the possible range (between 10 and 22 spoonfuls) or whether she needed to reconstruct the exact, original value. Sarita favored reconstruction, arguing that picking an average would not represent Paula's true solution. Ted countered that Paula probably could not reproduce her original solution, even if she tried. Steven then suggested that substituting the average would probably be a workable substitute. Lynne, the teacher, responded with the following statement (O'Connor & Michaels, 1993, p. 322):

> So then, you don't agree with Sarita that if she/
>
> picks a number halfway between/
>
> that that's not really making her first concentrate either//

In this intervention, the teacher is scaffolding not only a solution to the problem, but also a participant structure for reaching a solution that opens the floor for students to interact directly with each other. Her use of "so" indicates that her inference is warranted (i.e., a comment on issues raised in the discussion) and allows Steven to agree or not. By this means, she invites Steven to participate on an equal footing with her. (Notice that in the IRE model the teacher reserves the right to evaluate the response and leaves the student no opportunity to negotiate.) Simultaneously, she is creating the opposition between Steven and Sarita, casting them into discursive roles and inviting them to talk to each other. Finally, she has reintroduced and clarified the central content issue of the discussion—how to generate an acceptable value for the graph. Revoicing is a far more engaging and equitable participation structure than the IRE model, with the teacher still in control and still able to scaffold.

Instructional Conversations

The participatory structures previously examined, the IRE model and revoicing, are typically used with large groups, but they are also possible with small groups in which the teacher is a participant. In fact, one of the common disadvantages of educational practice is that teachers tend to use large group structures to control language in small group settings, rather than take advantage of their opportunity to teach students other participatory structures. Although instructional conversations are often modified for use with large groups (e.g., class discussions), they are more effective in small group settings.

There are at least two forms of instructional conversations. The first is a routinized set of procedures (a metascript) that can be used to deal with a variety of topics and texts. One example is Palincsar and Brown's (1984) reciprocal teaching method, in which students and the teacher take turns (a) asking questions, (b) making predictions about text, (c) clarifying whenever needed, and (d) summarizing cumulatively. The repetition of these behaviors creates a participatory framework that regulates the students' thinking as they play out their shifting roles from student to teacher to student. This form of routinized instructional conversation has many of the characteristics of control language, with one very significant difference: The students themselves, after repeated exposure to the method, learn to exercise the control (a phenomenon also related to the goals of other forms of strategy training). Reciprocal teaching has been successful in facilitating listening comprehension as well as reading comprehension and is more effective with students with language learning delays than with students who are making adequate progress in listening and reading. Student progress results from their having to make their knowledge and thinking processes, ordinarily hidden, explicit (Englert, 1992).

A second form of instructional conversation is less formal and more natural, although it is still different from conversations in other settings (e.g., instructional conversations are limited to the topic assigned, although Leamon's, 1997, work indicates that students frequently deviate from that rule). These types of exchanges are usually between or among students and are associated with forms of cooperative learning (see Dishon & O'Leary, 1994). Because they are more closely associated with everyday uses of language, they are typically used as the context for interventions for students with language disorders (Nelson, 1993; Owens, 1995). Furthermore, Ruiz (1995) found that language-diverse students blossomed during instructional conversations, because they had control over their own language structures and the ability to talk from personal experience (rather than being limited to providing information upon request). During these instructional conversations, their language became richer and more expressive and allowed them to display more highly developed cognitive and linguistic skills than participation in the IRE model permitted.

Summary

Careful analyses of the participation structures teachers create in schools—for example, the IRE model, revoicing, and instructional conversations—not only would reveal the strengths and weaknesses of our scaffolding techniques for bringing about achievement, but also would alert us to possible unintended outcomes such as the ones mentioned: disadvantaging students who are unfamiliar and unpracticed in using the particular participation structure, controlling students' responses in ways that lead to underestimation of their communicative competence and abilities, constructing power relations that establish the teacher as sole arbiter of "truth," and limiting the flow of social interactions among students. By becoming explicit in our thinking about and use of classroom interaction patterns, we can learn to use them more fairly and efficiently. Initially, we can define structures that match those that are culturally familiar to the students (see Au, 1980; Heath, 1986), while teaching them those that are unfamiliar but commonly used in schools.

Dialogic Interaction

Instructional dialogue is far better suited to enabling teachers to recognize and assess the dynamic, situation-specific behaviors and goals that occur throughout a lesson than are instructional interventions based on teacher presentations and control. By reading the constantly changing quality of students' state of knowledge through personal interactions either between themselves and students or between students and their peers, teachers have opportunities not only to offer carefully calibrated instruction but also to free themselves from rigid expectations of student behaviors. Often, teachers expect student behaviors to remain consistent across contexts and, through IRE instructional models, force them to fit these expectations. Such teachers are in danger of failing to move beyond what have become stereotyped conceptualizations of students' abilities and capabilities, especially those of students with special needs for whom highly controlled and highly contrived instruction is a common occurrence.

The Social Nature of Teaching and Learning

Reid and Leamon (1996) noted that what we have learned about the effects of various language-based, participatory frameworks in classrooms requires a reevaluation of the nature of the traditional teaching–learning interchange. Currently, many special educators and SLPs present students with simplified and isolated components of a task one at a time until each component has been learned. The assumption is that mastering the components enables students to coordinate and use them. This expectation, however, has not proven true (Brown & Campione, 1981, 1984; Gagne, 1965). Although recent texts for special educators and SLPs advocate more student initiated, socially embedded, and holistic practices (see Merritt & Culatta, 1998; Reid, Hresko, & Swanson, 1996), and procedures for average and gifted achievers have undergone significant changes in the last decade, interventions carried out by many special educators and SLPs are still entrenched in reductionist practices.

Unfortunately, many students with language differences and disorders continuously fail. Some are still practicing isolated basic skills or strategies in teacher-designed exercises during their high school years, especially in pull-out settings. Consequently, the essential nature of their schooling differs from that of their peers who are reading, writing reports, and otherwise engaging in context-embedded activities that enhance their knowledge acquisition abilities as well as their knowledge per se. Large numbers of these students drop out. Nearly all are unprepared for advanced academic or employment training. Most will say that they hate school. What they do know, they have learned outside of school and yet, ironically, having been dependent on others to structure their learning in school, few have learned how to learn independently.

A renewed interest in education among scientists in a wide array of disciplines has revitalized educational or instructional research (Bruner, 1996). Perhaps the two most important outcomes have been the pervasive, fundamental recognition that students are actively in control of what is learned and that educationists must study learning in context, the contexts created primarily through language. It is the students who give meaning to the activities in which they engage, because they spontaneously select what they will attend to, interpret what they notice, and actively seek to make sense out of information. But students' self-regulation depends on interactions with the physical and social world. A nurturant social environment can promote and provoke learning. Students learn by participating in events and activities with others, from comparing their own thoughts and solutions with those of others, from hearing arguments and perspectives of which they would not have thought, from having to explain or defend their own thinking, and from gradually adopting the ideas and strategies to which they are exposed—in short, from *engaging in activities and participating in dialogue* (Brown, Campione, Reeve, Ferrara, & Palincsar, 1991; Wansart, 1990).

Two legacies of both Piaget's and Vygotsky's work are particularly relevant to education. First is the importance of interactive, interdependent, and personalized dialogues between teacher and learner. For Piaget this dialogue occurred in the clinical method, and for Vygotsky in the zone of proximal development, which Vygotsky (1978, p. 86) defined as "the distance between the actual developmental level as determined by independent problem solving and the level of potential development as determined through problem solving under adult guidance, or in collaboration with more capable peers." A second important legacy from both Piaget and Vygotsky is the use of social interaction as a means to elevate levels of understanding (see especially Inhelder, Sinclair, & Bovet's, 1974, studies on learning, and also Forman, Minick, & Stone, 1993; Gallagher & Reid, 1983). Even with the most careful dialogic support, however, the student must still play an active role in selecting, interpreting, organizing, and reorganizing what is assimilated into background knowledge.

Wood, Bruner, and Ross (1976) were among the earliest to highlight the importance of dialogue for scaffolding instruction. As indicated earlier, scaffolding is a process of enabling students to solve a problem, achieve a goal, or carry out a task that would be beyond their ability if they were not given help. By scaffolding instruction, teachers enable students to operate within the zone of proximal development. Using several examples of classroom discussions that were collected using the reciprocal teaching metascript in which students-as-teachers summarize, question, predict, and clarify (for an example, see Table 1.4), Palincsar (1986) showed how the most effective teachers (a) are responsive to the students' contributions and comments, (b) keep the discussion focused, (c) build meaning by extending the students' current level of knowledge, (d) conduct ongoing diagnoses of the students' understanding, (e) adjust task difficulty in accordance with the students' momentary needs, and (f) give feedback and support for correct productions. This kind of interaction enables students to generate their own strategies, to express their own ideas, to relate what they are reading to their personal knowledge, and to share what they are thinking with others. This reciprocal teaching metascript and other forms of instructional conversations, therefore, invite students to develop their language of personal identity.

Duffy et al. (1987) also found that the most successful teachers did more than provide the explanations, modeling, and demonstrations characteristic of direct instruction. Throughout the lesson, they generated spontaneous explanations that were calibrated to the students' developing understandings. These qualitative differences in verbal interactions were important in creating an instructional environment that fostered achievement. Missiuna and Samuels (1989) also found this kind of dialogic—and, therefore, contingent and mediated—learning more effective with preschoolers who had language, learning, and behavioral difficulties. Other researchers have also studied the effects of dialogic instruction on content and process variables. Table 1.5 lists an illustrative, but not exhaustive, sampling of work done with students with language learning disabilities.

The Mechanisms of Change

Stone (1989, 1998; Stone & Conca, 1993; Wertsch & Stone, 1979) argued that *prolepsis* is an integral component of scaffolding, one that helps make sense of the dynamics occurring within dialogic interactions. The term refers to a speaker's assumption that a listener has some information that the speaker does not have to make explicit during communication. What remains unspoken requires the listener to construct an idea about the knowledge the speaker has

Table 1.4
Example of Effective Dialogue

READING the students' and teacher are discussing:

There are many different creatures in the sea. Many of the fish you see will be swimming in schools. They are looking for food. Most of them are friendly.

But you might see some unusual fish. You might see a big, flat fish. It looks as if it has wings. You might see a sea horse. It swims with its head up and its tail down. It carries baby sea horses in a pocket on its front.

1. T: I need someone to ask a question about the new information I just shared with you.
2. S2: How does the sea horses . . . carry their babies in their pouch?
3. T: Okay. Does someone remember the answer?
4. S5: Um, that's the only way they can carry them. They don't have any hands or anything.
5. T: Now, was he doing a little bit of predicting or figuring out how that sea horse is able to do that? Did the story really tell why they carry them in their pouches?
6. S5: Or they might drowned. They might not be able to swim and they might drowned.
7. T: You are right in all of your answers and thinking. Your question was a good question in that it got us thinking about why they did have pouches and why they carry their babies there, but, you were going a bit further than the written word. You were pretty smart to figure that out. Can anyone think of a question that they did give us the answer in the story?
8. S4: Um, what kind of animals are they?
9. S6: Um . . . sea horses.
10. T: What else did they see besides the sea horses?
11. S6: Um . . . crawfish.
12. T: See, what you might have wanted to ask, and C __ might have wanted to ask "Why were they called unusual fish or animals?" Why do they call a sea horse unusual? . . . Because they carry babies in a pouch. Most fish don't do that, right? That you could have asked using information here.
13. S3: Why do the fish go to school?
14. T: Great question. I did say that. Who could answer his question?
15. S2: Um . . . (pause) Maybe to keep safe, away . . .
16. S1: I know another way. A big pile, a school, a big pile of fish is called a school of fish.

(*continues*)

Table 1.4 *Continued.*

17.	T:	Do you think maybe R ___ wasn't quite sure what school meant in this story? Is it the kind of school that we are in? We come to school to learn, don't we? But in this story it does mean a big gathering of fish. But, I bet that they do learn how to get food, and it's also for . . .
18.	S1:	To protect them.
19.	T:	Very good. Okay, can someone summarize what we've learned in this part? What was the most important information that we've learned from this story already, M ___ ?
20.	S4:	Them going to school.
21.	T:	Who's them?
22.	S5:	The fish.
23.	T:	Do they go to school or are they living in schools? Do you think they have rooms like we do?
24.	S2:	Yeah.
25.	T:	They just gather together and that's how they make a school. And that might seem a little unusual. Now, let's see what other unusual creatures there might be. Do you know what I mean by creatures?

Note. From "The Role of Dialogue in Providing Scaffolded Instruction," by A. S. Palincsar, 1986, *Educational Psychologist, 21,* pp. 87–89. Copyright 1986 by Lawrence Erlbaum Associates. Reprinted with permission.

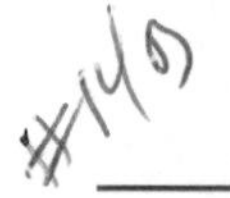

Table 1.5
Dialogic Instruction for Students with Learning Disabilities

Author(s) and Publication Date	Study Content
Burbules & Rice (1991)	Sharing different discourses
Chinn, Waggoner, Anderson, Schommer, & Wilkinson (1993)	Oral reading
Englert, Raphael, Anderson, Anthony, & Stevens (1991)	Writing
Hiebert & Wearne (1993)	Mathematics
Nieto (1994)	Promoting critical reflection
Perl (1994)	Fostering the growth of the self
Scruggs, Mastropieri, Bakken, & Brigham (1993)	Science instruction

taken for granted. If the speaker is more knowledgeable than the listener or if the ideas present a challenge, the act of constructing the speaker's message is very likely to lead to cognitive growth.

One of the best ways to support dialogic instruction is through instructional conversations. Contrary to what most of us believe, numerous researchers (e.g., Doise, Mugny, & Perret-Clermont, 1975; Forman & McPhail, 1993; Schunk, 1989) have demonstrated that a superior model is not necessary to progress in learning. For example, in cooperative learning settings in which students share responsibility for task completion, students with learning disabilities benefit most from student models who are similar or only slightly better in competence (see Forman & McPhail, 1993; Shunk, 1989). Furthermore, Shunk also found that having more than one model is only as effective as having a single model if that single model is also coping with the task. However, having multiple models is more effective than a single model who has already mastered the task, even if that model is the teacher! Schunk explained this finding by suggesting that students with learning disabilities do not think that they can attain a teacher's level of competence. It is also possible that the facilitative effect is related to similar, and therefore comprehensible, levels and strategies for information processing (Reid, 1989).

In a somewhat older but still very important study, Doise et al. (1975) found that groups achieve levels of performance that are superior to and cannot be accounted for by the performance of even the most advanced member. These sociologists explained that, in group efforts, one student's comments force the others to notice aspects of the problem under study that might have otherwise gone unnoticed. Then group members need to coordinate disparate points of view. Doise et al. referred to this phenomenon as a "conflict of communication," a mechanism that resembles prolepsis, but that also creates a contradiction (Piaget, 1977)—both of which require efforts at understanding. These studies suggest that learning is promoted by the social interaction itself and not, as some have suggested, by the copying of a model's performance.

Summary and Conclusions

Classroom discourse is the single most important variable in creating the classroom environment and, consequently, in students' school success. Despite official curriculum guides and interventionists' intentions, the actual curriculum is mutually created within the confines of the classroom by teachers, their students, and other members of the instructional team. What happens in classrooms is a function of attitudes and expectations that are often unarticulated, but that interact with and modify the culturally instantiated traditions with which students come to school. It is important to honor these traditions as educators inculcate "schooled" ways of using language. Both verbal and non-verbal communications can be used to build bridges from what students know to what they do not yet know.

The collaborative approach to assessment and intervention represents one of our best hopes for getting past the Catch-22 of not knowing how to interact appropriately with students whose cultural traditions vary from those of the mainstream and for designing appropriate instruction for students who are having genuine difficulties with language usage and development. As a group of professionals conscious of the disparity in students' home experiences and knowledgeable about a broad range of academic contents and strategies, the instructional team can collectively generate approaches to instruction that avoid unfair or ineffective practices. Having a variety of specialists (i.e., SLPs, special education teachers, bilingual teachers, or ESL teachers) jointly plan, instruct, and evaluate interventions moves the focus from lessons to students—where it belongs. The classroom teacher cannot possibly address the individual needs of a heterogeneous group of students. A team can. As language demands become increasingly decontextualized and complex, team members can provide supports and modify assignments that will enable all students to be challenged appropriately.

Clearly the essential character of teaching is changing. Teachers and specialists are no longer all-knowing dispensers of knowledge. They are instead "respected authorities" (Palincsar, 1986) who help students "exercise cognitive activities that are just emerging" (Brown et al., 1991) by asking leading questions, providing explanations, challenging responses, providing examples, and stirring up opposing viewpoints (Gallagher & Reid, 1983). To the extent that they are needed, teachers and specialists participate in joint problem-solving activities, scaffolding student behaviors with the goal of improving students' levels of participation until they become independent.

The research on dialogue tells us that teachers need to listen more carefully to what students say, to welcome their participation, and to use attempts at making sense and solving problems to diagnose students' shifting mental representations of the task. Teachers' verbalizations need to be responsive to the students' needs as they change over time. Students, therefore, need to talk as much as or perhaps even more than teachers (Mariage, 1995).

The cooperative learning research reveals that teacher–student interactions may be far less important than we have assumed, and that student–student interactions have a greater impact on social development and academic achievement (Johnson, 1980). The most common of these instructional arrangements include peer tutoring, traditional cooperative learning (students working together to attain a common goal, often by taking responsibility for different aspects of the task), and methods of interactive teaching (students and teachers participate as group members who perform instructional tasks jointly, as in reciprocal teaching). The teacher's role is to foster collaboration (rather than to make comparative judgments concerning students' progress and abilities), to scaffold, and to manage the establishment and operations of the groups. Collaborative learning environments, "through a nexus of social support, shared goals, modeling and incidental instruction, awaken new levels of competence in young" (Brown & Palincsar, 1989).

AND PERSONIFICATION IS A FORM OF INDIRECT COMPARISON...
IN WHICH HUMAN QUALITIES ARE...
•SIMILE
• METAPHOR
T.M. BALCHAK
9/98

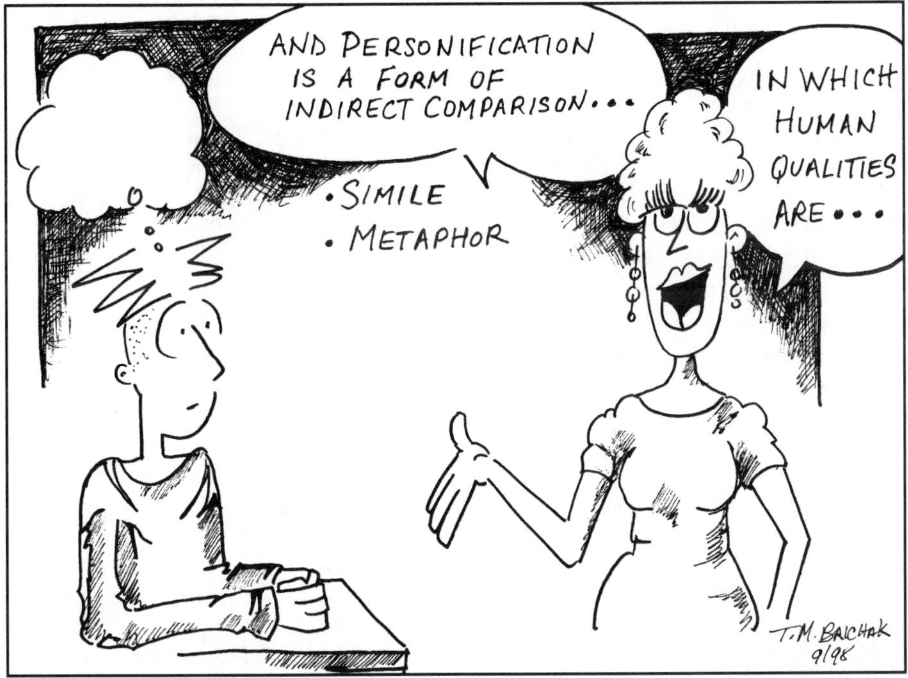

One of the most significant insights in education in recent decades is that teaching and learning are largely linguistic processes: Language is both the content of and the context for instruction.

References

Au, K. (1980). Participation structures in a reading lesson with Hawaiian children. *Anthropology and Education Quarterly, 11*, 91–115.

Bashir, A. S., & Scavuzzo, A. (1992). Children with language disorders: Natural history and academic success. *Journal of Learning Disabilities, 25*(1), 53–65.

Brown, A. L., & Campione, J. C. (1981). Inducing flexible thinking: The problem of access. In M. Friedman, J. P. Das, & N. O'Connor (Eds.), *Intelligence and learning* (pp. 515–530). New York: Plenum Press.

Brown, A. L., & Campione, J. C. (1984). Three faces of transfer: Implications for early competence, individual differences, and instruction. In M. Lamb, A. Brown, & B. Rogoff (Eds.), *Advances in developmental psychology* (Vol. 3, pp. 143–192). Hillsdale, NJ: Erlbaum.

Brown, A. L., Campione, J. C., Reeve, R. A., Ferrara, R. A., & Palincsar, A. S. (1991). Interactive learning, individual understanding: The case of reading and mathematics. In L. T. Landsman (Ed.), *Culture, schooling, and psychological development* (pp. 136–170). Hillsdale, NJ: Erlbaum.

Brown, A. L., & Palincsar, A. S. (1989). Guided cooperative learning and individual knowledge acquisition. In L. B. Resnick (Ed.), *Knowing, learning, and instruction: Essays in honor of Robert Glaser* (pp. 393–451). Hillsdale, NJ: Erlbaum.

Bruner, J. (1990). *Acts of meaning*. Cambridge, MA: Harvard University Press.

Bruner, J. (1996). *The culture of education*. Cambridge, MA: Harvard University Press.

Burbules, N. C., & Rice, S. (1991). Dialogue across differences: Continuing the conversation. *Harvard Educational Review, 61*, 393–416.

Bushman, L. (1995). Communicating in the language of mathematics. *Teaching Children Mathematics, 30*(2), 324–329.

Cazden, C. B. (1988). *Classroom discourse: The language of teaching and learning*. Portsmouth, NH: Heinemann.

Chinn, C. A., Waggoner, M. A., Anderson, R. C., Schommer, M., & Wilkinson, I. A. G. (1993). Situated actions during reading lessons: A microanalysis of oral reading error episodes. *American Educational Research Journal, 30*(2), 361–392.

Collins, J., & Michaels, S. (1986). Discourse and the acquisition of literacy. In J. Cook-Gumpertz (Ed.), *The social construction of literacy* (pp. 207–222). New York: Cambridge University Press.

Darder, A. (1991). *Culture and power in the classroom: A critical foundation for bicultural education*. Westport, CT: Bergin & Garvey.

Dewey, J. (1938/1963). *Experience and education*. New York: Macmillan.

Dewey, J. (1944). *Democracy and education*. New York: Free Press.

Dishon, D., & O'Leary, P. W. (1994). A *guidebook for cooperative learning: A technique for creating more effective schools* (2nd ed.). Holmes Beach, FL: Learning Publications.

Doise, W., Mugny, G., & Perret-Clermont, A. N. (1975). Social interaction and the development of cognitive operations. *European Journal of Social Psychology, 5*, 367–383.

Duffy, G. G., Roehler, L. R., Sivan, E., Rackliffe, G., Book, C., Meloth, M. S., Vavrus, L. G., Wesselman, R., Putman, J., & Bassiri, D. (1987). The effects of explaining the reasoning associated with using reading strategies. *Reading Research Quarterly, 22*, 347–368.

Edwards, J. R. (1989). *Language and disadvantage* (2nd ed.). London: Whurr.

Englert, C. S. (1992). Writing instruction from a sociocultural perspective: The holistic, dialogic, and social enterprise of writing. *Journal of Learning Disabilities, 25*(6), 153–172.

Englert, C. S., Raphael, T. E., Anderson, L. M., Anthony, H. M., & Stevens, D. D. (1991). Making strategies and self-talk visible: Writing instruction in regular and special education classrooms. *American Educational Research Journal, 28*(2), 337–372.

Forman, E. A., & McPhail, J. (1993). Vygotskian perspectives on children's collaborative problem-solving activities. In E. A. Forman, N. Minick, & C. Addison Stone (Eds.), *Contexts for learning: Sociocultural dynamics in children's development* (pp. 213–229). New York: Oxford University Press.

Forman, E. A., Minick, N., & Stone, C. A. (Eds.). (1993). *Contexts for learning: Sociocultural dynamics in children's development* (pp. 213–229). New York: Oxford University Press.

Friere, P. (1998). *Teachers as cultural workers: Letters to those who dare teach*. Boulder, CO: Westview Press.

Gagne, R. M. (1965). *The conditions of learning*. New York: Holt, Rinehart and Winston.

Gallagher, J. M., & Reid, D. K. (1983). *The learning theory of Piaget and Inhelder*. Austin, TX: PRO-ED.

Gallas, K. (1995). *Talking their way into science: Hearing children's questions and theories, responding with curricula*. New York: Teachers College Press.

Gee, J. (1985). The narrativization of experience in the oral style. *Journal of Education, 167*(1), 9–35.

Gee, J. P. (1989a). Literacy, discourse, and linguistics: Introduction. *Journal of Education, 171*(1), 5–19.

Gee, J. P. (1989b). Two styles of narrative construction and their linguistic and educational implications. *Discourse Processes, 12*, 287–307.

Gee, J. P. (1990). *Social linguistics and literacies: Ideology in discourse*. Bristol, PA: Falmer Press.

Heath, S. B. (1982). Questioning at home and at school: A comparative study. In G. D. Spindler (Ed.), *Doing the ethnography of schooling*. New York: Holt, Rinehart and Winston.

Heath, S. B. (1983). *Ways with words: Language, life, and work in communities and classrooms*. Cambridge, England: Cambridge University Press.

Heath, S. B. (1986). Sociocultural contexts of language development. In *Beyond language: Social and cultural factors in schooling language minority students* (pp. 143–186). Los Angeles: California State University, Evaluation, Dissemination and Assessment Center.

Hidalgo, N. M., McDowell, C. L., & Siddle, E. V. (1993). *Facing racism in education* (Reprint Series No. 21). Cambridge, MA: Harvard Educational Review.

Hiebert, J., & Wearne, D. (1993). Instructional tasks, classroom discourse, and students' learning in second-grade arithmetic. *American Educational Research Journal, 30*(2), 393–425.

Hymes, D., & Cazden, C. (1980). Narrative thinking and story-telling rights: A folklorist's clue to a critique of education. In D. Hymes (Ed.), *Language in education: Ethnolinguistic essays* (pp. 126–138). Washington, DC: Center for Applied Linguistics.

Individuals with Disabilities Education Act of 1990, 20 U.S.C. § 1400 *et seq*.

Individuals with Disabilities Education Act Reauthorization of 1997, 20 U.S.C. § 1400 *et seq*.

Inhelder, B., Sinclair, M., & Bovet, M. (1974). *Learning and the development of cognition*. Cambridge, MA: Harvard University Press.

Johnson, D. W. (1980). Group processes: Influences of student–student interaction on school outcomes. In J. H. McMillan (Ed.), *The social psychology of school learning* (pp. 123–168). New York: Academic Press.

Labov, W. (1972). *Sociolinguistic patterns*. Philadelphia: University of Pennsylvania Press.

Lazerson, M. (1983). The origins of special education. In J. G. Chambers & W. T. Hartman (Eds.), *Special education policies: Their history, implementation, and finance* (pp. 15–47). Philadelphia: Temple University Press.

Leamon, M. M. (1997). *An ethnographic study of narrative voice, institutional canon and discourse in middle school students in an urban school*. Unpublished doctoral dissertation, University of Northern Colorado, Greeley.

Luria, A. R. (1976). *Cognitive development: Its cultural and social foundations*. Cambridge, MA: Harvard University Press.

Macedo, D. (1994). *Literacies of power: What Americans are not allowed to know*. Boulder, CO: Westview Press.

Mariage, T. V. (1995). Why students learn: The nature of teacher talk during reading. *Learning Disability Quarterly, 18*, 214–234.

McCullum, P. (1989). Turn-allocation in lessons with North American and Puerto Rican students. *Anthropology and Education Quarterly, 20*, 133–156.

Mehan, H. (1979). *Learning lessons*. Cambridge, MA: Harvard University Press.

Mehan, H. (1984). Language and schooling. *Sociology of Education, 57*, 174–183.

Mehan, H. (1992). Understanding inequality in schools: The contribution of interpretive studies. *Sociology of Education, 65*, 1–20.

Merritt, D. D., & Culatta, B. (1998). *Language intervention in the classroom*. San Diego, CA: Singular.

Michaels, S. (1981). "Sharing time": Children's narrative styles and differential access to literacy. *Language in Society, 10*, 423–442.

Michaels, S. (1985). Hearing the connections in children's oral and written discourse. *Journal of Education, 167*, 36–56.

Michaels, S. (1987). Text and context: A new approach to the study of classroom writing. *Discourse Processes, 10*, 321–346.

Michaels, S. (1990). The dismantling of narrative. In A. McCabe & C. Peterson (Eds.), *Developing narrative structure* (pp. 303–351). Hillsdale, NJ: Erlbaum.

Michaels, S., & Collins, J. (1984). Oral discourse styles: Classroom interaction and the acquisition of literacy. In D. Tannen (Ed.), *Coherence in spoken and written discourse* (pp. 219–244). Norwood, NJ: Ablex.

Minami, M., & Kennedy, B. P. (1991). *Language issues in literacy and bilingual/multicultural education* (Reprint Series No. 22). Cambridge, MA: Harvard University Press.

Missiuna, C., & Samuels, M. T. (1989). Dynamic assessment of preschool children with special needs: Comparison of mediation and instruction. *Remedial and Special Education, 10*, 53–62.

Nelson, N. W. (1993). *Childhood language disorders in context: Infancy through adolescence*. New York: Macmillan.

Nieto, S. (1994). Lessons from students on creating a chance to dream. *Harvard Educational Review, 64*, 392–426.

O'Connor, M. C., & Michaels, S. (1993). Aligning academic task and participation status through revoicing: Analysis of a classroom discourse strategy. *Anthropology and Education Quarterly, 24*, 318–335.

Owens, R. E. (1995). *Language disorders: A functional approach to assessment and intervention*. Needham Heights, MA: Allyn & Bacon.

Palincsar, A. S. (1986). The role of dialogue in providing scaffolded instruction. *Educational Psychologist, 21*, 73–98.

Palincsar, A. S., & Brown, A. L. (1984). Reciprocal teaching of comprehension-fostering and comprehension-monitoring activities. *Cognition and Instruction*, *1*, 117–175.

Perl, S. (1994). Teaching and practice: Composing texts, composing lives. *Harvard Educational Review*, *64*, 427–449.

Philips, S. (1982). *The invisible culture: Communication in classroom and community on the Warm-springs Indian Reservation*. New York: Longman.

Piaget, J. (1977). *The development of thought: Equilibration of cognitive structures* (A. Rosin, Trans.). New York: Viking Penguin. (Original French edition published 1975)

Poplin, M. (1992). Educating in diversity. *Educating for Results*, *14*, 18–24.

Poplin, M. S. (1993). Making our whole language bilingual classrooms also liberatory. In J. U. Tinejero & A. F. Ada (Eds.), *The power of two languages: Literacy and biliteracy* (pp. 126–150). New York: Macmillan/McGraw-Hill.

Reid, D. K. (1989). The role of cooperative learning in comprehensive instruction. *Journal of Reading, Writing, and Learning Disabilities—International*, *4*, 229–242.

Reid, D. K. (1998). Scaffolding: A broader view. *Journal of Learning Disabilities*, *31*, 386–396.

Reid, D. K., & Button, L. (1995). Anna's story: Narratives of personal experience about being labeled learning disabled. *Journal of Learning Disabilities*, *28*, 602–614. Reprinted in M. S. Poplin & P. T. Cousin (Eds.). (1996). *Alternative views of learning disabilities* (pp. 333–356). Austin, TX: PRO-ED.

Reid, D. K., Hresko, W. P., & Swanson, H. L. (1996). *Cognitive approaches to learning disabilities* (3rd ed.). Austin, TX: PRO-ED.

Reid, D. K., Kurkjian, C., & Carruthers, S. S. (1994). Special education teachers interpret constructivist teaching. *Remedial and Special Education*, *15*, 267–280.

Reid, D. K., & Leamon, M. M. (1996). The cognitive curriculum. In D. K. Reid, W. P. Hresko, & H. L. Swanson (Eds.). *Cognitive approaches to learning disabilities* (pp. 401–432). Austin: TX: PRO-ED.

Ruiz, N. (1995). The social construction of ability and disability: II. Optimal and at-risk lessons in a bilingual special education classroom. *Journal of Learning Disabilities*, *28*, 491–502.

Schunk, D. H. (1989). Self-efficacy and cognitive achievement: Implications for students with learning problems. *Journal of Learning Disabilities*, *23*, 14–22.

Scruggs, T. E., Mastropieri, M. A., Bakken, J. P., & Brigham, F. J. (1993). Reading versus doing: The relative effects of textbook-based and inquiry-oriented approaches to science learning in special education classrooms. *Journal of Special Education*, *27*(1), 1–15.

Shapiro, H. S., & Purpel, D. E. (Eds.). (1993). *Critical social issues in American education: Toward the 21st century*. New York: Longman.

Stone, C. A. (1989). Improving the effectiveness of strategy instruction for the learning disabled: The role of communicational dynamics. *Remedial and Special Education*, *12*, 35–42.

Stone, C. A. (1998). The metaphor of scaffolding: Its utility for the field of learning disabilities. *Journal of Learning Disabilities*, *31*, 344–364.

Stone, C. A., & Conca, L. (1993). A social constructivist perspective on the nature and origins of strategy deficiencies in learning-disabled children. In L. Meltzer (Ed.), *Cognitive, linguistic and developmental perspectives on learning disorders* (pp. 23–60). Austin, TX: PRO-ED.

Tharp, R. G., & Gallimore, R. (1988). *Rousing minds to life: Teaching, learning, and schooling in social context*. New York: Cambridge University Press.

Vygotsky, L. S. (1978). *Mind in society: The development of higher psychological processes* (M. Cole, V. John-Steiner, S. Scribner, & E. Soulserman, Eds. and Trans.). Cambridge, MA: Harvard University Press.

Wansart, W. L. (1990). Developing metacognition through collaborative problem solving in a writing process classroom. *Journal of Learning Disabilities*, *23*, 164–170.

Wertsch, J. V. (1991). *Voices of the mind: A sociocultural approach to mediated action*. Cambridge, MA: Harvard University Press.

Wertsch, J. V., & Stone, C. A. (1979, October). *A social interactional analysis of learning disabilities remediation*. Paper presented at the International Conference of the Association for Children with Learning Disabilities, San Francisco.

Wilhelm, R. (1994). Exploring the practice–rhetoric gap: Current curriculum for African-American history month in some Texas elementary schools. *Journal of Curriculum and Supervision*, *9*, 217–233.

Wood, P., Bruner, J., & Ross, G. (1976). The role of tutoring in problem solving. *Journal of Child Psychology and Psychiatry*, *17*, 89–100.

Young, R. (1983). A school communication-deficit hypothesis of educational disadvantage. *Australian Journal of Education*, *27*, 3–15.

The Development of Discourse: Conversations, Stories, and Explanations

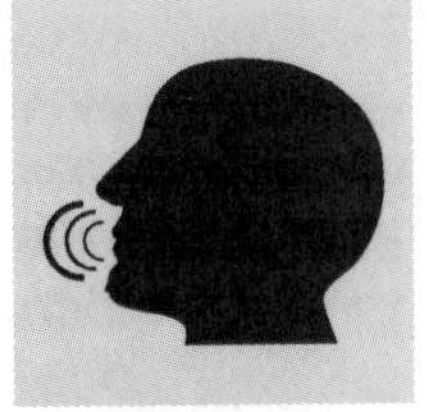

Chapter 2

D. Kim Reid

As the language samples in Chapter 1 made clear, when we communicate in schools (or outside them), we seldom use only individual letter sounds, syllables, or even single words. Instead, we communicate using chunks of utterances, usually groups of organized sentences. Also as noted earlier, we use the term *discourse* to refer to two or more oral or written, organized sentences. The three most common types of discourse are *conversation*, *narrative* (another word for story), and *exposition* (a term that refers to the setting forth of facts and ideas, such as explanations and definitions).[1] Each of these different discourse types has its own rules for combining sentences. For example, in Standard American English (SAE) (other dialects may differ) conversation requires taking turns talking about a specific topic; stories require a beginning, middle, and end; and exposition uses topic and detail-containing sentences. It is our knowledge of the way different discourses are structured that makes us part of a linguistic community whose members are able to discern and create a wide variety of discourse types (also called *genres*) and to use that structural information as an aid to comprehension and recall, especially when the content is somewhat unfamiliar (Roller, 1990).

Each discourse genre exists in both spoken and written language. Conversation is typically oral, but it can also be written—the informal, talk-like style of a friendly letter is a good example. Stories also may be either oral or written, and the same is true of expository texts (lectures are good examples of spoken, expository texts). In most schools, however, we put little or no emphasis on teaching oral discourse. Instead, we put our resources, with the exception of some speech or public speaking classes, into teaching written language, often

[1]These are only the most common. According to Faigley, Cherry, Jolliffe, and Skinner (1985), in the field of rhetoric, discourse is divided into narration, description, argument, and exposition.

referred to as *literacy*. What we have failed to recognize is that "oral language is as much a part of literacy learning and acquisition as written language" (Wallach & Butler, 1994, p. 5).

Being literate means being able to participate fully in our communities (Gee, 1990), and that means being able to traverse the oral-literate continuum in both spoken and written language. We tend to use an informal, clause-follows-clause oral style (e.g., "Maria left the office and then she went home right away because she wanted to talk to her daughter") when we share a context with our audience and a more formal, more syntactically complex and embedded literate style (e.g., "Maria, who wanted to talk to her daughter, went directly home from the office") when the topic is decontextualized (Halliday, 1987). Consequently, whether we use an oral or a literate style depends on the situation, our purpose, and our audience (e.g., chatting with a friend or giving testimony in court), not on whether we are writing or speaking. Oral-literate style may also vary with text genre—conversational, narrative, or expository.

In addition to using the term discourse to refer to structured texts, we also use it to refer to language that is associated with a particular culture, setting, or discipline. Chapter 1 addressed classroom discourse, but there are other kinds of discourse. For example, we use *dominant discourse* to refer to the way language is used by any sociopolitical group in a position to say what is right and what is not about language usage (e.g., SAE). Other terms, such as *banking discourse*, *home discourse*, *religious discourse*, and *medical discourse*, refer to the limited range of acceptable language structures and the specialized vocabulary that is used in banks, homes, churches, professions, and so on. Obviously, discourses are culturally based phenomena that carry all sorts of social and political overtones.

Children, too, must learn to create different types of spoken and written discourses that are consistent with the expectations of various language communities. Furthermore, children whose home discourse is other than SAE must learn that dominant discourse as well, if they are to have access to the goods and services of our society (Gee, 1990). Also, all children must learn to shift among the situation-specific discourses related to institutions, disciplines, and the major text genre.

Within the last decade, language professionals have begun to turn their attention to learning to foster and evaluate discourse development, primarily in the context of the child's home language (Westby, 1994). This chapter will focus on the development of the three types of discourse mentioned previously—conversation, narrative, and exposition. For nearly all children, the learning of conversational techniques begins practically at birth and narrative structure well before school entrance, but for many children, all but the most cursory forms of exposition await instruction in school.

Learning To Engage in Conversation

Conversation, the use of language for direct social interaction, has traditionally been thought to be the primary context for language learning (N. Nelson, 1993) and one that largely develops before schooling begins. Conversation seems easy to those of us who have been engaging in it for years, but in fact successful conversation requires quite a bit of knowledge about adapting language to various speakers and contexts (see Table 2.1) and integrating that knowledge with the rules for morphology, syntax, semantics, and so on (these terms are explained in Chapter 3). Even making a simple request necessitates (a) getting attention, (b) being clear, (c) maintaining a positive social

Table 2.1
Pragmatic Abilities Needed for Conversation

1. Selection, introduction, maintenance, and change of topic
2. Turn-taking functions
   - Initiating dialogue
   - Responding in a contingent way
   - Repairing/revising what was unclear
   - Pausing appropriately
   - Dealing with interruptions and overlaps
   - Giving feedback to the speaker
   - Maintaining concise, high-quality communication
3. Selection of precise, accurate vocabulary and the maintenance of cohesion across contexts
4. Variation of style to meet the needs of the listener
5. Monitoring intelligibility, vocal quality and intensity, prosody, and fluency
6. Judgment of nonverbal situational aspects
   - Physical proximity
   - Physical contacts
   - Body posture and movements
   - Gestures
   - Facial expression
   - Eye gaze

Note. Adapted from "A Clinical Approach to the Pragmatic Aspects of Language," by C. A. Prutting and D. M. Kirchner, 1987, *Journal of Speech and Hearing Disorders, 52,* pp. 105–119.

relationship, (d) being persuasive, and (e) making repairs when something has been misunderstood (Ervin-Tripp & Gordon, 1986).

Rubin (1990) noted that one way to characterize conversational talk is to recognize that it involves ever-widening circles of participants (Figure 2.1). At the center of the circles is talking with oneself, often referred to as *inner speech*. According to Vygotsky (1987), inner speech emerges at about age 7 and is essentially *dialogic:* in inner speech, children converse with themselves exactly as they had once conversed with others—they simply internalize the dialogue. The purpose of this kind of speech is to make conscious and regulate one's own behavior. People often use inner speech to keep track of themselves when they are trying to solve problems, to help them figure out what to do next, and so on. Inner speech is, therefore, very important to learning and has been used as an instructional tool in therapy (Meichenbaum, 1977) and in strategy training programs (Graham & Harris, 1993; Harris & Graham, 1992, 1996) for students with special needs.

The next larger ring of the conversational circle is usually known as *conversation* and includes talking to one or two other persons. Sometimes one-to-one

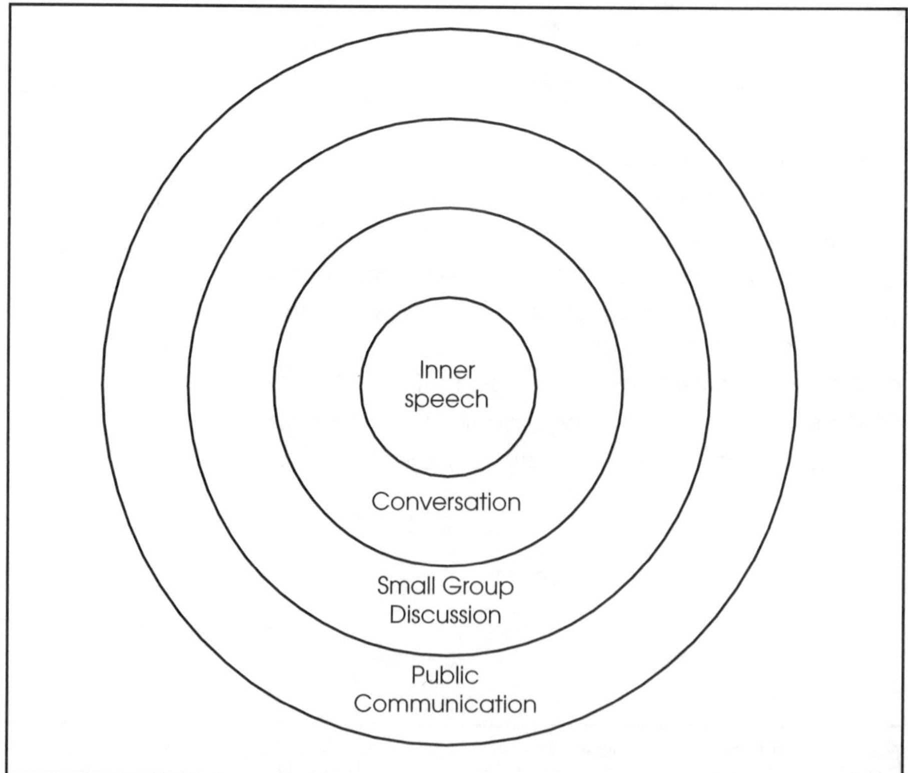

Figure 2.1. Conversational circles.

conversations take on a specific purpose and format, for example, that of an interview. The next larger ring includes conversations among four or more people, usually referred to as *small group discussions*. When we participate in still larger groups, the format of the interchange usually changes dramatically from one of more or less democratic turn-taking to one of inequality between the role of the speaker and that of the listeners—no longer conversational partners. Rubin calls this large-group format *public communication*. Most traditional classrooms rely on public communication models, such as the IRE (Initiate–Respond–Evaluate) model discussed in Chapter 1.

Because conversational abilities develop early and are universal, we sometimes fail to appreciate how complex they are and what a great achievement for growing children their mastery really is. Consequently, in the following text, I examine conversational abilities as normally developing people acquire them. Knowing about the normal course of development will prove useful when trying to understand the difficulties students with special needs experience in relation to discourse.

The Preschool Years

Owens (1984) summarized the work of researchers such as Bruner and his colleagues (1975, 1978; Ninio & Bruner, 1978), who have given us keen insight into the way infants learn to engage in conversation. Adults do very little direct, intentional language teaching. During the first 2 years of an infant's life, however, adults spontaneously model, cue, and prompt language behaviors in the natural course of caregiving. The style of language used by people who speak SAE (Crago, 1992) to interact with infants is so distinct that it has a name of its own, *motherese*, although it is characteristic of interactions with infants by all SAE speakers, not only mothers. Motherese tends to be high-pitched and slowed speech with exaggerated stress and intonation, basically "sing-songy." Relatively few words are used in short sentences (50% are single-word sentences) with long pauses after content words. Nearly 60% of these sentences are commands or questions.

Virtually from the moment of birth, mothers (and other caregivers) treat newborns as if they are already social beings, as if they already know how to participate in conversation. In fact, whether the mother is saying something like, "How are you?" or "Kutchi, kutchi, koo," she waits exactly the amount of time that adults in that culture pause for turn-taking before she says something else in her one-person "dialogue"—as did this mother in the following interchange with her infant:

MOTHER: Let's clean you up!

Turn-taking pause, during which time mother maintains eye contact with the baby.

MOTHER: Get this wet bib off.

Baby's smile is interpreted as her conversational turn.

MOTHER: Ah, nice and clean.

Turn-taking pause, after which mother again replies on behalf of the baby by saying,

MOTHER: Feeling better.

Thus, babies, almost from the minute of birth, are immersed in a sea of conversation that the mother and other caregivers wash over them, always pausing or actually filling in the baby's turn. As the baby begins to coo and babble, caregivers treat the baby's sound-making as a meaningful turn, as in this brief example:

MOTHER: It's bath time, Tracy. (putting baby in water)

BABY: Goooo.

MOTHER: Mm, nice warm water!

BABY: Kaaaa.

MOTHER: Yes, yes!

As babies' language further develops, their mothers up the ante, doing less and less of the conversational work and gradually, as their children become increasingly able, requiring them to participate more and more. It is through such *routinized* practice in highly constrained and repeated settings—at bath time, mealtimes, story times, bedtime—that parents scaffold, or support, their children's early language learning.

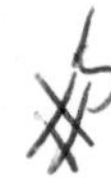

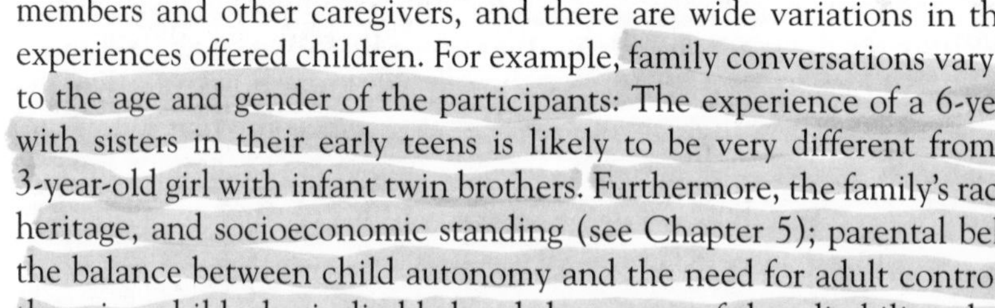

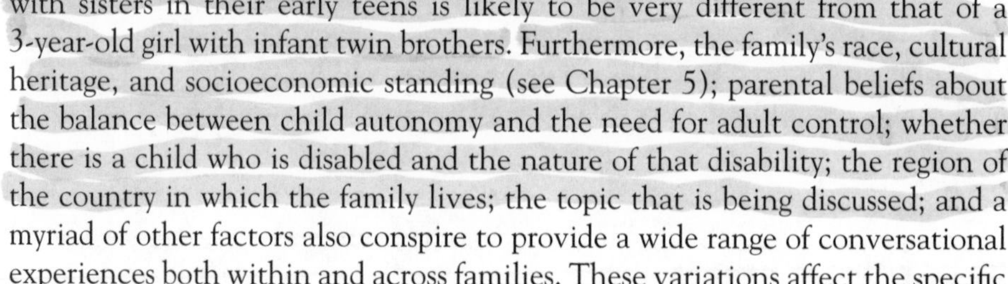

Most early language learning occurs through interactions with family members and other caregivers, and there are wide variations in the types of experiences offered children. For example, family conversations vary according to the age and gender of the participants: The experience of a 6-year-old boy with sisters in their early teens is likely to be very different from that of a 3-year-old girl with infant twin brothers. Furthermore, the family's race, cultural heritage, and socioeconomic standing (see Chapter 5); parental beliefs about the balance between child autonomy and the need for adult control; whether there is a child who is disabled and the nature of that disability; the region of the country in which the family lives; the topic that is being discussed; and a myriad of other factors also conspire to provide a wide range of conversational experiences both within and across families. These variations affect the specific vocabulary and dialect acquired, the duration of typical speaking turns and turn-taking pauses, standards of politeness, the types of question–answer interchanges practiced, and many other of the fundamental elements and techniques of language usage and acquisition.

Throughout children's preschool years, families also generate a wide variety of expectations specific to children's participation in conversations (Snow, 1991). For example, we as family members expect young children to initiate conversations and to be polite, especially in making requests. We expect them to learn to talk on the telephone, although the conversational partner is not visible. We expect them to tailor conversations for specific age groups and purposes, such as providing information to adults or entertaining themselves and their siblings on a long car ride. Gee (1988) has also shown that young children who are read to often will begin to "talk like books" during their conversations, using literate syntax and expressions such as "that dark, stormy night."

Finally, we expose even our youngest children to forms of nonliteral (sometimes also called *figurative*) language in conversations at home and in children's television shows, movies, songs, and storybooks. Pollio, Barlow, Fine, and Pollio (1977) estimated that people generally use nonliteral language about four times a minute in natural, conversational interactions. Our everyday language is so full of idioms (i.e., expressions in which the meaning is not equal to the sum of the meanings of the individual words), for example, that we do not even notice them and so we just naturally use them with children. Common idioms include "*Hold on* a minute!" or "*Get* in the car." Similarly, similes and metaphors, which are explicit and implicit comparisons, respectively, are common: "You're *like an angel*." "Oh, what a little *devil!*" Furthermore, we use instances of irony with children when we say one thing, but mean another. For example, a mother might say, "Oh, thanks a million!" when her young daughter comes home with a worm or even, "Nice going," when her son trips over his shoelaces. In these instances, children must ignore the meaning of the words and rely on cues, such as mom's grimace or smile, gestures, and her intonation to derive meaning.

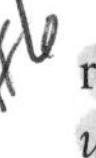

So, conversational discourse is far more complex than most of us ever realize and it is learned in only one way—through *interaction with other language users* (Sachs, 1989). Although it is the earliest form of discourse in which children engage—with, of course, the support of caregivers who can bear the burden of various aspects of the interchange until the children are able to do so themselves—it is fraught with all sorts of difficulties and takes a lifetime to learn. Conversation continues to play an important role in communication throughout life and becomes increasingly demanding during the school years.

The Elementary and Middle School Years

When students enter school, they typically must learn to use very different patterns of conversational interactions with their teachers (e.g., the scientific concepts discourse described in Chapter 1) than with their peers (i.e., underground discourse) and even different conversational patterns with peers under different circumstances (e.g., talking on the playground vs. working in reading pairs). Most often, classroom (sometimes also called *academic*) discourse differs from the natural conversations most students are used to when they enter school. It differs in many important ways, several of which were noted in Chapter 1, including the following: (a) there are usually many testlike questions, (b) students must keep their replies short and to the point, (c), students request a communicative turn by raising their hands, (d) discussion topics are frequently decontextualized, (e) the teacher usually reserves the privilege of initiating exchanges (97% of the time according to Shuy, 1988) and introducing new topics, and (f) there are different expectations for talking about mathematics and literature (Heath, 1978). Furthermore, students must simultaneously decipher the ongoing *social text* (equivalent to the language of control) in which teachers make clear the rules for participation—who can talk to whom for what purposes and under what circumstances—and the also ongoing *academic text* (i.e., the language of curriculum) that refers to the content and structure of the lesson (Cazden, 1988; Green, Weade, & Graham, 1988). Finally, and quite importantly, the teacher's direct and continual evaluation of the learner establishes a clear imbalance of power. (This power differential often occurs in adult experience between employer and employee, customer and salesperson, and service provider and client as well.)

Some of these differences are eliminated in alternative classrooms, such as those based on holistic and constructivist teaching models (Rubin, 1990). In such classrooms, students play an important role in deciding what they will learn and how they will learn it: Teachers do not hold exclusive gatekeeping power, students join in the rule-making for who participates when, collaborative projects foster much small group conversation, and the teacher becomes a consultant, facilitator, or coach. However, although there is considerable interest in alternative teaching models, most classrooms in both general and special education follow the traditional patterns of public communication described earlier (Staab, 1991).

Not only do students need to learn *how* to converse, but they also must learn to deal with teachers' increasingly sophisticated syntax and use of nonliteral language in academic contexts. Shuy (1988) reported that students must learn to be responsive to different patterns and styles of language usage across teachers. Even kindergarten children typically have a variety of teachers each day (e.g., parent volunteers or cross-age tutors; paraprofessionals and other teachers' aides; or art, physical education, and music teachers). Furthermore, as students progress through the grades, they

> must learn to listen, take notes, organize their own thoughts, follow classroom rules for talking and not talking, think about what they are hearing and relate it to what they already know, and imagine absent contexts and textbook authors as they try to understand classroom language. (N. Nelson, 1993, p. 452)

In addition, figurative language becomes increasingly common in the school curriculum—for example, the earth's *core* and presidential *landslides*—as well as in more general out-of-school settings. Milosky (1994) reported that nonliteral language was used over 10 times per minute of dialogue in "The Cosby Show" and is common in young people's magazines, storybooks, and instructional texts.

Students do not listen only to teachers, however. They also listen to other students who are engaged by the teacher or with whom they talk in small group discussions and projects. Morine-Dershimer and Tenenberg (1981) asked students watching classroom videotapes to report on what they heard "anybody" saying. The students reported most often on the comments of other students, especially the high-achieving ones and especially when the teacher asked a follow-up question (i.e., more than one question) either to the same student or on the same topic to a different student. Although teachers do the vast majority of talking in traditional classrooms, the students are more likely to notice what their peers say.

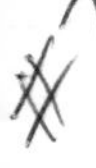

Furthermore, when Phillips (1985) studied peer group exchanges of 10- to 12-year-olds, he found that they typically began each session by negotiating the structure the conversational interaction would take: operational (a running commentary on what was happening), argumentational (articulating and evaluating different points of view), hypothetical (What about . . . ? What if . . . ?), experiential (I remember when I . . .), and expositional (answering implicit or expressed *wh* questions, such as Who? What? or When?). The nature of the conversation was not dictated by the subject matter. Surprisingly, question–answer, expositional discourse was rare, despite the frequency with which it typically occurs when teachers are in charge. What is important about Phillip's work is that the nature of the conversational discourse had an impact on the students' cognitive activity. Argumentation, for example, encourages thoughtfulness and the need to listen carefully to the propositions advanced by the other students.

In keeping with the earlier discussion of the oral-literate continuum, Hoskins (1990) pointed out that (a) reading and writing also share characteristics with conversational events and (b) helping students approach print literacy tasks from the perspective of engaging in conversation (because oral conversational discourse is so familiar) can be a quite useful strategy. Readers must use their intelligence and knowledge to "listen to," or interpret, the author's message, and writers must "speak to"—that is, design their text for—specific audiences, modifying their language to meet the needs of their (conversational) partners. Some classroom activities, such as the writing of dialogue journals (Swoger, 1989) and the passing of social notes (Lindfors, 1987), highlight the similarities between oral and written language.

Clearly, conversational abilities are integrally and causally related to learning. Students who cannot discern the rules for participation, who cannot accommodate to various teachers' styles and expectations, who cannot answer in concise and accurate statements, who cannot interact easily with their peers, who cannot adjust to the linguistic demands of various disciplines, and so forth, are at a distinct disadvantage in the classroom. Still, we devote little time in schools to helping students learn how to communicate. Staab (1991), for example, found that the amount of time third- and sixth-grade students were allotted to talk about content-related topics was somewhere around 7%, and about 93% of the time was devoted to teacher talk, quiet activities, and informal chatting among students during projects (i.e., underground talk). Her findings indicated that no significant change has occurred in at least 20 years. Despite the clear relationship of oral discourse to school success, teachers in North America generally are not concerned with providing their students with classroom opportunities to learn and practice oral discourse—perhaps because it is not graded and, therefore, not part of the accountability process.

With a little thoughtful planning, however, the teacher who is aware of the complex conversational demands of classrooms can provide students with opportunities for acquiring and practicing conversation, as well as expose them to modeling and coaching during extended discussion. Then that teacher will be able to both observe and intervene intelligently when difficulties arise. Scott (1994) suggested that teachers use a variety of verbal interactional patterns and styles, provide opportunities for students to talk at length both to each other and in interchanges with the teacher about the topics they are studying, and model the various types of small group exchanges—argumentational, hypothetical, and so on—described by Phillips (1985; see also Brown, Campione, Weber, & McGilly, 1992, for a discussion of ways to enhance classroom interactions).

The Later School Years

As students move into junior high, high school, and even college, much of what I have described about the early and middle school years still pertains, but conversational demands continue to become even more varied and complex. In the upper grades, what students need to know is highly decontextualized and almost entirely dependent on linguistic input. Teachers require their students to display greater independence in learning, especially with respect to reading, listening, and note-taking abilities. At the same time, because students have a variety of classes, they do not have any specific person to attend to and supervise their progress. Although language functioning is likely to be important to every aspect of classroom life, especially academic achievement (Ehren, 1994), few, if any, secondary school teachers assume responsibility for promoting students' overall language functioning or ensuring their language success (Larson, McKinley, & Boley, 1993).

The National Council of Teachers of English reported in 1976 that *listening* ability is correlated with overall language performance. Factors important to critical listening (Buttrill, Niizawa, Biemer, Takahashi, & Hearn, 1989) include the understanding of word meanings, relationships, and categories; active versus passive voice; the means for embedding and conjoining sentences; and knowledge of the ways that sentences can be transformed and segmented. Given that teacher utterances are typically longer and, as the student progresses through the grades, might sometimes approach hour-long (or longer) lectures or monologues, some attention to students' listening and note-taking abilities is increasingly important. Even teachers who do not directly teach listening skills can tailor their supportive materials (e.g., definition of vocabulary items, categories), oral delivery style (e.g., using active rather than passive sentences), and daily assignments in ways that foster students' listening abilities. Tasks that require students to supply missing information, abstract important information (vs. details), complete stories, or recognize absurdities in spoken information (Owens, 1995) can be very useful in helping students develop their listening skills. In each case, the instructional task requires the students to monitor and integrate information across an entire text.

Once students have listened to lectures or completed their readings and made notes about the information gleaned from them, they sometimes discuss the material or related problems in large or small groups. Most often, teachers expect these instructional conversations to occur at the literate end of the oral-literate continuum; that is, they expect students to use language structures more formal than those of typical conversation. The success of group work is based on that and other assumptions, such as students' understanding that they must limit their talk to the topic of the lesson. At the same time, they must be able to engage in a variety of different kinds of contextualized problem-solving and thinking processes and be able to negotiate the use of those that are most effective for the problem at hand.

Adolescence is a time of refining language and of understanding a broader range of characteristics of language usage. For example, although younger school-age students are aware of social class differences in language usage, adolescents are better able to identify the features of various dialects and registers. Sometimes they even use them and switch between them for different purposes (Romaine, 1984). Adolescence is also the time when registers become a more important focus of language acquisition. Young people need to differentiate among registers in order to respond to the demands of the more varied and formalized social contexts they come to experience during the teen years and in the use of the more complex language forms required from them (Gleason, 1993). Also, during adolescence, the relationship between communication abilities and acceptance in the peer group becomes stronger than at any other time in life (Gallagher, 1991).

No wonder it is at this time that the use of slang typically becomes a badge of peer group identity. It serves the purpose of denoting who holds membership in the group and of distinguishing them from outsiders. Today's adolescents, like those of every other generation, have adopted a unique vocabulary, including such terms as *phat* or *dude*, terms that would seem out of place or perhaps even funny if they were used by members of adult social groups. These terms mark teenagers as members of a particular subculture. Because slang terms change rapidly and frequently, sustained group membership requires the ability to learn and adapt language equally fast and often.

Gleason (1993) reported that it is not clear why some individuals choose, deliberately or unconsciously, to adopt a particular register. It may be that they identify with the group or that they have a particular facility for "picking up" words or accents and, therefore, find the adoption of various dialects and registers pleasurable or amusing. Some people, on the other hand, including many students with special needs, may have difficulty staying abreast of new terms and rapid changes in usage. Others, such as members of the African American community who refuse to use SAE or feminists in male-dominated professions, may demonstrate resistance or conflict by their failure to adopt a particular register. Meanwhile, those who participate in ritualized or technical situations, such as sports or computer programming, must learn the language associated with these fields or risk appearing as either a novice or an outsider.

Still, learning to communicate in ways that guarantee acceptance into the peer group is not sufficient. As they begin to move into advanced training or work, teenagers also need to be able to leave particular registers behind. Slang, for example, may be dysfunctional when disagreeing with a parent, asking a favor from an adult neighbor, or negotiating with an employer. What is appropriate is determined by both context and culture. For example, the ethnic jokes that were considered humorous 20 years ago are now considered offensive and boorish. In addition, mathematical, medical, legal, and other work-related *jargons* (i.e., technical languages associated with a particular field) may hinder communications rather than improve them. Consequently, selection among registers requires a great deal of reflection on experience ("I wish I'd said . . ." "Next time I'll tell her . . .").

Finally, characteristic of the demands of the later school years is an increased emphasis on nonliteral language: slang is often figurative; school textbooks contain approximately five figures of speech per page by the 11th grade (Pollio, Smith, & Pollio, 1990); and rapid, humorous conversational exchanges that turn on figurative uses of language become the social norm in many adolescent groups (Blalock, 1982). Older students can process and often prefer different types of figures of speech from those understood, used, and preferred by younger students—those that are conceptually, rather than perceptually, based (e.g., "She's as free as the wind"); those that are less familiar (e.g., "His rock star antics got him in trouble"); and those that can be expressed in a variety of syntactic and lexical forms (e.g., "her diamond eyes," "her eyes as bright as diamonds," "her flashing eyes"). They are also more adept at recognizing and interpreting irony, although irony often fails even among adults. Consider how often people feel the need to explain, "I was only kidding!"

Summary

Conversation, which begins nearly at the moment of birth for most children, has been considered the principal context for language learning. It begins with the caregiver's immersion of the newborn in routines that are repetitive and control the range of vocabulary. The primary source of modeling and teaching during the preschool years is the verbal interaction within the family, which varies in virtually every way that families vary. Consequently, children entering school at age 5 have already had significantly divergent language experiences. In addition, although most people think of nonliteral language as the domain of older students, even preschool children are regularly exposed to figures of speech.

When children enter school, the range of linguistic models expands to include teachers and peers; new demands surface with respect to vocabulary, complexity, and language usage; and adaptations to the school discourse become necessary—at least for those children not exposed to education-like discourse at home prior to entering school. Furthermore, school-aged children must learn to learn almost exclusively from text (both oral and written, literal and figurative), that is, by listening or reading, taking notes, monitoring comprehension, answering questions, initiating questions, and so forth.

During the transition to adolescence and later to college or employment, students must cope with still increasingly complex and varied conversational contexts. They must become adept at learning in situations that are either entirely or primarily linguistic. Level of facility with speech registers admits them, or not, to membership in the peer group, while, simultaneously, contexts in which such specific registers may be inappropriate become more numerous, more varied, and more formalized. Figures of speech become both more pervasive and more sophisticated.

Rubin (1990) summarized quite eloquently the important role that conversational abilities play in our lives:

> Speaking the word . . . is knowledge producing as well as ego affirming. . . . We internalize talk, and it becomes thought. We externalize talk, and it becomes our link to social reality. We elaborate talk, and it becomes our bridge to literacy. Like the sea, talk is the environment that first incubates and then nurtures our development. (p. 3)

Learning To Tell Stories

Narrative is not only a type of discourse, but also a way of knowing and an important context for language learning. Children begin to frame stories very early, as they reflect on roles and experience events in their natural environments, especially as they engage in symbolic play. As children enact and reenact familiar event sequences, their narratives become increasingly elaborated, with disruptions in the "going to the supermarket" story being caused by a car crash, a forgotten shopping list, or an invasion by monsters. Stories become gradually decontextualized as they are repeated, acted out with puppets or cutouts, and carried home to entertain the family at dinnertime.

Although we often associate stories with children, narratives play an important role in all our lives. Sharing experiences encoded in narrative form—such as stories about how Aunt Susan fared in her new job, the skirmish between the package delivery woman and Mr. Emery's dog, or the wonderful sequence of events that made mine a red-letter day—is constant in adult conversations. In fact, as Heath (1983) has shown, stories occur frequently in home discourse. Furthermore, stories abound in news reports and broadcasts; TV shows and movies; and adult (as well as child) reading materials, such as short stories and novels. Some form of narrative existed and continues to exist in every culture and in every period of history.

Although conversation and narrative have a good deal in common, they also differ in a variety of important ways (Owens, 1991):

> First, narratives are extended units of text. Second, events within narratives are linked with one another temporally or causally in predictable ways. Narratives are organized in a cohesive, predictable, rule-governed manner representing temporal and causal patterns of relating information not found in conversation. Third, the speaker maintains a social monologue throughout. The speaker must produce language that is relevant to the overall narrative while remaining mindful of the information needed by the listener. (p. 236)

This quotation from Owens also points to some of the demands inherent in producing well-formed narratives—the needs for cohesion, predictability, rule-governed structure, causal and temporal patterns, and monitoring of the listener's comprehension and the making of repairs as needed. Milosky (1990) elaborated them thus:

> The child must recall and organize content, take into account the listener by determining shared background, formulate new utterances, relate them to what has already been said, and introduce referents and distinguish unambiguously among them in subsequent utterances. The need to balance all these demands makes narration cognitively demanding and requires extensive mental resources. (p. 13)

There are four common genres of narrative discourse: recounts, eventcasts, accounts, and fictionalized stories (Owens, 1991). Their distribution, frequency, and degree of elaboration vary greatly across cultures. *Recounts*, descriptions of past experience that the person participated in, read about, or observed, most typically occur in middle and upper class families where the discourse of school permeates the family's everyday discourse. The recount is a narrative type frequently solicited in the lower grades of schools. Recounts, however, are less and less frequently requested as middle and upper class children achieve mastery over the other three forms of narration.

Eventcasts are verbal replays or explanations of current or future events and are the earliest form of narrative to which children in middle to upper class families are exposed. Caregivers often use eventcasts while nurturing, reading to, or playing with children. Notice that the interactions between the mother and her infant that were presented in the section on conversation took the form of eventcasts. Similarly, children often engage in eventcasts during play when they tell other children how they want them to act.

Accounts are simple, self-initiated, spontaneous narratives in which children share their experience ("You know what? My baby sister is getting heavy."). Although they are common in middle and upper class households, accounts are not used as frequently by members of some groups. Heath (1983) found that accounts were not used by Southern, white, working class children until they entered school. Furthermore, Asian American children learn early that it is appropriate to share accounts only within the family.

Finally, *fictionalized stories* have a variety of structures and contents that vary according to specific cultures (see Chapters 1 and 5). For example, in some cultures, the storyteller is expected to relate all of the relevant information; in other cultures, the listener is supposed to make sense of the events. In some cultures, anyone can tell a story; in other cultures, stories are the province of only a designated few, for example, the elders. In some cultures, stories tend to have happy endings; people from other cultures find such stories uninteresting.

Although narratives are used across all cultures and all four forms are expected to be acquired to some extent by white, middle class children by age 3, stories vary considerably in structural type and age of acquisition across cultures and subcultures. The lock-step, Eurocentric curriculum of North American schools, however, typically does not allow for cultural variations and, consequently, as noted in Chapter 1, many children from nonmainstream cultures have difficulties related to learning about the differences between their "home narratives" and narrative usage in school.

Narratives, however, are not merely about describing events or telling stories. Bruner (1990), among others (Ricoeur, 1981; Polkinghorne, 1988), argued that narrative is a form of knowing that stands in contrast to scientific knowing. Unlike science, narrative knowing is not about truth and prediction; it is instead concerned with the interpretation of meaning. Narrative knowing is a way of understanding and organizing events in our lives, so as to make sense of them and, through that sense-making, to construct our understanding of ourselves. Self, then, is a story-in-progress in which we serve as our own protagonist and which explains not only who we are and who we have been, but also who we have the potential to become. Hence, narrative discourse is highly interwoven with identity (Gee, 1990) and begins to develop shortly after the advent of language.

The Preschool Years

There is evidence that narratives begin to develop quite early. For example, by having her parents routinely put a tape recorder under Emily's crib at nap time and at bedtime beginning when Emily was 21 months old and continuing over a 15-month period, K. Nelson (1989) studied 2-year-old Emily's presleep monologues and bedtime conversations with her parents. These tapes were then analyzed not only by K. Nelson herself, but also by several other scholars of child language and cognitive development.

What was surprising to all was the distinct difference between the rich monologues in which Emily engaged night after night just before falling asleep and the comparatively short and sparse contributions she made to the conversational dialogues with her parents. Although the scholars were not consistent in their interpretations of the organization of these monologues, they all agreed that her monologues contained several different types of discourse, including (a) conversation (e.g., with her stuffed animals); (b) narrative (or proto-narrative, in which she recounts events in her young life, stories that have been read to her, or imaginary happenings); and (c) a problem-solving (i.e., posing problems, examining them in narrative terms, and coming to some resolutions), but less well-structured exposition-like text.

The importance of this work is that it yielded many new insights (cognitive, linguistic, social, and personality related) into the developing child's mind. Among them is the recognition that narrative (and to some minor extent perhaps exposition) is, in addition to conversation, an important and principal context for the development of child language. Furthermore, K. Nelson (1989) noted that narratives served the 2- to 3-year-old Emily in three general domains of experience:

> First, there is the world of people and things, activities in which Emily participates, past episodes and future anticipations. All of these she needs to understand if she is to take her part successfully within that world. . . . Second, there is the task of mastering the language itself through representing and interpreting in linguistic and narrative forms. . . . Emily has made great progress in this direction by the time our story opens, but she has far to go in making language work for her in constructing, interpreting, problem-solving, and fantasizing activities. And third, there is the discovery of herself as a thinking, feeling, acting person in the world of other people who think, feel, act, and interact with her. (p. 20)

Emily's monologues demonstrate not only how she uses narrative discourse to learn language, but also how she uses narrative to learn about herself.

To learn narrative, children need two kinds of experience: They need to know enough about how the world works to construct scripts or schemas about common events and they need to have had enough experience with hearing stories to know how stories are organized and used to reconstruct reality (N. Nelson, 1993). As Emily's presleep monologues have shown, narrative development begins as early as 2 years. By age 4, increased memory capacity enables children to recount the past and to tell simple stories of their own or others' authorship (Owens, 1984), but not until age 8 can children tell narratives really well (Owens, 1991).

Sutton-Smith (1986) described the development of young children's narratives. Children's earliest self-generated narratives in SAE have a vague plot associated with events, usually frightening or disruptive, in the child's life. Between 2 and 3 years of age, children do not realize the need for introductions or the provision of background information for the listener, so their narratives have no identifiable beginnings, middles, or endings. They are strings of statements following one another in "additive chains": "There birdie. Kitty mine. Tree birdy house." There is no plot or story line. There are no cause–effect relations, and the sentences can be rearranged in any sequence without changing their meaning. The children are more concerned with performance and text qualities, such as prosody, than with the structure of the text.

Between ages 3 and 5, children begin to relate narratives with logical sequences, but still with no plot or causality. These stories often include third-person pronouns, past-tense verbs, and temporal conjunctions. They have a beginning and an end. Here a 4-year-old tells about a bird she watched fly away to bring food to his chirping chicks: "The bird lived in the nest. Sometimes he flies away. And then he comes back with worms for the babies."

As noted in the introduction to this section, it is a rare home environment that does not expose preschoolers to some form of narrative, because sharing accounts, recounts, eventcasts, and stories is such a pervasive part of our daily lives. We come to know one another and keep up with what is happening to one another through the sharing of narratives. But, in some homes—mostly among the middle and upper classes—children have access to and are expected to learn to use all four forms of narrative. In other subcultures, however, children may not learn some forms of narrative until they enter school. Clearly, children who have facility with all narrative forms have an advantage when they begin school, because narratives dominate the curriculum of the first several years.

Children who also have experience with storybook narratives, however, have an even greater advantage. Preschool children who hear written language read aloud do better with reading and writing when they enter school and, according to the conclusions Cullinan (1989) reached when she reviewed the research in this area, also seem better able to understand the world. Children with little or no exposure to written narratives tend to do poorly throughout the school years, whereas those with thousands of hours of exposure tend to excel in school (Adams, 1990).

Why would this be true? First, children whose home language is not the SAE that is required in schools have an opportunity to become familiar with

SAE and to learn something about it in an interactive setting. Additionally, children engaged in storybook reading have the opportunity to learn the conventions of print (reading top to bottom and left to right, predicting from titles, matching words to pictures, etc.) and the vocabulary to talk about print (words such as *page*, *book*, *letter*, *picture*). They often learn to name the letters of the alphabet and to identify some words. Some learn that the letters are, at least to some extent, phonological representations. They are exposed to sentences that are more complex and more literate than those we typically hear in conversation, and repeated immersion in the discourse helps them come to expect stories to have a particular structure, to begin and end in certain ways (e.g., "Once upon a time . . ." and "They lived happily ever after"), and to be continuous with oral language.

Such students also have the opportunity to engage in warm and interesting dialogues with their parents (or preschool teachers) both about the books per se and about the content of the stories. However, they learn not only about the world, but also to enjoy reading and frequently to express themselves in print through spontaneous efforts at writing. Finally, through listening to written language read aloud, they have opportunities to experience vicariously many situations (e.g., a morning on the farm, a family holiday), events (e.g., bicycle races, boat trips), and beings or objects (e.g., lions, baobab trees, African baskets) that may not be directly available in their environment. Consequently, storybook reading may be particularly helpful as preparation for the still unknown world of schooling for children whose life experiences are either limited or chaotic.

The Elementary and Middle School Years

Like all other aspects of language acquisition, narratives go through a period of development (see Table 2.2) beyond the preschool years (N. Nelson & Friedman, 1988, cited in N. Nelson, 1993), when, in SAE, children's earliest oral stories are more or less collections of information that focus on whatever has caught their fancy. There is no overall structure to these stories and few, if any, relationships among the individual elements. These "stories" are often called *heaps*. As they grow older, children move through the telling of sequences of events to primitive narratives. The *event sequences* have a central character and a setting, but there are no explicit temporal relations or transitions. They follow a John does act 3, John does act 6, John does act 2 kind of format. The *primitive narratives* contain a central character, setting, and topic, but they are put together because they share a situation; abstract relationships are missing. Stories about school or family trips that include comments on the

Table 2.2
Narrative Development

1. **Heaps**
   - Text organization comes from whatever attracts attention
   - No story macrostructure
   - No relationship or organization among elements or individual microstructures
2. **Sequences**
   - Narrative has macrostructure with central character, setting, topic
   - Activities of central character occur in particular setting
   - Story elements are related to central macrostructure through concrete associative, or perceptual bonds
   - Superficial sequences in time
   - No transitions
   - May use format A does X, A does Y, A does Z; or A does X to N, A does X to O, A does X to P
   - No ending to narrative
   - Trip stories may be in this category if events lack logical sequence or trip theme
3. **Primitive Narratives**
   - Characters, objects, or events of narratives are put together because they are perceptually associated and complement each other
   - Elements of the narrative follow logically from attributes of the center
   - Attributes of the center are internal to the character, objects, events, and they determine the types of events that occur
   - May use inference in narrative
   - Narrative goes beyond perceptual and explicit information, but stays concrete, with links forged by shared situation rather than abstract relationship
   - May talk about feelings
   - Organized trip stories fall in this category if they include multiple comments on events, including interpretive feelings
4. **Unfocused Chains**
   - Events are linked logically (cause–effect relationship)
   - Elements are related to one another
   - No central theme or character, no plot or story theme
   - Lack of evidence of complete understanding of reciprocal nature of characters and events
   - True sequence of events

(*continues*)

Table 2.2 *Continued.*

5. **Focused Chains**
   - Organized with both a center and a sequence
   - Actual chaining of events that connect the elements
   - Does not have a strong plot
   - Events do not build on attributes of characters
   - Characters and events of narratives seldom reach toward a goal
   - Weak ending, no ending, or end does not follow logically from the beginning
   - May be problems or motivating events that cause actions
   - Transitions are used
   - More because–then chains are used
   - May be a trip story if the events follow logically from each other more than just occurring next on the same trip
6. **True Narratives**
   - Integrate chaining events with complementary centering of the primitive narrative
   - A developed plot
   - Consequent events build out of prior events and also develop the central core
   - Ending reflects or is related to the issues or events presented in the beginning of the narrative
   - Intentions or goals of characters are dependent on attributes and feelings

Note. From "Development of the Concept of Story in Narratives Written by Older Children," by N. W. Nelson and K. K. Friedman, in *Childhood Language Disorders in Context: Infancy Through Adolescence* (p. 430), by N. W. Nelson, 1993, Needham Heights, MA: Allyn & Bacon. Copyright 1993 by Allyn & Bacon. Reprinted with permission.

various events as well as interpretive feelings generally qualify as primitive narratives. The next level of story structure in the developmental continuum is an *event chain* with no central focus. In this phase of narrative development, events are logically linked to one another (e.g., by cause–effect relations), but there is no central theme or plot. At the following level, *focused chains* connect the elements into a whole, but the events are not dependent on the attributes of the character. The plot and ending are weak and neither the character nor the events lead toward a goal. Finally, *true narratives* have a central plot to which all events are related. Later events grow out of earlier ones and the goals are related to the character's attributes and feelings. In true narratives, the ending reflects the issues or events laid out at the beginning. In short, true narratives contain a setting and a problem or conflict to which the characters respond with some intention or goal, and, as they carry out their plan, their actions lead to some resolution, or ending (see Table 2.3 for the simplest topic-centered story format). Some narratives make use of other literary devices, such as foreshadowing, flashbacks, and so forth.

Around second grade, children begin to tell stories with the following structure: a beginning, a problem, a plan to overcome the problem, and a resolution (Sutton-Smith, 1986). As their storytelling abilities continue to develop, they learn to use multiple or highly elaborated plots. The construction of a plot is dependent on the ability to incorporate cause–effect relationships, rather than simply connecting events serially. Although 2- to 3-year-olds can use some causal expressions, the ability to construct coherent causal narratives—first with references to mental states and motivations (Kemper & Edwards, 1986) and, a bit later, to physical causality (McCabe & Peterson, 1985)—generally begins to develop at about age 5. In addition, by second grade (Sutton-Smith, 1986), children include beginning and ending markers

Table 2.3
Story Structure for a Single-Episode Story

1. **Setting:** introduces the protagonist(s) and the physical/social context.
2. **Initiating event:** introduces a change in the protagonist's environment.
3. **Character's internal response:** includes information about the character's goals (e.g., Mary wanted to cry), or feelings (e.g., Mary became very angry), or cognitions (e.g., Mary thought John was obnoxious), or plans (e.g., Mary decided to not play with John).
4. **Attempt:** the character's overt behavior.
5. **Consequences:** the direct results of the action are described.
6. **Reaction:** the character(s) respond to the consequences of the actions.

A Sad Playmate

Mary and John were playmates at school. John called Mary a brat. Mary wanted to cry. She stopped playing and ran away from John. Then John sat down on the grass and started to cry. Mary felt sorry that she had made her friend sad too.

Note. Adapted from "An Analysis of Story Comprehension in Elementary School Children," by M. L. Stein and C. J. Glenn, in *Multidisciplinary Approaches to Discourse Comprehension,* by R. Freedle (Ed.), 1979, Hillsdale, NJ: Ables.

("Once upon a time," "The end") and a greater variety of conjunctions (e.g., *and, then*), locatives (*in, on, next to*), comparatives (*biggest, almost as mean as*), and adjectives. Their stories become longer, their characters more consistent, and their event sequences true chronologies.

After age 8, the plot becomes clearer, with a definite resolution of the central problem (Peterson & McCabe, 1983; Sutton-Smith, 1986). Additionally, the presentation of the story is carried by the language (rather than the performance). Johnson (1982, cited in Owens, 1991) listed the characteristics of the narratives constructed by 10-year-old children as follows:

> Fewer unresolved problems and unprepared resolutions
> Less extraneous detail
> More overt marking of changes in time and place
> Greater concern for motivation and internal reactions
> More complex episode structure
> Close adherence to the story grammar model[2] (p. 240)

Narrative development varies with the types of stories individual children are asked to tell (e.g., accounts of personal events, stories recounted from television) and reaches its peak in the episode-embedded oral stories of 11- and 12-year-olds. Of course, those children who read and who hear written stories read aloud once again have an advantage, and there is some evidence that the structure of the stories children tell is related to the structure of the stories that are read to them (N. Nelson & Friedman, 1988).

An extensive literature correlates poor storytelling with low scores on standardized tests of oral and written language and elucidates the high likelihood of co-occurrence of poor storytelling (or retelling) and the labeling of students as having special educational needs (Culatta, Page, & Ellis, 1983). Gee (1989), however, presented two reasons why, in his estimation, such work is "rational nonsense." First, he argued that language development is not linear and, therefore, cannot be assessed properly with standardized or other linear measures that evaluate only a particular set of words and constructions typical of the dominant discourse. Second, nearly all humans, with the exception of only the most severely impaired, learn to both understand and use narrative

---

[2]The story grammar model described by Stein and Glenn (1979) has seven story elements. Stories usually being with a (1) description of the setting. An (2) initiating event that will promote some action on the part of the character(s) sets the plot in motion. The character(s) then react to the event. This is called the (3) internal response, which in turn leads to their formulation of (4) internal plans. The character(s) then engage in (5) overt action intended to bring about some resolution to the initiating event. Their attempts lead to (6) direct consequences. And, finally, storytellers tell us the (7) character(s)' emotional, cognitive, or behavioral responses to the outcome.

discourse. In interpreting the literature on narrative development, therefore, it is important to keep in mind that students' culture or race and socioeconomic backgrounds are key factors in determining who performs poorly on all of the measures we have mentioned. Low scores, then, may very well be related to structural or dialectal differences or the effects of poverty per se, rather than to any inability to learn to use narrative. For more in-depth descriptions of how story structures differ in other cultures and dialects, see Chapter 5.

The Later School Years

Storytelling abilities peak in the middle grades and narrative virtually disappears from high school and college curricula with the instructional transition to what Britton (1970) called *transactional* writing, that is, the more cognitively advanced rhetorical forms of analysis, argument, and exposition (Wanner, 1994). Once students arrive at junior high school, "story" takes on the connotation of literature and students' opportunities to learn through the familiar forms of narrative are lost. Wanner rues this loss, pointing out that literature is "material written by a stranger from another time and place, and presented, not as an event to be incorporated into one's life experience, but as an icon to be revered and analyzed" (p. 4). Through her own work, Wanner has shown how, in high school teaching, narrative can be partnered with the transactional forms of writing to great advantage.

N. Nelson and Friedman (1988) have shown that approximately 25% of college students do not write true narratives. Why this is the case, is not clear. It may be the result of deemphasizing narrative in secondary schools, but that is difficult to say, because, as Hedberg and Westby (1993) indicated, the research on narrative development among normally developing students typically ends with studies of 11- and 12-year-olds.

Summary

Narrative is both an important context for language learning and a way of knowing oneself. It is a discourse, like conversation, that is pervasive in all human cultures and, consequently, a discourse that virtually everybody learns. Narratives differ from conversation in that they are more extended and, therefore, require cohesion, predictability, rule-governed structure, causal and temporal relations, and monitoring and repairs. Narratives serve as vehicles for learning about the world (and vice versa), mastering language, and discovering oneself.

Narrative is context sensitive, in the sense that narratives take different forms and carry different meanings for people in different cultures. Sometimes, with our focus on SAE in classrooms throughout North America, students from nonmainstream homes are mistakenly judged to be narrative deficient, when in fact they are simply narrative different.

Narrative begins developing, at least, as early as 2 years of age and progresses from ill-formed heaps to well-formed stories that (a) are integrated and coherent, (b) are complete with respect to elements (setting, characters, plot, etc.), and (c) use a variety of literary devices (e.g., flashbacks, analogies). The ability to formulate narratives peaks at about 11 to 12 years of age. Although most children are exposed to some form of narrative in their homes, those who consistently hear written narratives read aloud during their preschool years have a decided advantage both at entrance to school and throughout their school years (Adams, 1990). By listening to stories, they both learn the structure of narrative discourse and expand their knowledge about the world. Furthermore, they gain first-hand knowledge about what reading and writing are like in much the same way that children learn a good deal about driving long before, as adolescents, they actually get behind the wheel of a car.

Constructing Expository Text

Exposition is the discourse that conveys sequenced or categorized factual or technical information—for example, explaining how to play a computer game or describing what a tiger looks like. Although there is some evidence that proto-exposition, at least, begins during the preschool years (recall K. Nelson's, 1989, study with Emily), expository text becomes more important in the later phases of language acquisition. We begin to emphasize expository discourse when children enter school, but especially after the third or fourth grade. Instruction in the structure of expository text is often more highly integrated with learning to read and write than are conversation and narrative. Most academic discourse in the later grades, especially that in lectures and textbooks, is expository.

Westby (1994) summarized the seven most commonly used types of expository text and diagrammed the structures typically associated with them in SAE (how these structures vary across cultures is addressed in Chapter 5). The types of exposition Westby defined include description (i.e., telling what something is), enumeration (i.e., providing a list that is related to a topic), sequential/procedural text (telling what occurred or how to do something), comparisons and contrasts (i.e., elucidating similarities and differences), problem solving (i.e., stating a problem and offering solutions), persuasion (taking and trying to justify a position), and cause–effect explanations (i.e., giving reasons why something happened).

The Preschool Years

The seeds of later expository development are sown during the preschool years. Parents may make explanations or read books to their children that are not only narrative in structure, but also, wholly or in part, expository. For example, the similarities between some forms of narrative (i.e., recounts and eventcasts) and forms of exposition are readily apparent, especially as the content becomes more impersonal and decontextualized. Furthermore, as their main focus or as subsections within stories, many books designed for young children describe objects and phenomena, list objects related to categories and activities, explain the sequence of events involved in building a house or making pudding, compare cars with airplanes, and so forth—all expository functions.

The Elementary and Middle School Years

Like conversation and narrative, then, students must learn both to understand explanatory texts produced by others and to produce such texts themselves. To produce expository text requires students to have control over information related to the topic, to select and organize information logically, to use cohesive devices (e.g., pronouns and repetitions) to interconnect components of the text, and to maintain fluency, in both cognitive processing and ongoing text formulation. The complexity of this genre probably accounts, at least in part, for its late development.

The early roots of exposition have not been well studied. Slater and Graves (1989), however, demonstrated that, beginning in the fourth grade, students use their knowledge of the structure of expository text to facilitate both comprehension and recall. One indication that text structure aids comprehension is that students remember more main ideas than supportive details. Slater and Graves also showed that those students who do not use their knowledge of text structure spontaneously can be taught to do so and that they benefit from such instruction, particularly when the content of the passage is unfamiliar.

Children who have difficulties with expository discourse are particularly at risk for school failure, because exposition is the coin of the educational realm. Teachers spend much of the school day giving directions; presenting information through lectures or mini-lectures; proposing hypotheses; explicating theories and procedures; making predictions, judgments, and generalizations; drawing conclusions; and describing people, events, and periods of history, literature, and so forth. Consequently, students must comprehend the orally presented exposition of the classroom as well as that presented in written form in their trade books and textbooks, handouts, and other written classroom materials. In addition, however, they may need to produce and monitor their own self-talk while doing mathematics problems, science experiments, or text editing. Furthermore, when their learning is tested, students often must read (or have already read) an expository selection, answer (or perhaps formulate) factual and inferential questions about it, and write a response that is itself expository.

There is no particular sequence for learning expository text structures. Traditionally, early literacy instruction has focused on narrative, but in recent years (see Calkins, 1983) scholars have begun arguing that exposition should be taught from the child's first days in school. In Table 2.4 is an example of the most common format for exposition in SAE, the typical five-paragraph essay. Other forms are introduced in Chapter 4, because exposition is closely tied to written language instruction. Often and especially for students having difficulties, graphic organizers (see Figure 2.2)—both displays and mapping—are useful aids in both comprehending (Gillespie, 1993; Hennings, 1993) and generating (Cooper, 1997) text.

The Later School Years

One complicating factor in determining students' levels of competence with exposition that is particularly important in the later school years is the nature of the expository presentations from which they are expected to learn. Clearly, not all teachers' lectures are well organized; neither are all textbooks. Roller (1990) and Ohlhausen and Roller (1988) recommended that teachers consider the level of difficulty of particular texts before making judgments about what students can and cannot do. They showed that texts that contain the same information but are organized differently vary in how difficult they are to comprehend. Texts that are structured in a way that makes the content relations explicit, for example, are much easier to read than those that do not—contrary to the assumptions underlying most "readability" formulas. As students become more and more responsible for learning independently, however, the quality of the texts, oral or written, to which they are exposed becomes a central factor in enabling or prohibiting their acquisition of knowledge.

Furthermore, listening and reading are *interactive* processes. The ability to make sense of text depends on what one already knows with respect to both content and discourse structure and is able to relate to the text at hand. In their

Table 2.4
Structure of Expository Text

Introduction: Topic 1, Topic 2, Topic 3, summarizing statement and/or bridge to the following paragraph

Topic 1: Supporting detail 1, Supporting detail 2, Supporting detail 3, summarizing statement and/or bridge to the next paragraph

Topic 2: (repetition of Topic 1 structure)

Topic 3: (repetition of Topic 1 structure)

Summarizing statement: Reiteration of Topic 1, Topic 2, Topic 3, concluding statement

Cowboys

Cowboys are strong men who are good at riding horses. They round up cattle into herds and drive them from Texas to the North. Cowboys sleep outside when they are on the trail. Because of their hard life, they need special clothing. Cowboys are the heroes of the West.

The trip North is a long and dangerous one. The cattle seem to know that they will soon be made into meat and leather. They try over and over again to run away. Sometimes the whole herd stampedes. Cowboys must watch the cattle both day and night to keep them from running away.

Cowboys sleep outside on the ground, so that they are always close to the cattle. They sleep on bedrolls that they carry on their saddles. Their food travels with them in a chuckwagon. They usually make a big circle around the campfire and sing songs to cheer themselves up after a hard day's work.

The cowboy must wear nearly everything he needs. Most cowboys carry a six-shooter to stop a stampede or to blast a rattlesnake. Their boots protect them from snakebites and keep their feet from slipping through the stirrups. The cowboy's hat is his sunshade and his umbrella too. Without these clothes, a cowboy would be in real danger.

A cowboy's life is hard and lonely. He must guard the cattle very carefully. Sleeping outside is cold and uncomfortable. It is a good thing the cowboys have hats to use for pillows. No wonder there aren't many cowboys anymore.

---

study using social studies texts, Ohlhausen and Roller (1988) found that students in seventh and ninth grades did better than fifth graders in determining unspecified content relationships, not because they read better, but because they had had more experience studying nations and knew the types of categories of

A. A Formal Outline

Playing Golf

I. Selecting Equipment
   A. Clubs
      1. Length relative to height
      2. Handedness
      3. Full or short set
      4. Steel or graphite
   B. Other Accessories
      1. Golf bag
      2. Shoes
      3. Gloves
      4. Balls
      5. Tees, ball marker, repair device, towel
II. Learning To Play
   A. The Swing
      1. Stance
      2. Body rotation
      3. Weight distribution
      4. Ending position
   B. Putting
      1. Reading the green
      2. Lining up to the ball
      3. Holding the club
      4. Estimating speed and direction
III. Keeping Score
   A. Counting strokes
   B. Par
   C. Penalties

Note. Adapted from "Independent Study Skills," by D. K. Reid and W. P. Hresko, in *Teaching the Learning Disabled: A Cognitive Developmental Approach* (pp. 435–463), by D. K. Reid (Ed.), 1988, Boston: Allyn & Bacon.

(*continues*)

Figure 2.2. Types of graphic organizers.

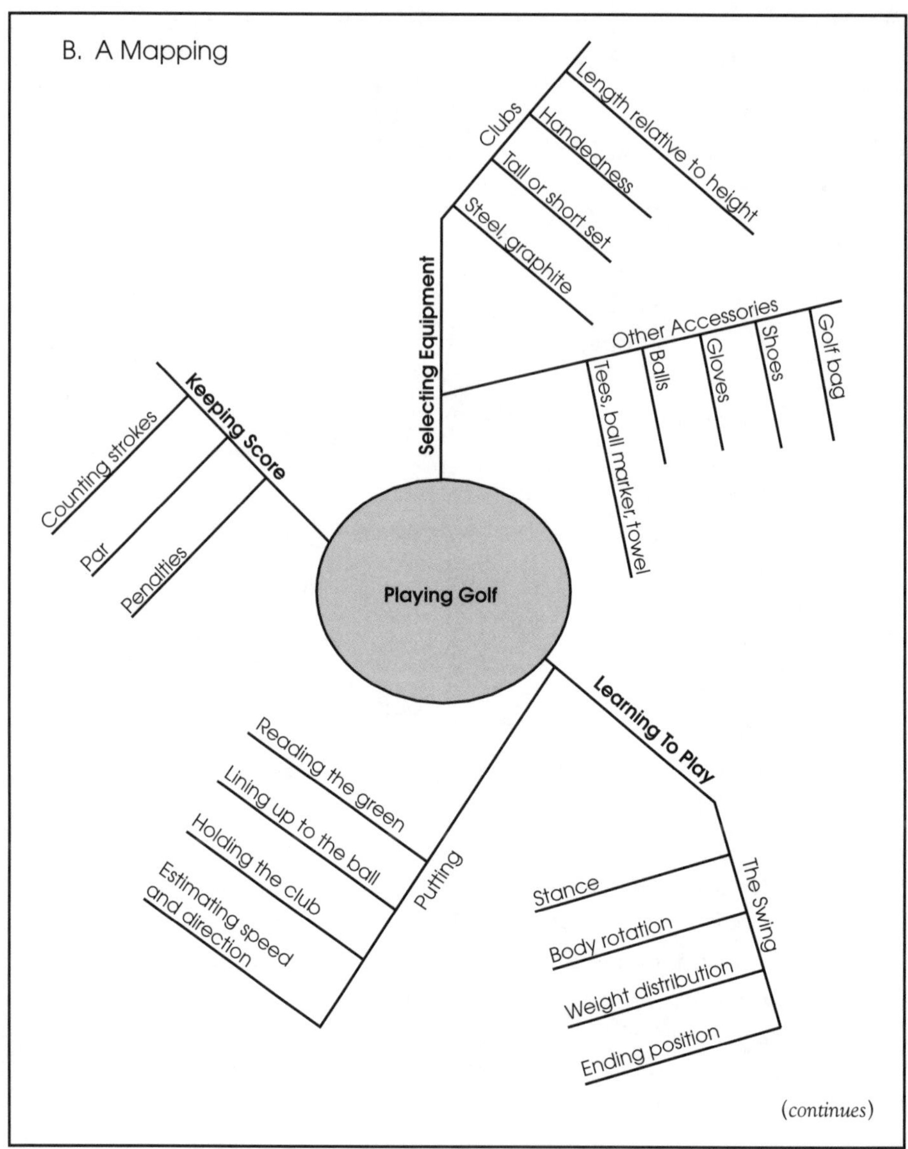

Figure 2.2. *Continued.*

description (e.g., their typography, climate, location, and major exports) that are important to such an endeavor.

Also to be able to bring meaning to texts, students need to be familiar with the differences in the types of discourse that are related to the various

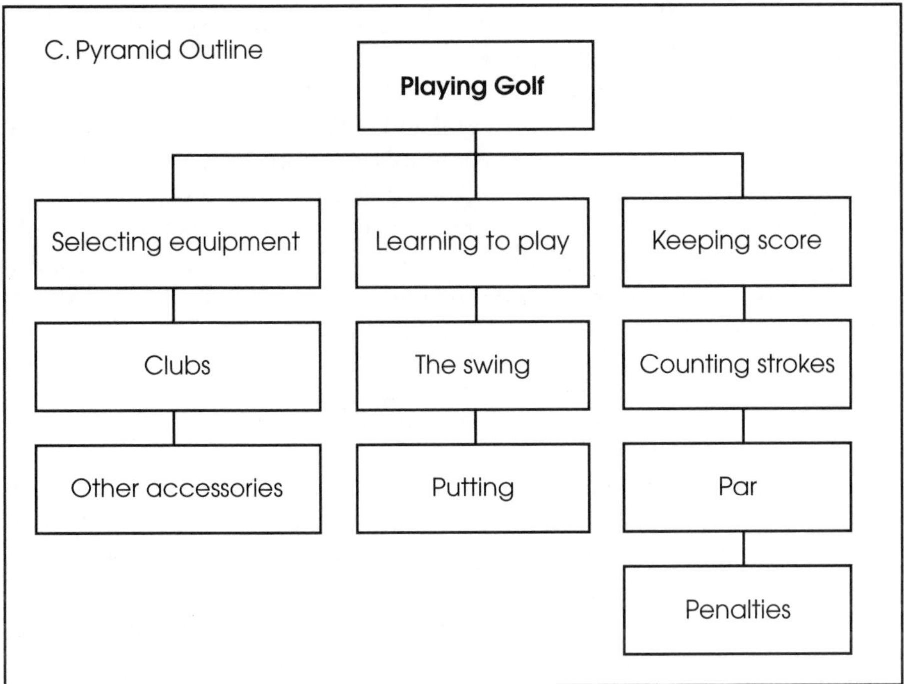

Figure 2.2. *Continued.*

disciplines they are studying. Hennings (1993) demonstrated that, because the key ideas of history are time, place, causation, and ultimate meaning, students must learn to engage the text actively to organize historical figures and events into a meaningful timetable, to locate the events in a specific geographic region, to compare and contrast these with other events in other cultures and locations, to hypothesize about the relations among various causes and effects, and to assess the accuracy and validity of the "facts" included in the passage. Analysis and comprehension of textbooks and lectures in mathematics and English would require very different types of activity.

Finally, in the upper grades, much important information may be omitted from textbooks. Beck, McKeown, Sinatra, and Loxterman (1991) discovered that textbooks often make unrealistic assumptions about what students know. In a unit about the French and Indian War, the textbooks failed to provide information about such crucial issues as why the war began and its relationship to the Revolutionary War. The students had only vague ideas. When the researchers revised the textbooks to include the missing pieces, the students both comprehended and remembered more.

Particularly in the upper grades and college, then, students must learn to learn independently from text, both oral and written. What they bring to that text in terms of their knowledge of content and the structure of both text and the discipline will have an impact on what they are able to learn. The way the text is structured will, in addition, interact with what students know to facilitate or inhibit their learning. Consequently, especially for older students, it is important to evaluate the text for its comprehensiveness, well-formedness, and explicitness before attempting to evaluate students' levels of competence.

Summary

In sum, expository text is probably the most dominant form of discourse used in classrooms. The preponderance of both what teachers say and what students read and write is in expository form, especially after the primary grades. Like conversation and narrative, the complexity demands of exposition increase throughout the school years as teachers impose higher and higher expectations for longer and more sophisticated reports and presentations using more sophisticated language systems. Students must learn to recognize and use several different expository formats (e.g., cause–effect, compare and contrast) to address the content of instruction appropriately and thoroughly.

Although exposition is the *sine qua non* of education, both conversational and narrative abilities have been taken for granted after the primary grades and left to flourish, or not, on their own. Despite the increasingly complex demands for performance in both types of discourse, little instructional effort has been expended toward developing them. However, there are a few hopeful signs in the new standards-based education. At least in some regions, such as the state of Colorado, attention is now being paid to helping students develop competence in oral as well as written discourse.

Discourse Development and Other Factors

Language is complex. It exists at myriad levels and in unlimited variation. There is no set of skills that can be taught to make students proficient language users. Language acquisition, therefore, cannot be facilitated through task analyses and skills practice. It needs to *develop through use and in interactions with competent language users*. That means that language is acquired best in the context of meaningful, higher order units of text (i.e., discourse structures)—conversation, narrative, and exposition.

However, although language is learned in the context of discourse functions, those functions are affected by the levels of competence students attain in each of the language systems. These systems are described in Chapter 3. They include articulation and phonology, suprasegmentals, semantics, morphology and syntax, pragmatics, and metalinguistics. In discourse, students must coordinate and integrate the use of those systems.

Discourse also interacts with cognitive, affective, and social as well as other linguistic proficiencies and deficiencies. Although problems with discourse structures are commonplace among students with special needs, there is no way to predict from a particular disability category the type of discourse difficulties a student is likely to demonstrate. In fact, it is likely that students with special needs will have some problems related to all discourse structures and the more severe the disability, the more severe the disruption in discourse processes is likely to be.

Language Problems Associated with Discourse Development

Students whose disabilities affect language learning and learning through language constitute a heterogeneous group. Students with phonological difficulties are at risk in conversations and with oral narratives and exposition because speech sounds are the vehicle for transmitting meaning or semantic knowledge (Hoffman, Schuckers, & Daniloff, 1989). In fact, conversation and storytelling are preferred contexts for treating phonological disorders (Owens, 1995): When the emphasis is on communication success, improvements in phonological performance and expressive language occur simultaneously (Hoffman, Norris, & Monjure, 1990). In addition, there is no longer any doubt that phonological awareness and the ability to segment phonemes are important to the acquisition of reading and writing (Blachman, 1987; Bryant & Bradley, 1985; Catts, 1986; Liberman & Shankweiler, 1985; Snowling & Hulme, 1989; Stanovich, 1986a, 1986b, 1988a, 1988b; Tallal & Stark, 1982) and hence the development of understandings related to narrative and exposition.

Because the connections among ideas in both oral communication and written texts are signaled by syntactic devices, students with deficits, or even differences, often experience lack of clarity in comprehension (Byrne, 1981; Conte, 1993; Liles, 1985a, 1985b, 1987; Wiig & Semel, 1984). The structures that tend to be particularly problematic are passive voice, pronouns that refer back to previously stated referents, causal relationships expressed by prepositions, embedded clauses, and compound and complex sentences (N. Nelson, 1998; Owens, 1999).

Semantic knowledge is obviously key to discourse success. Students must be able to store and retrieve words to understand and convey thoughts, make meaningful connections between concepts, understand the various forms of figurative language that are used frequently in every form of oral and written text and in adolescence become the badge of peer identity (Nippold, 1998), and construct language in a variety of social and academic situations (Larson & McKinley, 1995). In fact, the entire school day is focused on students' acquisition and application of meaning.

Language Differences Associated with Discourse Development

Students who are limited English proficient or who speak nonstandard dialects of English often come from nonmainstream cultures. Their English may deviate from SAE with respect to all or some of the language systems. Students with first languages other than English may have distinctive accents. Whether a different language or a nonstandard dialect, syntactic and morphological cues may be affected and semantic knowledge will reflect the world view and discourse structures associated with the student's culture. The particular suprasegmental features of the native language may also differ from SAE, making the students' production of English sound markedly different. Along with phonemic differences, suprasegmental features explain why speakers of nonnative or nonstandard dialects do not easily develop the prosodic characteristics of SAE. In addition, the way language is used—the rules for conversational interchanges, preferred idioms and other tropes, for example—vary across linguistic cultures.

Consequently, although there is no language disability, the students' home language may simply not match the language that is used in school. The consequences are often disastrous. Students from nonmainstream backgrounds, especially those who are poor and have different dialects, are likely to be overrepresented in special education or to be low achievers in school. Although students with more obvious language differences are now protected by law from placement in special education classrooms, some misdiagnoses still occur.

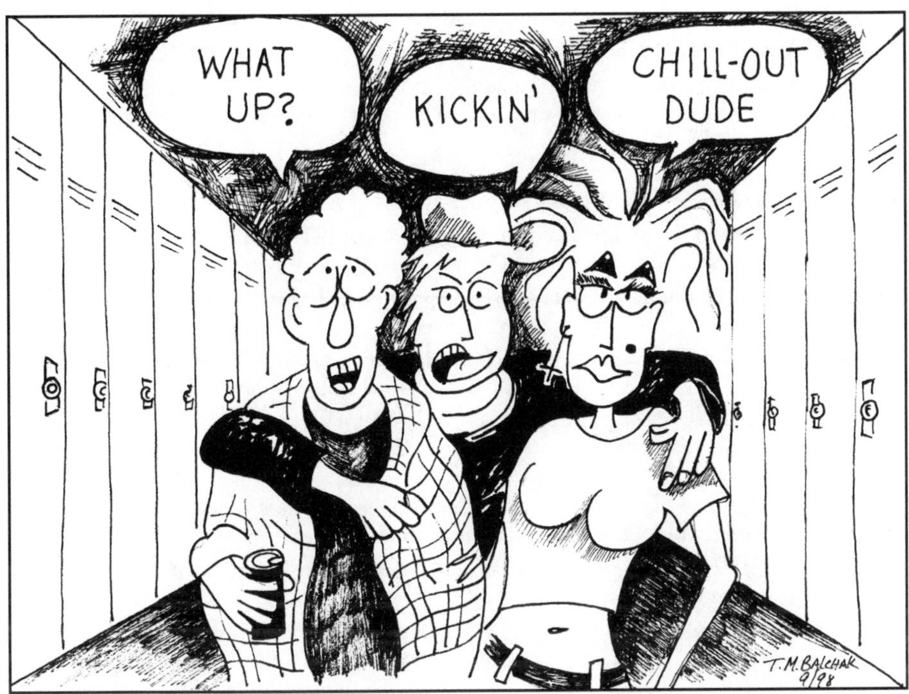

During adolescence the use of slang typically becomes a badge of peer group identity. It serves the purpose of denoting who holds membership in the group and of distinguishing from outsiders.

References

Adams, M. J. (1990). *Beginning to read*. Cambridge, MA: MIT Press.

Beck, I. I., McKeown, M. G., Sinatra, G. M., & Loxterman, J. A. (1991). Revised social studies text from a text-processing perspective: Evidence of improved comprehension. *Reading Research Quarterly*, *26*(3), 251–276.

Blachman, B. A. (1987). An alternative classroom reading program for learning disabled and other low-achieving children. In R. Bowler (Ed.), *Intimacy with language: A forgotten basic in teacher education* (pp. 29–37). Baltimore: The Orton Dyslexia Society.

Blalock, J. (1982). Persistent auditory language deficits in adults with learning disabilities. *Journal of Learning Disabilities*, *15*, 604–609.

Britton, J. (1970). *Language and learning*. London: Penguin Press.

Brown, A. L., Campione, J. C., Weber, L. S., & McGilly, K. (1992). *Interactive learning environments: A new look at assessment and instruction*. Berkeley: University of California, Commission on Testing and Public Policy.

Bruner, J. S. (1975). The ontogenesis of speech acts. *Journal of Child Language*, *2*, 1–20.

Bruner, J. (1978). On prelinguistic prerequisites of speech. In R. N. Campbell & P. T. Smith (Eds.), *Recent advances in the psychology of language* (pp. 242–256). New York: Plenum.

Bruner, J. (1990). *Acts of meaning*. Cambridge, MA: Harvard University Press.

Bryant, P., & Bradley, L. (1985). *Children's reading problems*. New York, Basil Blackwell.

Buttrill, J., Niizawa, J., Biemer, C., Takahashi, C., & Hearn, S. (1989). Serving the language learning disabled adolescent: A strategies-based model. *Language, Speech, and Hearing Services in Schools, 20*, 185–204.

Byrne, B. (1981). Deficient syntactic control in poor readers: Is a weak phonetic memory code responsible? *Applied Psycholinguistics, 2*, 201–212.

Calkins, L. M. (1983). *Lessons from a child: On the teaching and learning of writing*. Portsmouth, NH: Heinemann.

Catts, H. W. (1986). Defining dyslexia as a developmental language disorder. *Annals of Dyslexia, 39*, 50–64.

Cazden, C. B. (1988). *Classroom discourse: The language of teaching and learning*. Portsmouth, NH: Heinemann.

Conte, B. (1993). *The effect of genre, vocabulary, and syntax on the comprehension of expository text in language impaired and non-impaired adolescents*. Unpublished doctoral dissertation, Boston University, Boston, MA.

Cooper, C. S. (1997). Using collaborative/consultative service delivery models for fluency intervention and carryover. *Language, Speech, and Hearing Services in Schools, 22*, 152–153.

Crago, M. B. (1992). Ethnography and language socialization: A cross-cultural perspective. *Topics in Language Disorders, 12*(3), 28–39.

Culatta, B., Page, J., & Ellis, J. (1983). Story retelling as a communicative performance screening tool. *Language, Speech, and Hearing Services in Schools, 14*, 66–74.

Cullinan, B. E. (1989). *Emerging literacy: Young children learn to read and write*. Newark, DE: International Reading Association.

Ehren, B. J. (1994). New directions for meeting the academic needs of adolescents with language learning disabilities. In G. P. Wallach & K. G. Butler (Eds.), *Language learning disabilities in school-age children and adolescents* (pp. 393–417). Needham Heights, MA: Allyn & Bacon.

Ervin-Tripp, S., & Gordon, D. (1986). *Language competence: Assessment and intervention*. Austin, TX: PRO-ED.

Faigley, L., Cherry, R., Jolliffe, D., & Skinner, A. (1985). *Assessing writers' knowledge and processes of composing*. Norwood, NJ: Ablex.

Gallagher, T. M. (1991). Language and social skills: Implications for assessment and intervention with school-age children. In T. M. Gallagher (Ed.), *Pragmatics of language: Clinical practice issues* (pp. 11–41). San Diego: Singular.

Gee, J. (1988, June). *Perspectives on literacy: Cultural and social diversity*. Workshop presented at the Emerson College LLD Institute, Boston.

Gee, J. P. (1989). Two types of narrative construction and their linguistic and educational implications. *Discourse Processes, 12*, 287–307.

Gee, J. P. (1990). *Social linguistics and literacies: Ideology discourses*. London: Falmer Press.

Gillespie, C. S. (1993). Reading graphic displays: What teachers should know. *Journal of Reading, 36*(5), 350–354.

Gleason, J. B. (1993). *The development of language*. New York: Macmillan.

Graham, S., & Harris, K. R. (1993). Self-regulated strategy development: Helping students with learning problems develop as writers. *Elementary School Journal, 94*(2), 169–181.

Green, J. L., Weade, R., & Graham, K. (1988). Lesson construction and student participation: A sociolinguistic analysis. In J. L. Green & J. O. Harker (Eds.), *Multiple perspective analysis of classroom discourse*. Norwood, NJ: Ablex.

Halliday, M. A. K. (1987). *Comprehending oral and written language*. San Diego: Academic Press.

Harris, K. R., & Graham, S. (1992). *Helping young writers master the craft: Strategy instruction and self-regulation in the writing process*. Cambridge, MA: Brookline Books.

Harris, K. R., & Graham, S. (1996). *Making the writing process work: Strategies for composition and self-regulation*. Cambridge, MA: Brookline Books.

Heath, S. B. (1978). *Teacher talk: Language in the classroom*. Washington, DC: Center for Applied Linguistics.

Heath, S. B. (1983). *Ways with words: Language, life and work in communities and classrooms*. London: Cambridge University Press.

Hedberg, N. L., & Westby, C. E. (1993). *Analyzing storytelling skills: Theory to practice*. Tucson, AZ: Communication Skill Builders.

Hennings, D. G. (1993). On knowing and reading history. *Journal of Reading, 36*(5), 362–370.

Hoffman, P. R., Norris, J. A., & Monjure, J. (1990). Comparison of process targeting and whole language treatments for phonologically delayed preschool children. *Language, Speech, and Hearing Services in Schools, 21*, 102–109.

Hoffman, P. R., Schuckers, G., & Daniloff, R. (1989). *Children's phonetic disorders: Theory and treatment*. San Diego: College-Hill.

Hoskins, B. (1990). Language and literacy: Participating in the conversation. *Topics in Language Disorders, 10*(2), 46–62.

Kemper, S., & Edwards, L. (1986). Children's expression of causality and their construction of narratives. *Topics in Language Disorders, 7*(1), 11–20.

Larson, V. L., & McKinley, M. S. (1995). *Language disorders in older students: Preadolescents and adolescents*. Eau Claire, WI: Thinking Publications.

Larson, V. L., McKinley, N. L., & Boley, D. (1993). Service delivery models for adolescents with language disorders. *Language, Speech, and Hearing Services in Schools, 24*, 36–42.

Liberman, I. Y., & Shankweiler, D. (1985). Phonology and the problems of learning to read and write. *Remedial and Special Education, 6*, 8–17.

Liles, B. (1985a). Cohesion in the narratives of normal and language disordered children. *Journal of Speech and Hearing Research, 28*, 123–133.

Liles, B. (1985b). Production and comprehension of narrative discourse in normal and language disordered children. *Journal of Communication Disorders, 18*, 409–427.

Liles, B. (1987). Episode organization and cohesive conjunctives in narratives of children with and without language disorder. *Journal of Speech and Hearing Research, 30*, 185–196.

Lindfors, J. W. (1987). *Children's language and learning* (2nd ed.). Needham Heights, MA: Allyn & Bacon.

McCabe, A., & Peterson, C. (1985). A naturalistic study of the production of causal connectives by children. *Journal of Child Language, 12*, 145–160.

Meichenbaum, D. (1977). *Cognitive behavior modification: An integrative approach*. New York: Plenum Press.

Milosky, L. M. (1990). The role of world knowledge in language comprehension and language intervention. *Topics in Language Disorders, 10*(3), 1–13.

Milosky, L. M. (1994). Nonliteral language abilities. In G. P. Wallach & K. G. Butler (Eds.), *Language learning disabilities in school-age children and adolescents* (pp. 275–300). Needham Heights, MA: Allyn & Bacon.

Morine-Dershimer, G., & Tenenberg, M. (1981). *Participant perspectives of classroom discourse. Executive summary of final report*. Syracuse, NY: Syracuse University Division for the Study of Teaching.

Nelson, K. (Ed.). (1989). *Narratives from the crib*. Cambridge, MA: Harvard University Press.

Nelson, N. W. (1993). *Childhood language disorders in context: Infancy through adolescence*. Needham Heights, MA: Allyn & Bacon.

Nelson, N. W. (1998). *Childhood language disorders in context: Infancy through adolescence* (2nd ed.). Needham Heights, MA: Allyn & Bacon.

Nelson, N. W., & Friedman, K. K. (1988). *Development of the concept of story in narratives written by older children*. Unpublished paper, Western Michigan University, Kalamazoo.

Nelson, N. W., & Friedman, K. K. (1993). Development of the concept of story in narratives written by older children. In N. W. Nelson (Ed.), *Childhood language disorders in context: Infancy through adolescence*. Needham Heights, MA: Allyn & Bacon.

Ninio, A., & Bruner, J. S. (1978). The achievement and antecedents of labeling. *Journal of Child Language*, *5*, 1–15.

Nippold, M. A. (1998). *Later language development: The school-age and adolescent years*. Austin, TX: PRO-ED.

Ohlhausen, M., & Roller, C. (1988). The operation of text structure and content schemata in isolation and interaction. *Reading Research Quarterly*, *23*, 70–88.

Owens, R. E. (1984). *Language development: An introduction*. New York: Merrill.

Owens, R. E. (1991). *Language disorders: A functional approach to assessment and intervention*. New York: Macmillan.

Owens, R. E. (1995). *Language disorders: A functional approach to assessment and intervention* (2nd ed.). Needham Heights, MA: Allyn & Bacon.

Owens, R. E. (1999). *Language disorders: A functional approach to assessment and intervention* (3rd ed.). Needham Heights, MA: Allyn & Bacon.

Peterson, C., & McCabe, A. (1983). *Developmental psycholinguistics: Three ways of looking at a child's narrative*. New York: Plenum Press.

Phillips, T. (1985). Beyond lip-service: Discourse development after the age of nine. In G. Wells & J. Nicholls (Eds.), *Language and learning: An interactionist perspective* (pp. 148–173). London: Falmer Press.

Polkinghorne, D. E. (1988). *Narrative knowing and the human sciences*. Albany: State University of New York Press.

Pollio, H., Barlow, J., Fine, H., & Pollio, M. (1977). *Psychology and the poetics of growth*. Hillsdale, NJ: Erlbaum.

Pollio, H., Smith, M., & Pollio, M. (1990). Figurative language and cognitive psychology. *Language and Cognitive Processes*, *5*, 141–167.

Prutting, C. A., & Kirchner, D. M. (1987). A clinical approach to the pragmatic aspects of language. *Journal of Speech and Hearing Disorders*, *52*, 105–119.

Reid, D. K., & Hresko, W. P. (1988). Independent study skills. In D. K. Reid (Ed.), *Teaching the learning disabled: A cognitive approach* (pp. 435–463). Needham Heights, MA: Allyn & Bacon.

Ricoeur, P. (1981). *Hermeneutics and the human sciences* (John B. Thompson, Trans.). Cambridge, England: Cambridge University Press.

Roller, C. M. (1990). Commentary: The interaction of knowledge and structure variables in the processing of expository prose. *Reading Research Quarterly*, *25*(2), 79–89.

Romaine, S. (1984). *The language of children and adolescents*. Oxford: Blackwell.

Rubin, D. L. (1990). *Perspectives on talk and learning*. Urbana, IL: National Council of Teachers of English.

Sachs, J. (1989). Communication development in infancy. In J. Berko-Gleason (Ed.), *The development of language* (pp. 35–58). Columbus, OH: Merrill/Macmillan.

Scott, C. M. (1994). A discourse continuum for school-age students. In G. P. Wallach & K. G. Butler (Eds.), *Language learning disabilities in school-age children and adolescents* (pp. 219–248). Needham Heights, MA: Allyn & Bacon.

Shuy, R. W. (1988). Identifying dimensions of classroom language. In J. L. Green & J. O. Harker (Eds.), *Multiple perspective analysis of classroom discourse* (Vol. 28, pp. 115–134). Norwood, NJ: Ablex.

Slater, W. H., & Graves, M. F. (1989). Research on expository text: Implications for teachers. In K. D. Muth (Ed.), *Children's comprehension of text* (pp. 140–166). Newark, DE: International Reading Association.

Snow, C. E. (1991). Diverse conversational context for the acquisition of various language skills. In J. Miller (Ed.), *Research on child language disorders* (pp. 105–124). Austin, TX: PRO-ED.

Snowling, M. J., & Hulme, C. (1989). A longitudinal case study of developmental phonological dyslexia. *Cognitive Neuropsychology*, 6, 379–401.

Staab, C. F. (1991). Teachers' practices with regard to oral language. *The Alberta Journal of Educational Research*, *37*(1), 31–45.

Stanovich, K. E. (1986a). Cognitive processes and the reading problems of learning disabled children: Evaluating the assumption of specificity. In J. K. Torgeson & B. Y. W. Wong (Eds.), *Psychological and educational perspectives on learning disabilities* (pp. 67–96). New York: Academic Press.

Stanovich, K. E. (1986b). Matthew effects in reading: Some consequences of individual differences in the acquisition of literacy. *Reading Research Quarterly*, *21*, 360–407.

Stanovich, K. E. (1988a). Explaining the differences between the dyslexic and the garden variety poor reader: The phonological-core variable-difference model. *Journal of Learning Disabilities*, *21*, 590–604.

Stanovich, K. E. (1988b). The right and wrong places to look for the cognitive locus of reading disability. *Annals of Dyslexia*, *38*, 154–177.

Stein, M. L., & Glenn, C. J. (1979). An analysis of story comprehension in elementary school children. In R. Freedle (Ed.), *Multidisciplinary approaches to discourse comprehension* (pp. 53–120). Hillsdale, NJ: Ables.

Sutton-Smith, B. (1986). The development of fictional narrative performances. *Topics in Language Disorders*, *7*(1), 1–10.

Swoger, P. A. (1989). Scott's gift. *English Journal*, *78*, 61–65.

Tallal, P., & Stark, R. E. (1982). Perceptual/motor profiles of reading impaired children with or without concomitant oral language deficits. *Annals of Dyslexia*, *32*, 305–317.

Vygotsky, L. S. (1987). *The collected works of L. S. Vygotsky: Vol. 1. Problems of general psychology* (R. Rieber & A. Carton, Eds., & N. Minick,. Trans.) New York: Plenum.

Wallach, G. P., & Butler, K. G. (1994). *Language learning disabilities in school-age children and adolescents: Some principles and applications*. Needham Heights, MA: Allyn & Bacon.

Wanner, S. Y. (1994). *On with the story: Adolescents learning through narrative*. Portsmouth, NH: Boynton/Cook.

Westby, C. E. (1994). The effects of culture on genre, structure and style of oral and written texts. In G. P. Wallach & K. G. Butler (Eds.), *Language learning disabilities in school-age children and adolescents* (pp. 180–213). Needham Heights, MA: Allyn & Bacon.

Wiig, E. H., & Semel, E. M. (1984). *Language assessment and intervention for the learning disabled* (2nd ed.). New York: Merrill/Macmillan.

The Development of Oral Language

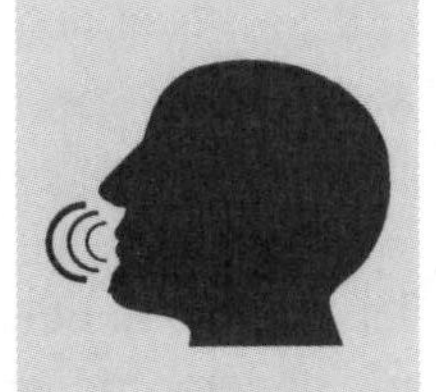

Chapter 3

Kathleen R. Fahey

Language is the primary means people use to express ideas, learn new information, and establish and maintain social relationships. As noted in previous chapters, its development is central to academic achievement and social competence. An understanding of normal language development during the preschool, elementary, and high school years allows general and special education teachers to interact efficiently and effectively with each other and with speech–language pathologists (SLPs), as well as to plan curricula based on students' prior knowledge and to foster new ways of learning for future social and academic opportunities.

This chapter focuses on the development of Standard American English (SAE) as the first language in native speakers. Chapter 5 focuses on the characteristics of other languages and dialects (i.e., Ebonics, Hispanic American, Asian American, and Native American) and their impact on children's acquisition of English as a second language.

Language Competence and Performance

Successful communication and learning in our schools is dependent on both language competence and performance. *Language competence*—the large body of knowledge that children acquire from everyday experiences in their environment—allows people to interact with others in functional and productive ways. People are language competent when they know what social-communication rules are appropriate in common situations, what vocabulary is appropriate for the topic and setting, how to engage appropriately in turn taking during exchanges, how to respond to commands and directions, and how to acquire new information during interactions (Gleason, 1997; Owens, 1992). *Language performance*, on the other hand, refers to one's ability to use language in meaningful ways and in a variety of situations. Students speak about their ideas and experiences using expansive vocabulary and the grammar of their native language to participate in meaningful dialogue with other students and teachers and to use language as a tool for reasoning, problem solving, and developing writing (Gleason, 1997; Owens, 1992).

When students do not have either the expected language competence or the performance capabilities upon entry to kindergarten or higher grades, teachers face the problem of a mismatch between the level of the child's language and the curriculum to be taught. One common example of such a mismatch occurs when a kindergarten student is not able to label colors, numbers, or the alphabet, or to play verbal rhyming games. Such a student may require many experiences and much time to develop the concepts that his or her peers have upon school entry. Although such mismatches present challenges for both teacher and student, as well as for classmates who must adjust to individual differences as they interact with each other, the classroom environment can and should be the place for bolstering a student's language competence and performance.

Prior to entry in kindergarten, some schools complete initial observations (variously referred to as screenings, readiness testing, kindergarten roundup, or developmental testing) of students' language and other areas of development (i.e., hearing acuity, social maturity, fine and gross motor skills), which provide teachers with an estimate of students' performance abilities in these areas. Students who "pass" the established criteria are enrolled in kindergarten, whereas those who do not demonstrate sufficient abilities are sometimes channeled into developmental kindergartens or preschools, or are referred to special education for further evaluation. Students with severe developmental problems may be placed into special education programs. I take exception to the term *readiness* because it denies the fact that children normally have different experiences, backgrounds, and opportunities that contribute to their development (i.e., language, social-emotional growth, fine and gross motor skills) and their knowledge of school (i.e., literacy, school discourse, school culture). We should expect such differences and kindergarten teachers should address them. We cannot assume a given set of skills or knowledge base. Instead, we must recognize the variety of levels and interests that students bring to school and be ready to teach them where they are.

Experienced teachers have a sixth sense about what children understand and produce at various age levels, so it is not surprising that it is the teacher who refers specific children for evaluation of speech, language, or learning abilities. Often, teachers can describe what they see or hear that causes them concern. Such descriptions are very helpful to the SLP or other special educators in selecting classroom-based assessments or norm-referenced tests to determine the nature and extent of a child's language or learning problem. It is through an understanding of where each student is in language development that teachers can support and nurture further language growth.

The Development of Oral Language Systems

Oral language development occurs gradually across several years as children interact first with their families, and later with teachers and peers in school. Oral language systems include (a) articulation and phonology, (b) prosody or suprasegmentals, (c) morphology and syntax, (d) semantics, (e) metalinguistics, and (f) pragmatics. *All of these develop simultaneously, with interactions occurring between and among them*. Although the divisions among the language systems are artificial, they enable us to talk about the complexity of language in manageable units.

Articulation and Phonology

The knowledge and use of the sound system of the native language develops gradually from infancy through high school, with the predominant attainments occurring from a few months of age to about 7 or 8 years. The developmental process is fairly predictable, yet children show an amazing range of variability (Bernthal & Bankson, 1998). The trends guide us in our observations of children and help us determine whether development is on target or delayed.

The Preschool Years

Articulation, probably the most familiar term to parents and teachers, refers to the production of speech sounds in a speaker's native language. Because children typically learn the language of their families first, it is important that parents talk frequently to their infants and children during routines such as bathing, dressing, and feeding. Although the child cannot verbally participate, such talk establishes early links between sounds and meanings. Although children perceive and learn to produce speech sounds at an early age, it takes several years for speech to be used completely and correctly in conversation. The biological system develops slowly and affects the motor control of the speech mechanism. Thus, children require time and practice to integrate the production of speech sounds with emerging vocabulary and sentence structure. Table 3.1 shows the common trends in speech sound perception and production from infancy through the preschool years (Weiss, Gordon, & Lillywhite, 1987).

Table 3.1
Developmental Trends in Speech Perception and Production: First 4 Years

Age in Months	Speech Perception and Production
1 through 5	Discrimination of speech sounds
	Reflexive vocalizations such as crying, squeaking, vowel-like sounds
	Production of many vowels and consonants, including /l, h, k, g, m, n, b, p, j, ŋ, r, t, v, z, θ/
	Vocal play and babbling with syllable repetition
6 through 12	Use of changing pitch during babbling
	Babbling reaches its peak
	Imitation of sounds made by others
	Continued development of vowels, diphthongs, and consonants
	Sequences of syllables with the prosody of the native language (jargon)
	Repetition of babbling or words heard from others (echolalia)
	Understanding of a variety of words in context
	Use of invented words and true words
	Simplification of difficult words
13 through 24	Development of word combinations
	Refinement in the production of speech sounds within old and new words
	Individual preferences for sound use
	Use of pitch changes to influence meaning
	Speech production is typically 25% to 50% intelligible
25 through 36	A variety of consonants and vowels used accurately
	The prosody of the native language is used for conveying intentions
	Speech production is intelligible 60% to 80% of the time

(*continues*)

Table 3.1 *Continued.*

Age in Months	Speech Perception and Production
37 through 48	Consonants continue to be learned in the production of more difficult words including /f, s, z, ʃ, tʃ, dʒ, ʒ, ð, r/
	Speech intelligibility increases to 90% or higher

Note. Adapted from *Clinical Management of Articulatory and Phonologic Disorders* (2nd ed.), by C. E. Weiss, M. E. Gordon, and H. S. Lillywhite, 1987, Baltimore: Williams & Wilkins. (See Appendix 3.A for the International Phonetic Alphabet.)

Notice that by the time most children enter preschool and kindergarten, the sound system is used for functional and intelligible communication.

Phonology, a more inclusive term, refers to the knowledge speakers have about sounds and the rules for putting sounds together in any particular language. Children learn the appropriate sound combinations through exposure to their language via the social interactions parents and others engage them in. The similarity between articulation and phonology is that both describe the speech sound system. The differences can be thought about in terms of competence and performance. Consider the preschool child learning to produce speech sounds, who for several years produces words as best she can with sound omissions, substitutions, or distortions. For example, a 3-year-old may produce *thumb* as "fum" or *rabbit* as "wabbit." These pronunciations do not cause alarm, because adults know that most young children hear the 'th' and 'r' sounds but have difficulty producing them accurately. Thus children attempt words with these sounds but end up producing sounds they can say easily. The child knows the sounds but lacks the motor sophistication to produce them, because sounds require precise coordination of the speech mechanism (tongue, lips, soft palate, etc.). On the other hand, understanding how language develops enables us to recognize that 3-year-olds who consistently omit all or most final consonants in words may be demonstrating a lack of knowledge about the role these consonants play in establishing word meanings. Simplifying words this way can drastically affect meaning (e.g., "*bo*" for *boat, bowl, bone*). A child who simplifies words may be able to put many different sounds on the ends of words, but does not do so because she fails to recognize an important rule in speech production (i.e., final consonants). The omission of final sounds is much more serious than pronunciation difficulties because it often results in poor intelligibility. It also reflects a problem in the child's knowledge of phonological rules, which is a symptom of an underlying language development problem.

The simplification strategies children use during the preschool years, also known as *phonological processes*, are normal as they learn the sound system. These simplification strategies, common between 1 and 4 years, are listed in Table 3.2 (Bernthal & Bankson, 1998; Lowe, 1994; Weiss et al., 1987). For instance, it is common for children even after 3 years of age to attempt words with consonant clusters by producing only one of the consonants within the cluster, such as when the word *tree* is pronounced "tee." Most simplifications are replaced by mature production of sounds in words after age 3 or 4. Their continued use beyond age 4 is an important factor in determining whether a child has a delay in the phonological system. Particularly, a child's level of intelligibility during conversation with adults and other children often concerns parents and preschool teachers; thus, we encourage them to refer the child to an SLP who will complete an assessment of the sound system.

Another challenge for preschoolers is the development of the use of units of meaning. These are called *morphemes* and are described at length later in this chapter. For now, note that morphemes reflect changes in tense (present, past, future), number (singular or plural), ownership (possessive), and so forth. These are relevant to our discussion here because when morphemes are added to words, the pronunciations of the words change. For example, notice the pronunciation changes in *walk–walked*, *bag–bagged*, and *react–reacted*. The suffix is produced as a 't,' 'd,' or 'ed' depending on the sound immediately preceding it. These variations occur naturally as speakers connect speech sounds into meaningful units. The relationship between the units of meaning and the phonemes to express the units is called *morphophonemics*. Students who are delayed in phonology or in the development of the grammar itself may omit or distort these word endings (Gleason, 1997; Owens, 1992).

The Elementary and Middle School Years

Parents and educators alike use terms such as *speech* and *pronunciation* to talk to young children about producing speech sounds. For school-age children, however, we refer to our English alphabet to label and think about speech sounds, such as when students ask how words are spelled or when we highlight sounds during phonics activities or rhyming games. SLPs use the International Phonetic Alphabet (IPA) so that the unique aspects of each sound are represented by a particular symbol. Familiarity with the IPA (Appendix 3.A) can help general and special education teachers understand specific problems described in assessment reports. The SLP can provide a translation key using standard dictionary symbols for sounds to make it easy for others to interpret reports.

By age 8, elementary students are quite mature in producing sounds during connected speech. Local (1983) suggested that such maturity may be the result

Table 3.2
Common Word Simplification Strategies (Phonological Processes) in Toddlers and Preschoolers

Prior to Age 3		After Age 3	
Phonological Process	**Example**	**Phonological Process**	**Example**
Unstressed syllable deletion	"mato"—tomato	Cluster reduction	"poon"—spoon
Final consonant deletion	"bo"—boat	Epenthesis	"saleep"—sleep
Doubling (reduplication)	"tata"—tiger	Gliding	"yike"—like
Diminutization	"banki"—blanket	Vocalization	"wheo"—wheel
Consonant assimilation	"noon"—soon	Stopping	"dut"—juice
Velar fronting	"doat"—goat	Depalatalization	"fis"—fish
Prevocalic voicing	"bat"—pat		

of having mastered the intricate production of sound combinations. The slight modifications that sounds undergo as they are influenced by surrounding sounds are called *allophonic variations*. Say "pumpkin" slowly as if you were having students spell it. Now say it rapidly in the sentence "Carve the pumpkin for the October party." Notice how the individual sounds become modified (e.g., "pungkin"). Word pronunciations are also altered through regional dialects (e.g., "punkin"). In spite of the modifications, as long as the meaning of the word is unchanged, speakers of the language recognize the word being said. As students encounter new words and try to modify old ones, they experiment with the precision with which they say the sounds and begin to master the complicated syllable arrangements of longer words.

Elementary students continue to apply the morphophonemic pronunciation rules as they add or omit prefixes and suffixes to words. Words are also altered in various ways to communicate nuances in meaning. Refinement of analytical skills used to understand systematic alterations in words occurs over time. Not until age 8 to 10 do children notice the changes that occur when derivations are created. For example, we *divide* two numbers through an operation called *division*. This vowel shift rule (i.e., second 'i' from long to short) is an example of changes in pronunciation when nuances of meaning are added to words (Grunwell, 1986).

Reading and writing instruction also help to accelerate oral language development and awareness of phonological rules as children gain knowledge about how speech sounds function in words. Likewise, *phonological awareness* (the ability to recognize and manipulate sounds in words) and *metalinguistics* (the ability to think about the components of language) provide students with insights about how the language is constructed. These abilities allow students to spell words, add prefixes and suffixes in writing, make up poems that rhyme, engage in word play (e.g., pig latin), and understand jokes that rely on understanding subtle manipulations of sounds and other components of language.

The Later School Years

As students advance through adolescence and become young adults, they continue to add new words to their listening and speaking vocabulary. They try new words, refining their articulation through practice, and reflect on old and new knowledge about the sound system. For example, a new word from a science lesson (e.g., *disproportionate*) may be segmented into syllables for ease in pronunciation and spelling, divided into units of meaning for understanding (i.e., *not in proportion*), and practiced in various sentences for correct usage in semantic and syntactic contexts. Students appreciate word similarities and differences as they manipulate sounds and units of meaning in speaking and writing.

Students must also adjust to the increased demands that the curriculum imposes, such as lectures spoken with increasingly complex sentence types (e.g., compound, complex) that convey complex ideas. As language complexity increases, so too do the subtleties of meaning through devices such as contrastive word stress, speaker's attitude, social dialects, and style variation—all of which are discussed in the next section.

Summary

The development of the sound system of SAE involves a complex process that spans many years. During the preschool years, children establish and use speech sounds to produce words and sentences to communicate with others. Through experience and modeling, they learn about sound combinations and implicit rules for using sounds in words and for adding sounds to change tense, number, ownership, or so forth. They also accrue knowledge about how words sound and begin to recognize, manipulate, and play with sounds. During the elementary school years, knowledge of speech sounds becomes an important base for learning to read and write within the curriculum. Although the speech sounds are usually produced accurately by most children, all children continue to apply speech production principles to new words and words that change through additions of prefixes, suffixes, and derivational forms. This fine-tuning of speech continues throughout the elementary years and is facilitated by continued development of reading and writing. Older students and adults use their knowledge of sounds and morphemes to attempt to produce unknown words, refine their pronunciations, and reflect on the construction of words containing several morphemes. They recognize subtleties in meaning conveyed by speaking characteristics such as formal and informal styles, dialect, and attitudes.

Suprasegmental Aspects

Our ability to produce speech sounds allows us to articulate individual words, whereas our knowledge of sound boundaries in words allows us to separate one word from another. *Suprasegmentals* refer to (a) pauses between words, phrases, and sentences; (b) pitch contours and loudness levels allowing us to ask questions, make statements, or put emphasis on words; (c) stress on particular syllables within words or words within phrases; and (d) rhythm, including the timing of sounds and words across utterances. Suprasegmental characteristics are sometimes referred to as "the music" or *prosody* of a language.

The Preschool Years

The development and use of the suprasegmental aspects of speech, which develop prior to and along with speech sounds, are important in the perception and production of the native language. Prior to 6 months of age, babbling is not distinguishable from one language to another. After 6 months, however, babbling contains the suprasegmental characteristics of whatever language a child hears in his or her environment (Bernthal & Bankson, 1998; de Boysson-Bardies, Sagart, & Durand, 1984), especially through the engaging prosodic features of motherese (Fernald & Kuhl, 1987; Fernald & Simon,1984). Gradually, children learn to use prosodic features in babbling. For example, children babble the sounds "da, ta, da, ba, da" into the telephone with rising and falling intonation (da↑ta↑da↘ba↑da↘) because they observe this use of language from family members. *Jargon* is the term used to describe the very early (at 10 to 14 months) joining of syllables and the use of the natural melody of the language. Children often use jargon when they are alone. For example, before they fall asleep many children hold conversations with stuffed animals in their cribs or beds.

Suprasegmental aspects reveal the moods and feelings behind what we say. Parents can, for instance, know what their child is thinking or feeling by the way he says "no." The meaning of this word can reveal frustration, uncertainty, unwillingness, denial, or negation, depending on how it is said and in what social context it is used. It takes several years for children to learn how to control suprasegmental aspects, such as their rate of speech and their tone, when addressing parents and other adults. Often, adults convey displeasure when children express bossy, excessively loud, or whining utterances. Gradually, through cues from others, children learn how to express their ideas in socially acceptable ways.

The Elementary and Middle School Years

During the elementary school years, further understanding, control, and selectivity in the use of suprasegmental aspects occur. One such development is the grammatical use of prosody. Contrastive stress is used in English to highlight new information (e.g., "I have *five* marbles now"), distinguish pronoun importance or reference (e.g., "Sharon called Mary and then Linda called *her*"), emphasize particular words for meaning (e.g., "What did she *tell* you?"), and distinguish noun compounds from noun phrases (e.g., "blackboard," "black board") and nouns from verbs (e.g., "′defense, de′fense"). Because use of contrastive stress is determined by grammatical structure, learning to use appropriate stress is a gradual process that can continue into later childhood (Grunwell, 1986). Teachers use contrastive stress frequently as they convey information to students; however, some children as old as 12 may still be learning stress placement rules. Teachers can assist children in this development by saying the same thing several different ways so that the meaning of contrastive stress is conveyed through other forms.

Another avenue involving prosodic development is described by Grunwell (1986) as *sociophonology*. Here, social situations determine the style of speech patterns used. Even very young children modify speech style according to different listeners and situations (e.g., speaking to an animal, role-playing parent style). During the elementary years, students become skilled at using different voices for characters (E. Clark & Andersen, 1979) and varying word and grammar choices according to situational differences (Brenneis & Lein, 1977; Cook-Gumperz, 1977).

The Later School Years

As older students are presented with more variety by the social settings they encounter (e.g., travel, part-time employment, competing in sports or music), they recognize social dialects and the prestige differences between dialects. They also acquire the ability to adjust their pronunciation and grammatical patterns to reflect common (lower prestige) or more formal (higher prestige) styles (Day, 1982; Giles, Harrison, Creber, Smith, & Freeman, 1983; Reid, 1978). This flexibility allows them to fit in socially with particular groups.

Suprasegmental aspects of speech are often incorporated into the instruction of literary style. For example, if persuasion is being addressed in drama class as one form of argument, students practice using the intonation and stress attributes to influence someone else's thinking about a topic. The way a message is conveyed can be as powerful as (or more powerful than) the words used. Students learn to manipulate these characteristics in a variety of ways in both social and academic settings (Owens, 1992). Middle school students become masters of sarcasm, whereas upper level high school students adopt an air of superiority. No matter what the age of the speaker, listeners readily recognize whining, begging, sarcasm, evasiveness, disinterest, anger, or playfulness. These meanings are communicated through the suprasegmental aspects of speech.

Summary

The prosody of our language includes features such as pausing, pitch contours, stress, and rhythm that speakers use to convey ideas, emotions, and attitudes.

As infants hear the language of their households, which contains particular prosodic features, they incorporate such features into their babbling. With the acquisition of the sound system, vocabulary, and grammar of the native language, they use prosodic features to convey intention and mood. School-age children gradually learn how to vary prosodic features and to use such features in appropriate contexts so that they convey nuances in meaning. In particular, students use contrastive stress to emphasize grammatical units in order to highlight meanings. They also begin to appreciate and use stylistic variations depending on the social situations they encounter. Older students expand their knowledge and use of different dialects and styles, especially as they find acceptance in different social groups. They more easily adjust to social situation differences and use prosodic features in more refined ways.

Morphology and Syntax

During the first year, youngsters acquire speech sounds and prosody through babbling and jargon. They already understand many words that family members say, and they express their intentions through gestures. This foundation paves the way for the development of words, word combinations, and sentences. The gradual development of grammar allows speakers to elaborate their ideas and to convey them effectively to others.

The Preschool Years

Sometime between 10 and 14 months, toddlers produce their first words. The utterances sound like words in the native language and are produced in specific contexts for specific purposes. Family members recognize these words and respond by meeting the request or acknowledging the comment, and providing praise and models for pronunciation. Gradually, word variations and combinations form as children expand on the type and number of words they know how to say. For instance, saying "up" is very functional for a 1-year-old, but "mommy up" provides a more powerful request.

Morphemes are units of meaning conveyed through speech. A *free morpheme* is an independent unit (word) that stands alone, such as *toy, dog, catch,* and *eat* (Owens, 1992). *Bound morphemes* can also be added to words to alter meanings. One type of bound morpheme *inflects* words through the addition of phonemes that change tense, number, or ownership, or to make comparisons. For example, we add the 's' sound to *house* to make it plural *(houses)*. Another type of bound morpheme creates *derivations* through the addition of prefixes and suffixes as when the verb *fasten* is changed to *unfasten* (Owens,

1992). Refer to Table 3.3 for examples of inflectional and derivational morphemes.

The development of free and bound morphemes permits children to convey intentions through single words. Yet, children quickly move beyond using single words to combining them in creative ways in order to communicate with others. Children use a combination of gestures, single words, and word combinations as they develop language. They listen to others and model what is said but also experiment with new words and new combinations. Parents scaffold these utterances so that their children hear new uses and combinations for their language.

Table 3.3
Morpheme Types

Free Morphemes—units of meaning that exist as whole words.

Examples:	dog	swing	play	surprise
	bed	happy	blue	donut

Bound Morphemes—units of meaning that are added to free morphemes to change their meanings. They are inflectional or derivational.

Inflectional morphemes change the state or increase the precision of free morphemes by altering tense, pluralization, or possession, or by creating comparatives and superlatives.

Examples:	play + past	=	played
	dog + plural	=	dogs
	dog + possessive	=	dog's
	happy + more	=	happier, happiest

Derivational morphemes change classes of words by changing beginnings **(prefixes)** or endings **(suffixes)** of words.

Examples:

Prefixes		**Suffixes**	
un + do	= undo	revive + al	= revival
in + direct	= indirect	remark + able	= remarkable
pre + washed	= prewashed	teach + er	= teacher
non + functional	= nonfunctional	beauty + ful	= beautiful
trans + atlantic	= transatlantic	floral + ist	= florist
dis + band	= disband	slow + ly	= slowly

For example, a 15-month-old child may make a request for juice by saying, "Mama juice?" The mother may respond by saying, "Becky wants juice? Okay, here is juice."

Preschoolers continue to develop grammatical elements through lengthening of their utterances. Brown (1973) delineated stages based on *mean length of utterance* (MLU), which is the average number of morphemes produced in utterances within language samples. A typical language sample contains about 100 utterances (so that the average utterance length is representative of a particular child's language production). To determine the developmental stage, one counts the number of morphemes in each utterance, sums them across the 100 utterances, and divides by the total number of utterances (i.e., 100). The MLU is then matched to the stage that corresponds to morphological growth (Table 3.4). One- to 2-year-old children use single words and two-word combinations, whereas 2- to 3-year-olds use three- and four-word combinations. During the fourth year or later, children use combinations of four or more words. Although MLU is used as an estimate of grammatical development, it does not determine the range of utterance length, grammatical forms, or sentence types being used.

One analysis that allows us to determine the extent and complexity of grammatical development is to compare a child's MLU stage with the type of morphemes used within the sample. Table 3.5 shows 14 grammatical morphemes children develop as they expand utterance length. These morphemes occur in a predictable order (de Villiers & de Villiers, 1973) that relates to both semantic and syntactic complexity of the morphemes (Gleason, 1997). Other morphemes not included in the table (e.g., pronouns, negatives, questions) occur in sentence form development during MLU stages III (2.5 to 3.0 morphemes) through V (4.50+ morphemes).

Table 3.4
Mean Length of Utterance (MLU) Stages

Age Range (Months)	Mean Length of Utterance	MLU Stage
12 to 26	1.00 to 2.00	I
27 to 30	2.00 to 2.50	II
31 to 34	2.50 to 3.00	III
35 to 40	3.00 to 3.75	IV
41 to 46	3.75 to 4.50	V
47+	4.50+	V+

Table 3.5
Acquisition Sequence of 14 Grammatical Morphemes

Sample	Grammatical Morpheme
1. Me eat*ing*.	present progressive verb
2. No *on* Mommy.	preposition
3. More *in* cup.	preposition
4. Read *books* daddy.	plural
5. Daddy *came* home!	irregular past
6. That is *doggie's* bone.	possessive
7. Jimmy *was* at school.	uncontractable copula (main) verb
8. I got *the* blue ball.	article
9. Mommy *cooked* my cereal.	regular past
10. Annie *barks* too much.	regular third person
11. He *has* a big nose.	irregular third person
12. Who is hiding? We *are*!	uncontractable auxiliary verb
13. *We're* happy today.	contractable copula (main) verb
14. *I'm* tired now.	contractable auxiliary verb

Note. Adapted from "A Cross-Sectional Study of the Acquisition of Grammatical Morphemes in Child Speech," by J. G. de Villiers and P. A. de Villiers, 1973, *Journal of Psycholinguistic Research, 2,* pp. 267–278.

Along with the development of morphemes, preschoolers continue to expand utterance length through their use in noun and verb phrases, allowing them to engage in meaningful well-constructed dialogue with others. Detailed examples of noun and verb phrase expansion are available in several texts on language development (Gleason, 1997; Hoff-Ginsberg, 1997; Hulit & Howard, 1997; Owens, 1992).

Preschoolers develop noun phrases by learning to add articles (i.e., *a, an, the*), possessives (e.g., "Daddy's hat"; "My ball"), quantifiers (e.g., "all blocks"), descriptors (e.g., "hot stove," "big dog"), and pronouns during MLU Stages I and II. During Stage III, they use such grammatical forms to modify subjective and objective nouns. For example, the sentence "*The* dog has *black* nose" shows the use of the article to modify the subjective noun and a descriptor to modify the objective noun. Children also use demonstratives (e.g., *this, that, these, those*) during Stage III to modify nouns (Owens, 1992). By Stage IV, children use more pronouns than nouns in the subjective position of sentences and incorporate new modifiers into simple sentences. They also develop the ability to modify nouns after the noun occurs in the sentence (postnoun modification), such as when a prepositional phrase is used (e.g., "The girl in the chair"), an adjectival phrase occurs (e.g., "The girl next door"), or an adverb is added (e.g., "This one here"). Stage V changes occur when children begin to use relative clauses that modify nouns, such as "That lady who walks funny" (Owens, 1992).

Verb phrase development during Brown's stages allows children to express action, state, time, reference, mood, attitudes, and abilities (Owens, 1992). Within the first two stages, children develop verbs that take direct objects (transitive verbs), verbs that do not take direct objects (intransitive verbs), and those that determine state (e.g., *is, was, am*). Gradually, children use verbs to express action, to indicate action in progress through the use of the progressive tense marker *-ing,* as a negative helping verb (also known as an auxiliary) (e.g., *can't, don't, won't*), or as a semi-infinitive (e.g., *gonna, wanna, hafta*). Changes within Stages III and IV allow children to use positive helping verbs (e.g., *can, do, will*) and various forms of "to be," although its use as a helping verb may not correctly match the verb tense or the singular or plural noun or pronoun (e.g., "She are," "They is"). It is common during these stages that children overuse forms such as the regular past tense *-ed* marker on irregular verbs. Modal auxiliaries (e.g., *can–could, will–would, shall–should, may–must,* and *might*), which develop during Stage V, convey mood, ability, permission, intent, possibility, and obligation (Owens, 1992). They are used in statements and questions in both positive and negative forms. Even with greater sophistication of verb use, children within this stage still overgeneralize past tense forms and noun–verb agreement; however, they master them during Stage V and beyond. Additionally, Stage V advances allow children to use verb forms in inverted positions to ask wh-questions (e.g., "Where is he going?"), questions that begin with *do* (e.g., "Do you have anything to drink?"), and questions involving inversion of the subject and auxiliary verb (e.g., "Is Mom coming to pick us up?").

Grammatical development occurs simultaneously with development of sentence types, allowing children to convey declarative, interrogative, and imperative intentions. Sentence type development occurs gradually and coincides with the development of the noun and verb phrase elaborations described earlier.

Another way that youngsters expand their utterance length and complexity is through embedding and conjoining of phrases and clauses. This process begins early (Stages I and II) as children develop prepositions and semi-infinitives, but it is not until Stage IV and beyond that embedding of phrases such as noun complements, infinitives, relative clauses, and gerunds, as well as embedding and conjoining of subordinate clauses, occurs (Owens, 1992).

The Elementary and Middle School Years

By the time children enter kindergarten, they are able to create and comprehend well-formed declarative, imperative, and interrogative sentences. Their native language becomes a powerful tool for socialization and learning. However, elementary students are still refining their language and learning to use more complex forms. In particular, they need time and practice with morphological relationships (e.g., irregular verbs, noun–verb agreement); modality expressed through verbs, adverbs, adjectives, and nouns; correct use of subjective, objective, and reflexive pronouns; the sequential rules for ordering adjectives; and the ability to distinguish between mass nouns (e.g., *sugar, water, air*) and count nouns (e.g., *table, book, banana*) and to use the appropriate quantifying modifiers (e.g., *much, little, many, few*) (Owens, 1992). All of these developments occur gradually throughout the elementary years. For instance, it is not uncommon to hear students overgeneralize the past tense *-ed* rule to irregular verbs, producing *felled, buyed,* and *builded,* or to use the plural verb with a singular noun or vice versa, as in "The *monkeys is* all swinging from the trees." Some students have difficulty using *anaphoric reference*, which is the use of the correct pronoun following a noun (e.g., "The *lady* at the pool was laughing so hard *she* spilled the drink all over the towel").

Along with morphological changes, school-age students learn to interpret passive sentences as well as to use them in speaking and writing. This sentence type is difficult because its understanding and production require different processing than that used for active sentences. Most passive sentences contain a form of *be*, a past tense marker, and a prepositional phrase where the noun functions as an agent or instrument (e.g., "The flower was picked by the girl; The flowers were ruined by the hail; The hole was dug with the shovel"). Most school-age children use this sentence type by 8 years of age.

Sentence complexity continues to develop during the elementary grades, with students acquiring flexibility with embedding phrases in sentences. They use prepositional phrases (e.g., "The sun was bright *in the western sky*"), participial phrases (e.g, "The *light-hearted* girl skipped across the field"), gerunds (e.g., "I like *painting* at the river"), and infinitives (e.g., "My grandfather wanted *to wash his car*") in speaking and writing contexts.

Elementary students also expand grammatical complexity through compound and complex sentences, which require the use of conjunctions and embedding of clauses. Conjunctions allow speakers and writers to join simple sentences to make compound ones (e.g., "Mice like cheese and cats like mice") and to create dependent clauses for complex sentences (e.g., "When it became too dark for softball, we went home to watch TV"). Some conjunctions develop early (e.g., *and, then, but*), whereas others (e.g., *if, so, because, although, unless*) continue to develop from second through fifth grades (Emerson, 1979; Wing & Scholnick, 1981). In addition, students must use new strategies to interpret clauses when they are embedded at the end or in the middle of the sentence. Based on research, Owens (1992, p. 389) provided five examples of embedding from the easiest to the most difficult for students to understand:

1. The boy *who* lives next door gave me a present. (parallel central embedding: the same subject—boy—serves both clauses)
2. He gave me a present *that* I didn't like. (parallel ending embedding: the same object—present—serves both clauses)
3. He gave me the present *that* is on the table. (nonparallel ending embedding: the object of one—present—is the subject of the other)
4. He hit the girl *who* lives next door. (nonparallel ending embedding in both sentences: the object of the main clause—girl—is the subject of the embedded clause)
5. The dog *that* was chased by the boy is angry. (nonparallel central embedding: the subject of the main clause—dog—is the object of the embedded clause)

Students beyond age 12 continue to grow in the comprehension and use of coordinating and subordinating conjunctions in speaking and writing. Sentence length continues to increase and varies depending on the type of discourse genre used. For example, sentences in the persuasive mode are longer than in the descriptive, narrative, or conversational mode (Crowhurst, 1980; Crowhurst & Piche, 1979; Leadholm & Miller, 1992). Educators can enhance comprehension and use of conjunctions in speaking and writing through explicit teaching of their meanings and allowing plenty of opportunities to recognize and practice the types and functions of conjunctions in literacy activities (Geva & Ryan, 1985; Nippold, 1998).

Another attainment in syntactic growth involves the use of *intersentential* cohesive devices to join sentences together. Prior to about age 13, adverbial conjuncts are not very frequent in spoken language and only a few are used to connect sentences logically (e.g., *then, so, though*) (Scott, 1984). In fact, less common adverbials, such as *moreover, nevertheless*, and *similarly* develop with age and are somewhat easier to comprehend and use during reading than in writing tasks (Nippold, Schwarz, & Undlin, 1992). The development of adverbials is likely the result of exposure to these forms in literate contexts and can be facilitated through explicit teaching and practice, along with experience in reading academic texts (Nippold, 1998).

The Later School Years

During the adolescent and young adult years, students encounter many forms of literature and styles of spoken language, which vary in formality, discourse genre, and purpose. As noted in Chapter 2, most students are able to write in narrative and expository style to fulfill classroom assignments or personal communications with others (see also Chapter 4). The practice and feedback they receive during elementary school positions them to use grammatical devices effectively. This foundation also allows for continued refinement of grammar and the development of linguistic devices to relate clauses logically to each other in speaking and writing activities.

Nippold (1998) discussed two additional cohesive devices that high school and older students develop to minimize redundancy, provide variety, and generate a binding force between sentences. *Synonyms*, words with the same or nearly the same meaning, provide the speaker or writer with flexibility in word choice, which makes the message more interesting and reduces the need for repetition of words (e.g., "The *shrubs* were ruined by the hail. The leaves were shredded, especially on the *bushes* on the south side of the house"). *Word associations* that are opposites (e.g., *hot–cold*), categorical (e.g., *fruit–vegetable*), superordinate (e.g., *animal–dog*), whole–part (e.g., *car–engine*), or sequential (e.g., *fall–winter*) allow speakers and writers to relate ideas from one sentence to another and one paragraph to another. Both devices can be developed through exposure and practice, especially through reading and writing. However, it is not uncommon for students and adults to make syntactical errors when speaking and writing. Factors such as the type of discourse in use, the social situation, the complexity of structures, and the time taken to formulate the message can influence syntactic accuracy.

Summary

From their use of first words, young children begin a long journey in the development of morphology and syntax. During the preschool years, language learning involves the acquisition of thousands of words, which children learn to combine in increasingly longer and more complex utterances. They learn to use units of meaning within the noun phrase, such as articles, adjectives, prepositions, and plurals. Similarly, they learn the units within the verb phrase, such as present tense, present progressive, past tense, negation, and mood. As children continue to develop such morphemes, they learn to use statements, commands, and questions through simple sentences at first, then through more complex sentence types containing simple conjunctions and embedded phrases and clauses. It takes many years for elementary school children to understand

and correctly use various parts of speech, passive voice, later-developing conjunctions, and embedding of clauses within complex sentences. During middle school and high school, students learn to employ cohesive devices that serve to tie sentences together through the use of adverbials, synonyms, and word association strategies.

Semantics

The language system involving words, their meanings, and the relationships between words is known as *semantics*. It encompasses the development of vocabulary, knowledge of concepts and meanings, comprehension, and use of figurative forms, and is the driving force for the development of syntax. It is tied to the development of thinking and reasoning, developing slowly and in relation to the other language systems.

The Preschool Years

Infants recognize and form early understandings of simple words during the 4th month of life and the intentionality to interact with others by 6 months. They show particular wants and needs through cries and gestures and seek opportunities to interact with others through eye gaze, pointing, reaching, and facial expressions. The routines established in daily life encounters with adults and other children encourage turn-taking, exploration of the environment, and the social basis for communication.

As babbling emerges from 4 to 10 months, infants add gestures and gradually learn to express wants and needs. Babbling is typically highly reinforced by family members, and this attention sets the stage both for giving meaning to the child's babble and for providing models of words. Gradually, as infants comprehend the meaning of words and begin to say some of them, new opportunities emerge for them to convey intentions. Once first words emerge, the pace of development is remarkable.

Vocabulary Growth. It is fascinating to observe children during their first 2 years. Although they seem to learn language at a phenomenal rate, their first 50 words of vocabulary and vocabulary growth beyond single-word utterances are often quite unpredictable. Recall the earlier discussion about competence and performance. What children understand is not always demonstrated by their verbal productions. This is as true in the area of semantics as it is in phonology, suprasegmentals, and syntax. Because early words are often inseparable from the contexts in which they appear (K. Nelson, 1985), factors such as familiar routines in the home and the nature of interactions that family members have with their children (e.g., positive or negative, frequent or infrequent, interactive or functional) play a role in the development of first words.

It is common for young children to use several types of words to convey intentions, such as social words (e.g., *hi*, *bye-bye*) and functional words (e.g., *up*, *more*); however, some children are more inclined to use nouns than others, particularly when referring to common objects or family and pet names. Other factors contributing to the acquisition of words include the phonological composition of a word (Ferguson & Farwell, 1975; Leonard, Schwartz, Folger, & Wilcox, 1978; Stoel-Gammon & Cooper, 1984), the tendency of adults to label particular objects and request names of particular objects (Gentner, 1988; Goldfield, 1993), and the linguistic complexity of verbs, which may cause children to rely on general purpose verbs (E. Clark, 1993). Other individual differences include learning style (analytical or holistic), risk-taking, social nature of individual children, phonological memory (Hoff-Ginsberg, 1997), and particular contexts that occur in speaking environments (Barrett, 1995), such as routines or language games (Caselli et al., 1995; H. Clark, 1979).

By about 18 months, the first 50 words in a child's vocabulary generally emerge. This 50-word benchmark provides a glimpse of the development of grammatical categories (i.e., nouns, verbs, adjectives), phonology, and word meanings. Typically beyond this stage, children begin to combine words into meaningful phrases (Brown, 1973; Hoff-Ginsberg, 1997; Owens, 1992).

Other categories of words combine with nouns to make the first 50 words a very functional tool for a child's developing communication. Action words comprise the second most common category. Often they are highly functional words to satisfy needs, such as *go* and *eat*. Modifiers (e.g., *mine*, *hot*) and personal social words (e.g., *thank you*, *hi*) are often present but do not occur in abundance (K. Nelson, 1973). Keep in mind that the expressive vocabulary of a child at this age may be only about one fourth of the words the child understands. Large variation also occurs in the receptive and expressive vocabularies of individuals in the 12- to 18-month age range. The first 50 words in combination with gestures make it possible for children to make requests, refuse items or assistance, make statements, express pleasure or discontent, and answer yes–no questions. These communicative functions provide very direct social rewards and serve as the foundation for continued development.

A common occurrence during word acquisition is the overextension or underextension of word use as children explore their vocabulary in various situations. Children *overextend* word meanings when they apply a familiar word to a new situation. For example, a whale may be called "fish" because other creatures living in water are called fish. Children *underextend* word meanings when they do not generalize a word to new situations. For example, a child who has learned that daddy drives a car may not use the word to name other similar vehicles or may call them something else. As children gain experience and acquire more words, they decrease and ultimately eliminate over- and underextensions (Hoff-Ginsberg, 1997; Owens, 1992).

Preschoolers continue to add new words to their vocabularies and establish meaningful connections among the words and concepts they know based on how they are used (Gleason, 1997). Furthermore, when they encounter gaps in their vocabulary or forget words, they invent words by adding suffixes or creating compound words (Becker, 1994). For instance, a 4-year-old anxious to help dad cut the grass might say, "I can help you daddy with grass scissors." This creativity shows that children strive for simplicity, meaning, and productivity by using innovative, yet regular principles (E. Clark, 1993; Gleason, 1997).

As noted earlier, children who attend preschool or are exposed to preschool-type instruction develop words for concepts, including colors, numbers, rhyming, and literacy concepts (e.g., letters, the alphabet, words) that will make entry to kindergarten fairly easy. Such children have the vocabulary necessary to engage in school activities. Others may require explicit teaching of the concepts and words to participate fully in the classroom.

Figurative Language. Another aspect of semantic development, figurative language, begins during the preschool years. As noted in Chapter 2, such development requires the learner to understand meanings from the social contexts and cues, not from the typical (literal) ones (N. Nelson, 1993; Strand & Fraser, 1979). Several types of figurative forms exist, including jokes, metaphors and similes, idioms and slang terms, and proverbs and fables (Nippold, 1998; Owens, 1992). It is not uncommon, in the midst of a conversation about bravery on the high seas, for someone to say, "Hey, that reminds me of a joke. What did one skeleton say to the other? You have no guts." Figurative language pervades spoken and written language. It provides humor, provokes thought, and encourages analytical thinking.

Preschoolers encounter figurative forms in social situations with family and other caregivers or teachers. They delight in word play with others as they use language to be silly or entertain others. Early inventive figures of speech are concrete in nature and based on physical attributes. When my nephew Matthew was 4, he liked to deny what family members said. For instance, when asked if he was a creeper, he would respond, "No, I'm not a creeper. You're a creeper." Of course, the statement "You're a nice boy" evoked "No, I'm not a nice boy." At age 5, Matt enjoyed creating new names in the name calling game. What started as "You're a tomato head" progressed to "You're a broccoli head," "You're a swing head," "You're a spaghetti head," and so on. These routines were fun for all the participants and reflect this preschooler's creativity in language use.

The Elementary and Middle School Years

With increasing age, students undergo transitions in thinking and reasoning. Preschool children rely on visual-perceptual input to understand and relate to their world. Their thinking tends to be concrete, literal, and based on personal experience. School-age children move toward a stronger reliance on linguistic input that allows abstract, figurative, and categorical ways of viewing the world; thus, the semantic development of children in elementary school is significant.

Vocabulary and Word Definitions. Classrooms provide extensive opportunities for students to acquire new words. Through study in content areas, field trips, reading and writing activities, and interaction with peers and adults, students encounter new and previously acquired words in a variety of contexts. They learn that words have different meanings depending on their use. For instance, *pound* can be a weight, an action, or a place for homeless dogs and cats. School-age students increase understanding and use of spatial, temporal, familial, disjunctive, and logical relationships (Owens, 1992), as well as ability to describe and recognize psychological states of others (Peevers & Secord, 1973). They can, for example, use specific terms to designate the relocation of furniture in their room (e.g., next to the closet; on top of the desk). They also can relate to periods of time during each day, week, and month and can tell time on a clock or digital watch.

Another change during the school years is in the way students associate old and new words. Younger children think about words in relation to their experiences and how words go together syntactically (e.g., *cat–meows*, *airplane–flies*), which is called a *syntagmatic relationship*. Older children pair words with others from the same semantic class called the *paradigmatic relationship* (e.g., *orange–apple*, *tree–leaves*). These associations reflect a reorganization and refinement of the meaningful features of words and may allow for figurative uses of language (McNeill, 1966; Owens, 1992). Definitions also become more elaborate, dictionary-like, explicit, constrained, and contain more super- and subordinate categories (Owens, 1992).

Figurative Language. The ability to understand nonliterate forms and creatively express them develops most impressively during the elementary school years. Riddles, metaphors and similes, idioms, and proverbs and fables appear in stories, plays, textbooks, and classroom discourse, and during playground chants, rhymes, and taunts. Students gradually develop such understandings and continue to gain new understandings into adulthood.

RIDDLES. The understanding of riddles during the elementary years (Horgan, 1981; Shultz, 1974) requires recognition of incongruity, unexpected elements, multimeaning words (Hulit & Howard, 1997), and the ambiguous use of phonology, word meanings, and linguistic contexts (Nippold, 1998). Consequently, school-age children develop understandings of riddles across several years. For example, students understand riddles, which depend on the phonological similarity of words, between 6 and 9 years (Lund & Duchan, 1988), whereas they understand syntactic ambiguity created from multimeaning words after 9 years and as late as 15 years (Hulit & Howard, 1997; Muus & Hoag, 1980, as cited in Nippold, 1998; Shultz & Horibe, 1974, as cited in Nippold, 1998). The riddles below use several devices for manipulating meaning.

- What two states have the most ducks?
  North Dakota and South Dakota (Phonological similarity—Duck-oda)
- What's a hen weigh?
  A road chickens walk on (Homonyms—highway)
- What is smarter than a talking horse?
  A spelling bee (Analogy)
- Why did the skeleton jump off the cliff?
  Because he had no guts (Double meaning)
- What is an ooah bird?
  One that lays a square egg. OH-AH! (Onomatopoeia—painful)
- Did you ever eat at the broken drum?
  You can't beat it. (Play on words)

METAPHORS AND SIMILES. As noted in Chapter 2, metaphors and similes are figurative expressions that make comparisons between two items distinct in meaning. Metaphors are implied comparisons (e.g., "The dancer was a deer"), whereas, in similes, the comparison takes the form of an analogy (e.g., "The situation was like a house of cards"). School-age children understand metaphors and similes when they use their semantic knowledge of words and concepts, when concrete versus abstract nouns are included, and when they contain physical and sensory versus psychological (e.g., emotion, mental state, personality) comparisons (Nippold, 1998). Young school-age children use common metaphors more than personally created ones in their written language; however both types decline in frequency from third to sixth grade (Nippold, 1998; Pollio & Pollio, 1974). This decline is thought to occur because they learn to be more conventional in writing with age and experience. After sixth grade an increase in metaphor use occurs during descriptive prose (Polanski, 1989).

IDIOMS. Idioms are common verbal expressions that vary in meaning depending on the situational context and the intent of the speaker. For example, "She threw him off the track" can literally mean the heroic young girl rescues a clumsy boy who fell on the railroad tracks with an oncoming train bearing down. Figuratively, it often means that one person deceives the other in order to divert attention from himself. For instance, a roommate might blame the dog for a broken vase by saying, "The dog must have hit that vase with its tail." Studies investigating comprehension of idioms in children ages 5 through 13, and in young and older adults, show that performance steadily improves with age, that idioms vary in difficulty, and that context and experience help students interpret idioms (Nippold, 1998).

PROVERBS AND FABLES. The values and beliefs of a culture are reflected in its proverbs and fables. *Proverbs* are statements offering encouragement, advice, or warning when used in appropriate situational contexts. For example, "A stitch in time saves nine" is appropriate when immediate attention to a matter will save the person time and energy in the long run, such as changing the car oil at 3,000 miles rather than waiting until serious engine problems occur. *Fables* are short stories often about animals providing perspectives about human behavior. They teach lessons about daily life based on the choices characters make and end in a moral teaching that can be applied to daily situations. For instance, the "Tortoise and the Hare" teaches that steady progress toward a goal is often more profitable than a quick accomplishment.

Comprehension of proverbs also develops steadily with increasing age and educational experiences. By age 8 children understand some proverbs within stories and this ability continues to develop into adulthood. Proverbs are more difficult to explain than understand; a child may offer a literal interpretation at age 8 but understand the figurative meaning at age 12 to 14, yet even adults have difficulty explaining them. Some factors influencing comprehension and explanations of proverbs include their syntactic and semantic complexity, contextual support from sentences or stories, concreteness as aided by visual images, and familiarity with the culture (Nippold, 1998).

Slang. Slang is informal language that occurs in the spoken language of people within generations and within particular subcultures defined by age, region, and culture. Often, the slang term is created from a common word, but is given a different meaning, such as when *dude* is used by middle schoolers to refer to someone of the same age. Terms can also be created, such as when *rad* meant that something was good. Students acquire more slang terms as a function of grade level, and boys and girls show different knowledge of such terms depending on the topic of interest (Nelsen & Rosenbaum, 1972). In classrooms, students might use slang when making side comments to others (i.e., during underground exchanges) or during small group time.

Students are exposed to figurative forms as part of Western culture through family interactions, storybooks, television, classroom discourse, and textbooks. Elementary teachers can increase comprehension and enjoyment of these forms by (a) embedding them in situations rich with contextual support, (b) offering simple examples of form use in daily situations, (c) providing explanations of meanings, and (d) increasing experiences with forms in classroom activities.

The Later School Years

The changes in semantic knowledge characteristic of high school students reflect their increasing ability to invoke critical and logical thinking. Thus, students engage in thoughtful study and dialogue about topics, with attention to subtle differences in meaning that reflect precision, passion, and economy in word use. They become aware of nuances in meaning and are more adept than their middle school counterparts at understanding and using figurative language.

Vocabulary and Word Definitions. It is not surprising that high school students expand their vocabulary; they will continue to do so throughout life. Each new content area (e.g., algebra, U.S. history, French, biology) provides exposure to new words, definitions, and topics. In fact, participation in literate activities facilitates word learning and offers readers the opportunity to witness complex relationships between concepts. They encounter rare and abstract words in formal written contexts and develop understandings of connectives (e.g., *because, before, during*), double-function terms (e.g., *bright, dull, sour, straight*), and words conveying psychological states (e.g., *effervescent, blue*).

Older students define words very specifically and develop various definition types, including dictionary, operational, negation, comparison, and example (Nippold, 1998). They also advance in the use of devices such as synonyms, explanations, and categorizations of the word (Al-Issa, 1969, as cited in Owens, 1992; Litowitz, 1977, as cited in Owens, 1992; Storck & Looft, 1973, as cited in Nippold, 1998).

Figurative Language. Most acquisition studies of figurative forms are of elementary school and adolescent populations and show that understanding and use of figurative forms increase with age. In fact, studies suggest that development continues into adulthood (Brasseur & Jimenez, 1989; Nippold & Martin, 1989; Prinz, 1983). High school students and adults produce greater varieties of explanations of metaphors, show greater awareness of multimeaning words

(Gardner, 1974), and produce more metaphors than elementary students in formal writing tasks (Polanski, 1989). Young adults surpassed 12-year-olds and younger students in comprehending idioms (Lodge & Leach, 1975). Explanations of idioms become more sophisticated into adulthood (Prinz, 1983). Ackerman (1982) suggested that older students and adults require little to no contextual support in interpreting the meaning of common idioms. However, a recent study by Nippold and Martin (1989) revealed that adolescents found idioms easier to interpret in context (following a two-sentence story) than in isolation (i.e., "What does it mean to . . ."). The use of slang terms is an important aspect of later language development. As is true of other figurative forms, slang terms increase as a function of grade level, with some topics evoking more terms than others (Nelsen & Rosenbaum, 1972).

Because complete understanding of figurative forms occurs throughout high school and beyond, teachers should provide exposure to these forms through lecture and discussion, and in literacy activities. By asking students to recognize these forms, provide explanations, and incorporate them into speaking and writing activities, further development of the forms will occur. Students who struggle with understanding and using figurative forms may experience difficulties in social interactions resulting in alienation, frustrations, hurt feelings, and low self-esteem (Donahue & Bryan, 1984; Larson & McKinley, 1995). In the classroom, poor understanding of figurative forms can affect overall comprehension of lectures, discussions, and readings. When students demonstrate difficulty understanding and using word meanings and relationships, it is important that teachers refer them to an SLP for assessment and intervention planning.

Summary

The two focus areas of semantic development that preschool, elementary school, and high school students experience are vocabulary expansion and understanding of figurative forms. The development of vocabulary begins in infancy as children learn some social and functional words, the names of objects and people, the names of actions, and words that describe attributes as they interact with people in their environments. Because children learn in different environments and with differing types of experiences, the words children use vary greatly. As preschoolers use their vocabularies in many different contexts, they learn about new words that are related, often through scaffolding techniques from parents. They also learn to be creative when they do not know what word to use in a particular situation. Students in elementary and middle school continue to expand their vocabularies as they study content areas, participate in field trips, and engage in reading and writing activities.

They learn that some words have several meanings and expand knowledge of words that represent spatial, temporal, familial, disjunctive, and logical relationships. As new word relationships occur, students reorganize how they store them for understanding and use. High school students acquire new vocabulary with each content area under study. They also become more aware of the meanings of some conjunctions and adverbials (refer to the previous discussion about the development of syntax), as well as words conveying psychological states. Older students develop the ability to consider word meanings in a variety of ways (e.g., comparison, negation, operational).

Figurative language development in preschool children is exciting because its use often involves humor. Family members encourage children to play with language by using sound effects, teasing, facial expressions, and banter. During the elementary years, students develop understanding of several different forms of figurative language, including riddles, metaphors and similes, idioms, proverbs and fables, and slang. Both advancement in age and experience with these forms account for increases in the comprehension and production of figurative expressions. High school students not only comprehend figurative forms more accurately, but provide better explanations of meanings to others, especially when the figurative form is considered within the situational and linguistic context.

Considering the importance of vocabulary growth and the prevalence of figurative language in daily interactions, teachers must be concerned with students' development of the semantic aspects of language. Delayed acquisition in these areas can greatly affect students' comprehension of oral and written language, leading to poor achievement.

Pragmatics

Children become aware quite early that language is a social tool to get things done. Hulit and Howard (1997) define *pragmatics* as the study of functions, purposes, or intents of communication. Competence in pragmatics is tied directly to the social situation in which speakers and listeners participate, because the nature of the interaction between them is determined by the setting, mood and attitude, who is talking to whom, and their purposes. Thus, pragmatics involves not only the development of social communication rules, but also the flexibility to modify the rules situationally.

The Preschool Years

The importance of communication functions for infants is to get wants and needs met; for caregivers it is to foster the children's participation within the social context of the family. Parents and siblings use several techniques to participate in mutual routines with infants, and it is these daily routines that establish the social and cultural contexts for further interactions and language learning. N. Nelson (1993) referred to the balanced interaction in routines as *reciprocation;* the natural turn-taking phenomenon so vital to human discourse. Three-and 4-month-olds incorporate these early "dialogues" into the routines and games of their households, while family members respond with vocalizations, facial expression, eye gaze, and attempts to engage the infant in imitation. Soon after, infants are able to express their own intentions and get others to satisfy their goals through pointing and other gestures, looking, and vocalizations (6 to 8 months). Four prelinguistic functions in infants identified by Halliday (1975) include (1) satisfying needs and wants, (2) controlling the behaviors of others, (3) interacting with others, and (4) expressing emotion or interest. They use gestures and vocalizations to give commands as well as statements, to actively elicit the aid of others when they desire something, and to use objects to gain adult attention (Bates, Camaioni, & Volterra, 1975).

During the acquisition of first words, communication functions expand. Dore (1975), Halliday (1975), and Roth and Spekman (1984) identified several communicative functions typical of the first word period (Table 3.6), which is when the first 50 words are expressed. Although few words are in youngsters' repertoires, they are able to convey these many intentions through intonation patterns used with the words (Hoff-Ginsberg, 1997).

Table 3.6
Communicative Functions Conveyed by Single-Word Utterances as Categorized by Three Authors

Dore (1975)	**Halliday (1975)**	**Roth & Spekman (1984)**
Labeling	Exploring	Naming
Repeating	Categorizing	Protesting
Answering	Imagining	Rejecting
Requesting action	Pretending	Attention seeking
Requesting information	Informing	
Calling		
Protesting		
Practicing		

The two-word stage allows for more specific intentions to be expressed, such as regulating conversations and producing statements and exclamations (Roth & Spekman, 1984). At the same time, symbolic and pretend play allows children around 17 to 20 months of age to engage in interactive experiences with people and objects while exploring language. For example, these young children initiate topics, take one or two turns with a topic during established routines, and imitate words and phrases of others (Foster, 1986; Hoff-Ginsberg, 1997; Owens, 1992). Vocabulary growth is rapid as toddlers practice new vocabulary in novel combinations. However, it is not uncommon during this period for communication to break down between toddlers and caregivers, and they have difficulty making repairs when this occurs (Golinkoff, 1986).

Beyond the two-word stage, children continue to acquire vocabulary and expand word combinations in their utterances, doing better in spontaneous monologues than in dialogues with others. Turn-taking in dialogues is common and children under age 2 gradually talk more fully about objects, people, or events in their immediate view and experience (Gleason, 1997).

Young children beyond age 2 develop the ability to modify their speech in relation to social situations, such as when in the presence of dolls, younger children, children with developmental disabilities, or pets (Dunn & Kendrick, 1982; Guralnick & Paul-Brown, 1989; Shatz & Gelman, 1973). They adopt a style known as motherese, which is slower and contains more prosody than their regular speech style. This ability to *code switch* (switching from one language, dialect, or style in the course of conversation) shows that preschoolers are aware of how language can vary with situations and how to modify their speech to respond appropriately to the social situations and within multilingual environments.

Preschoolers also can make simple repairs when communication breaks down, such as when mispronunciations make family, friends, or preschool teachers ask for repetition of a word or phrase. Another awareness during these years is that much information in the immediate environment is shared by others, thus decreasing the amount of information that is new. This knowledge is called *presupposition*. Presupposition helps speakers determine what they need to say and what they can leave out. For example, a child who is crying while coming into the house may say, "Mommy, I fell down and hurt my knee." The parent would not fully understand a statement like "Mommy, I hurt it." Of course, this statement would be appropriate if on the same day the child said, "Mommy, I hurt it *again*."

The Elementary and Middle School Years

Pragmatics involves more than conveying intentions and understanding the intentions of others through speaking and listening. It involves flexibility in how language is used in various social interactions (Durkin, 1986). *Social cognition* refers to "the child's intuitive or logical representation of others, that is how he characterizes others and makes inferences about their covert, inner psychological experience" (Shantz, 1975, p. 258). This knowledge allows elementary school students to expand their own social roles and appreciate the roles afforded to others. They recognize language differences based on gender roles within the family, the peer community in the neighborhood and at school, and teacher language. They become adept at allocating roles to one another in pretend play and can easily manipulate vocabulary, accents, and phrase use.

Students in early grades (ages 7 and 8) change the way they view and talk about others, from physical appearance descriptions to those that include observations of motives, attitudes, or needs. They are, of course, influenced in their social perceptions of others by the people in their immediate environment. Words used by others to evaluate other people or groups negatively, for example, contribute to the child's frame of reference and may shape his or her attitudes and use of negative words. As they enter teenage years, students adopt several verbal and nonverbal strategies to communicate effectively in different social situations (Table 3.7). They learn to recognize and control suprasegmental aspects (e.g., intonation, stress), stay an appropriate physical distance from others (proxemics), and regulate discourse style situationally. Nonverbal language, such as facial expression and body language, is adjusted as well, depending on social and language contexts (Larson & McKinley, 1995).

Another factor in the development of pragmatics is the adjustments students must make to the nature and complexity of classroom language. For example, N. Nelson (1993) enumerated four uses of classroom language: (1) instructing reading and writing, (2) talking about language forms and

Table 3.7
Verbal and Nonverbal Communication Strategies for Teenagers

- Detecting, displaying, or controlling emotion through facial expression
- Detecting, displaying, or controlling gestures, body language, and eye contact
- Detecting, producing, and modifying intonation, stress, and rate
- Recognizing the impact of distance and maintaining socially acceptable distance
- Understanding and using situationally appropriate discourse styles and structures (e.g., classroom, baseball field, street corner)

Note. Adapted from *Language Disorders in Older Students: Preadolescents and Adolescents,* by V. L. Larson and M. S. McKinley, 1995, Eau Claire, WI: Thinking Publications.

meanings, (3) using language to convey procedures, and (4) using language to convey content. Flexibility in coping with different uses of language and different teacher styles can be a challenge for students, particularly when preschool experience is lacking or when a student's native language or dialect is different from the one(s) used in school. Furthermore, classroom settings also require students to use language in many different ways and for different purposes. Students learn to recite, tell about, explain, answer, discuss, listen, write, read, and apply information in individual, small group, and large group situations. They also learn to employ self-regulatory techniques such as inner speech and self-appreciation strategies (Lepper, 1983; Pellegrini, 1984).

Social interactions of students during the late elementary and middle school years are important for peer acceptance and establish each student within the social culture of his or her group. Preadolescent girls engage in cooperative performances consisting of chants and rhymes, sometimes accompanied by hand clapping or dancing. Girls tend to perform individually (e.g., jump rope routines), where each adds a creative element to the activity (Gilmore, 1986). The groups tend to be homogeneous in age and social status and are typically not competitive. Girls do, however, compete for exclusive friendships by sharing secrets, and break friendships by telling secrets (Lever, 1976; Maltz & Borker, 1982).

Maltz and Borker (1982) described the social world of boys as a status hierarchy, where language is used to assert dominance, attract and maintain an audience, and assert oneself when others have the floor. Preadolescent and adolescent boys engage in ritual insults or "verbal duels" that (a) refer to someone else who is different from the person receiving the insult, such as a mother; (b) refer to appearance, age, poverty, or sexual promiscuity; (c) are not true, are extreme, or are literally impossible; (d) are exchanged in dyads or triads and in front of an audience; and (e) are not denied by the recipient but rather are countered with a related one (Hoff-Ginsberg, 1997). See Chapter 5 for more extensive discussion of gender and cultural variation in language usage.

The Later School Years

The verbal bantering described during the elementary years continues through much of the high school years. Peer acceptance in a group and use of language that fosters peer solidarity is important for teenagers. However, the social circles of high school students broaden as they develop more independence and explore their interests. They adjust to part-time work situations, begin to date other students, and take on responsibilities in the home, school, and other settings. These expanded opportunities afford teenagers experience assuming social roles and shaping new beliefs and attitudes. Many students begin to plan for the future in apprentice positions or for college. All of these maturing factors foster individuality rather than group identity as students transition into adulthood. They move away from the language behaviors that identify them with their peers by adopting a more prestigious form of speech used by adults in formal situations (Labov, 1970).

Teachers are particularly attuned to the social behavior of children and adolescents, noting when some do not relate well to peers and adults, are left out of activities, and suffer ridicule from peers. These problems may signal the existence of language difficulties. In fact, some children with language delays seek the companionship of younger children whose language level more closely matches their own. The academic and social consequences of language delay make referral for assessment and intervention important and necessary. Teacher observation regarding a student's flexibility in the uses of language is helpful and appreciated in the evaluation process.

Summary

Language acquisition involves learning not only the segments (phonology, morphology, and syntax) and the suprasegments (stress, intonation, and pausing) of the native language, but also the interactional nature of the language. Infants learn to interact with parents who use vocalizations, facial expressions, and eye gaze to establish mutually engaging dialogue. As infants begin to express their own intentions through looking, vocalizing, and gesturing, family members model words and phrases that interpret the infants' intentions. Gradually, preschool children learn to convey their intentions by using words and sentences. They practice language through familiar routines and use the information that others provide during such experiences. Preschoolers also learn to modify how they speak according to particular social situations, such as when speaking to younger children, and they learn to adjust what they say depending on whether information is new or previously shared.

During the elementary and middle school years, students increasingly develop an understanding of the roles of others and can manipulate vocabulary, dialects, and phrase use to assume the interactional differences of social roles. They also adjust to the nature and complexity of classroom language by learning to express language for specific classroom purposes (e.g., reciting, answering, retelling) that differ from home interactions. Peer identity, being especially important during middle school, requires participation in new social routines and verbal interactions, which are defined by the particular group. Thus, the elementary and middle school years require a great deal of flexibility in language use.

The pragmatic development that characterizes the later school years reflects the broadening of experiences in new social realms and the gradual shift from being a part of the peer group to becoming an independent individual. Older students adopt adult-like styles, which become more refined with continued education.

It is important for teachers to observe students in interaction with others within the classroom environment as well as outside it. Students who find interactions difficult are often not accepted into their own peer group. Such students may have pragmatic language difficulties that limit their social competence. Early identification and intervention for pragmatic difficulties is discussed in Chapter 10.

Metalinguistics

The language systems can be thought about, manipulated, and studied, as when we recognize that someone spoke a very long sentence, that rhymes are created by altering first consonants in words (e.g., *big, dig, fig*), or that prepositional phrases modify nouns. This conscious attention to language is called *metalinguistic ability* (Gleason, 1997; Owens, 1992).

The Preschool Years

Children learn the language of their families from hearing it within everyday social interactions and through the amazing capabilities of the human brain. Researchers who study speech perception find that 1- to 4-month-old infants discriminate differences in speech sounds. For example, through body responses (e.g., sucking rate) infants demonstrate their perception of differences between sounds made by different articulation positions, such as the /b/, /d/, and /g/, and by 6 months they babble using the intonation of their native language. The ability to perceive speech sounds and other systems of language is a strong force in the rapid development of language (Bernthal & Bankson, 1998).

As early as 2 or 3 years, preschoolers begin "to deliberately reflect on and manipulate the structural features of spoken language, treating the language system itself as an object of thought, as opposed to using the language system to comprehend and produce sentences" (Tunmer & Cole, 1991). They monitor their own utterances and make repairs; practice sounds, words, and word combinations; and make adjustments depending on their communication partner (E. Clark, 1978). Such awareness is likely the result of both innate characteristics and direct experience with language.

Preschoolers also monitor their own utterances, checking to be sure their communication partner has understood them, and repairing utterances when necessary. They comment directly on their own utterances and on the utterances of others. For example, a child might respond to a nonsense statement with "Hey, that's not how you say it; that's silly." Preschoolers also deliberately practice new words, sentences, and social roles (E. Clark, 1978).

Phonological awareness, the ability to recognize and analyze sounds and sound patterns that make up words, is another type of metalinguistic knowledge that preschoolers develop (Hoff-Ginsberg, 1997). They show, for example in sound play, the notion of syllable change through onset and rime (e.g., *ips, pips, bips, fips*) and can detect sound and syllable changes in verbal tasks (MacLean, Bryant, & Bradley, 1987). Picture dictionaries and cause–effect alphabet toys help preschool children to learn a key word for each letter of the alphabet (e.g., *a–apple, b–banana, c–cat*). Some preschoolers have been taught to write their first names, produce letters and numbers, and even read simple stories. The extent to which preschool children pay attention to and manipulate sounds is tied to the amount of experience and explicit instruction they receive at home or in day care or preschool settings. This is important because research shows that phonological awareness is highly predictive of reading ability (Bradley & Bryant, 1983; Felton & Brown, 1990; Liberman & Shankweiler, 1985; Mann, 1993).

The Elementary and Middle School Years

The most growth in metalinguistics occurs in the elementary years as students use language as a tool for learning about many topics including the language itself. Elementary students refine the use of inflectional and derivational morphemes, judging their appropriateness in relationship to the other grammatical forms within sentences. They also judge utterances according to the setting and situational appropriateness. For example, they recognize when a fellow student is disrespectful when addressing a teacher. The progressive ability to evaluate what they hear shows the development of *comprehension monitoring*, an important metalinguistic ability during the school years and beyond, and one implicated significantly in reading as well as in language use. Kindergarten students have difficulty recognizing when listeners misunderstand them, and do not always know when messages from others are ambiguous, contradictory, or incomplete. After second grade, students are better able to recognize misunderstandings and engage in repair or requests for clarification (Beal, 1987; Beal & Flavell, 1983; Flavell, Speer, Green, & August, 1981; Karabenick & Miller, 1977).

School-age students engage in a high amount of reflection about specific linguistic units and can explain why forms are not correctly used within sentences. They provide various types of definitions for words and construct a variety of figurative language forms (E. Clark, 1978).

Phonological awareness increases rapidly upon entry to school and its relationship to reading acquisition is strong; children with high levels of phonological awareness tend to be strong readers. Conversely, poor readers and illiterate adults have poor phonological awareness. Some suggest that phonological awareness is a consequence of reading instruction (Wimmer, Landerl, Linortner, & Hummer, 1991), whereas others suggest that the relationship is reciprocal, with early phonological awareness being important for beginning reading, and the development of reading resulting in continued development of phonological awareness (Perfetti, Beck, Bell, & Hughes, 1987).

Some examples of phonological awareness activities present in early elementary curricula include tapping out the sounds in spoken words and syllables, identifying words that begin or end with particular consonants, identifying words containing particular vowels, producing alliterations (e.g., "Lily likes licking lemon licorice"), naming the first letter in words from its sound (e.g., *beach–b*, *Jason–J*), and so on. These and other activities alert students to the predictability and regularity of spoken and written language. Ongoing instruction in reading, writing, and language arts during elementary grades expands on students' knowledge of the various systems of language.

Larson and McKinley (1995) discussed several other aspects of meta-abilities appropriate for children past age 10. *Meta-ability* is "awareness of strategies and mental activities which carry out various cognitive processes such as memory, comprehension, learning, and attention" (van Kleeck, 1987, p. 114). These abilities include metalinguistics, metapragmatics, metacognition, and metanarrative skills. Students expand their awareness of these as they learn through social, academic, and vocational realms.

The Later School Years

Whenever students learn new information and apply what is known from previous learning, metalinguistic abilities come into use. It is not surprising then that students continue to expand their knowledge of the structure and function of language, noting the similarities and differences of spoken and written language. High school students recognize that past experience in listening, speaking, reading, and writing is useful for predicting and discovering new information. They essentially know what they know and know where to find unknown information. For instance, to write a two-page report on waste management, a high school student might first try the encyclopedia, but then seek waste management trade magazines or textbooks on the subject. As the student researches the topic, she determines unfamiliar words and concepts that interfere with her comprehension and then analyzes them phonologically, morphologically (e.g., *toxicology*, *ecological*), and for meaning.

Metalinguistic abilities also assist high school students in proofreading and editing their own writing or the writing of peers. These tasks involve being able to analyze sentence structure for grammatical form, recognize spelling errors, and determine whether information is appropriate to the paragraph structure.

Summary

As children develop the various systems of language, they also learn to recognize the components that make up words, phrases, and sentences. Even at very early ages, infants distinguish between spoken phonemes and come to understand that words have particular meanings. As preschool children acquire vocabulary and grammar, they also think about their own productions of words, as well as the language spoken by others. This developing awareness allows preschool children to make repairs when others do not understand them, practice sounds and words, and recognize when other speakers say something that lacks semantic sense. Preschool children also acquire the ability to manipulate sounds and syllables within words to create rhymes, and to associate written letters with sounds.

During the elementary and middle school years, metalinguistic abilities develop dramatically as students recognize semantic, syntactic, morphological, and phonological deviations in the speech and language production of themselves and others. They use a strategy called comprehension monitoring to evaluate what they hear so that they can repair their own utterances or ask other speakers to clarify their utterances. Phonological awareness develops rapidly as students begin to read and write. They not only use previous knowledge, but also develop new information through explicit instruction and experience with reading and writing activities.

Older students use metalinguistic abilities to critically analyze spoken and written language. Their knowledge of the systems of the language help them to predict information, discover new information, and interpret meaning. They learn how and where to find certain types of information (e.g., definitions, explanations, research) and gain access to such information. In addition, metalinguistic abilities assist students to proofread and edit their own writing.

Summary and Conclusions

The oral language system is made up of a complex set of subsystems that develop simultaneously and progressively from infancy to adulthood. Articulation and phonology, suprasegmental aspects, morphology and syntax, semantics, pragmatics, and metalinguistics develop steadily with age, but each child progresses on a journey that results from unique influences from his or her environment. Trends in communication development during the preschool, elementary and middle school, and later school years, are useful guidelines for teachers. These guidelines promote reflection about what students usually know about language, the level of language complexity provided in classroom discourse and curricular activities, and how mismatches in student and classroom language levels can present challenges for students and teachers.

A checklist of common language development characteristics during the toddler and preschool years is provided in Appendix 3.B, elementary and middle school years in Appendix 3.C, and high school and adult years in Appendix 3.D (based on Hedrick, Prather, & Tobin, 1975; Meacham, 1971; Sparrow, Balla & Cicchetti, 1984). These tools can be used by teachers, SLPs, and parents during observation of particular children for estimating language development and as a guide for making referrals for assessment by the school SLP or for charting student progress. General and special education teachers and SLPs need to work closely together with parents and students to identify language strengths (as well as weaknesses) and to provide timely and effective interventions, so that each student can participate fully in classroom learning.

Appendix 3.A
English Sounds in Key Words and International Phonetic Alphabet Symbols

Consonants

baby	/b/	nose	/n/	yellow	/j/
cracker	/k/	popcorn	/p/	zoo	/z/
deer	/d/	quick	/kw/	shower	/ʃ/
funny	/f/	rose	/r/	ring	/ŋ/
gopher	/g/	salt	/s/	thimble	/θ/
hammer	/h/	tiger	/t/	those	/ð/
joy	/dʒ/	violin	/v/	pleasure	/ʒ/
love	/l/	walrus	/w/	choose	/tʃ/
mommy	/m/	xray	/ɛks/	glottal stop	/ʔ/

Vowels and Diphthongs

beat	/i/	book	/ʊ/	bow	/aʊ/
bit	/I/	boat	/o/	bay	/eɪ/
bait	/e/	bought	/ɔ/	bow	/oʊ/
bet	/ɛ/	bottom	/ɑ/	but	/^/ (stressed)
bat	/æ/	bite	/aɪ/	Bert	/ɝ/ (stressed)
boot	/u/	boy	/ɔɪ/	remember	/ɚ/ (unstressed)
				about	/ə/ (unstressed)

Appendix 3.B
Language Development Checklist for Toddlers (Birth to 2 Years) and Preschoolers (3 to 4 Years)

Articulation and Phonology

Toddlers

______ Turns eyes and head toward sounds

______ Looks toward source of different sounds

______ Listens momentarily when spoken to

______ Cries and laughs aloud

______ Vocalizes for enjoyment

______ Imitates sounds made by others

______ Babbles and uses jargon to interact with self and others

______ Produces many vowels and consonants

______ Echoes a few words

______ Uses first names of family members and others

______ Simplifies single words and words used in combinations

______ Is intelligible 25% to 50% of the time

Preschoolers

______ Continues to add consonants and use them correctly in words

______ Refines the pronunciation of old and new words

______ Gradually uses fewer simplifications of words

______ Coordinates speech sounds in the use of morphemes

______ Is intelligible 60% to 80% of the time

Suprasegmental Aspects

Toddlers

______ Responds to pitch and loudness changes in voices of others

______ Responds to voice of others from other background noise

______ Uses changing pitch during babbling

______ Produces babbling with the prosody of the native language

______ Uses pitch change to signal meaning

______ Conveys intentions through the use of prosody

______ Develops use of several prosodic features (pitch, stress, rate) to signal meaning

Preschoolers

______ Develops use of several prosodic features (pitch, stress, rate) to signal meaning

______ Adds new words continuously to receptive and expressive vocabulary

______ Understands word meanings and concepts

______ Invents words in novel situations (e.g., "grass scissors")

______ Understands 1,000 words

______ Matches and identifies colors

______ Understands adjectives such as hard, rough, smooth

______ Recognizes penny, nickel, and dime

______ Counts items by number

______ Understands questions about the present

______ Retells a story or fairy tale

______ Relates experiences in sentences

______ Recites songs, nursery rhymes, or poems

______ Uses pictures to retell stories in books

______ Expands expressive vocabulary to 1,500 words

______ Appreciates humor and invents words to convey humor

Pragmatics

Toddlers

______ Smiles in the presence of caregiver

______ Responds to familiar and unfamiliar voices

______ Lifts arms to command "come" or "up"

______ Vocalizes for enjoyment

______ Uses gestures for "no," "yes," or "I want"

______ Makes choices between two objects

______ Takes vocal turn through babbling and early words

______ Uses object to gain attention of adult

______ Uses adult to get desired object

______ Conveys several communicative functions at one-word level

______ Expands on communicative functions with word combinations

Preschoolers

______ Uses language creatively in interactive experiences

______ Adjusts speech style to situations

______ Uses polite language forms to request ("please"), interrupt ("excuse me"), or thank others

______ Experiments with role playing through modification of speech style

______ Adjusts speech to the amount of shared knowledge between speakers (presupposition)

______ Uses language for many functions including communication, play, and learning

Metalinguistics

Toddlers

______ Discriminates differences in speech sounds

______ Listens intently to speech of others

_____ Practices sounds through babbling and jargon

_____ Practices words and word combinations

_____ Makes adjustments in speaking style for the listener

_____ Detects simple rhymes

Preschoolers

_____ Monitors own utterances and makes simple repairs

_____ Practices words and word combinations

_____ Adjusts speech style for speaking role or for listener

_____ Comments on own utterances and those of others

_____ Detects rhyming patterns

_____ Rhymes words

_____ Learns patterned phrases in songs (e.g., "B-I-N-G-O, and Bingo was his name-o")

_____ Appreciates humor and invents words to convey humor

_____ Associates letters with key words

_____ Draws with pencil or crayon

_____ Writes first name, letters, numbers, and simple words

_____ Begins to read simple words, phrases, or stories

Appendix 3.C
Language Development Checklist for Elementary (Kindergarten to 5th Grade) and Middle School (6th to 8th Grade) Years

Articulation and Phonology

Elementary School

______ Articulates clearly

______ May have a few sound distortions (e.g., /r, r-blends, θ, dʒ/)

______ Makes slight speech sound modifications as influenced by surrounding sounds

______ Alters speech to reflect dialect or language differences

______ Experiments with pronunciations of new words

______ Masters complicated syllable arrangements of long words

______ Refines pronunciations of words with inflectional or derivational morphemes

______ Increases awareness of how speech sounds function in words (phonological awareness)

______ Recognizes and manipulates sounds in words

______ Recognizes when others err in speech sound pronunciation

______ Repairs own pronunciation errors

Middle School

______ Articulates clearly with no distortions

______ Masters pronunciation of words with inflections and derivations

______ Code switches easily from dialects or other languages

______ Understands figurative language based on phonological manipulations

______ Recognizes when others err in speech sound pronunciation

______ Imitates various speaking patterns, including disordered speech (e.g., hypernasality)

Suprasegmental Aspects

Elementary School

______ Experiments with prosodic features (pitch, stress, rate, inflection) during interactions

______ Learns to match prosodic features to the social situation

______ Practices the use of prosody during reading of stories and plays and when reciting poetry

______ Uses prosody to influence others (e.g., whining, begging, politeness)

______ Uses contrastive stress to highlight new information

______ Modifies prosody according to social situations

______ Uses different voices for character roles

Middle School

______ Increases ability to describe and recognize psychological states of others

______ Understands spatial, temporal, familial, disjunctive, and logical relationships

______ Creates more elaborate dictionary-like definitions

______ Recognizes syntactic ambiguity in riddles

______ Increases metaphor use in descriptive prose

______ Increases understanding of idioms in situational contexts

______ Explains the meaning of some proverbs

______ Uses slang terms with peers

______ Plans future action

Pragmatics

Elementary School

_____ Infers about the psychological states of others

_____ Appreciates social roles of self and others

_____ Recognizes language differences based on gender, age, and situation (e.g., school, church)

_____ Allocates roles in pretend play

_____ Manipulates vocabulary, phrase use, and accent in pretend play

_____ Makes observations of others' motives, attitudes, or needs

_____ Begins to regulate suprasegmental aspects in situations

_____ Learns the social rules for situations (e.g., loudness level, vocabulary, polite forms)

_____ Learns appropriate physical distance from others (proxemics)

_____ Adjusts nonverbal language situationally

_____ Develops flexibility in the use of language during school (e.g., recite, tell about, explain)

_____ Employs self-regulatory speech

_____ Enjoys cooperative play with peers

_____ Develops assertive status through verbal duels

Middle School

_____ Adopts verbal and nonverbal strategies to adjust to social situations

_____ Recognizes the effort required for assignments requiring language use

_____ Develops skill in altering roles for drama and other creative works

_____ Continues to improve in manipulating the various systems of language

_____ Refines the use of suprasegmentals in situations

_____ Increases flexibility in the uses of language during school

_____ Becomes more independent in the use of self-regulation and other cognitive strategies

_____ Perfects peer interactions including cooperative play and verbal duels

Metalinguistics

Elementary School

_____ Recites the alphabet from memory

_____ Identifies letters, numbers, and words by sight

_____ Writes letters, numbers, and words

_____ Attempts to read and write unknown words

_____ Increases phonological awareness

_____ Reads common signs and instructions

_____ Reads stories and increases reading by grade level each year

_____ Reads on own initiative

_____ Alphabetizes by first letter(s)

_____ Writes sentences, notes, or messages

_____ Makes purchases by mail or advertisement

_____ Reads books, magazines, and newspapers

_____ Thinks about language to construct well-formed spoken or written messages

_____ Judges the appropriateness of grammatical morphemes

_____ Judges utterances according to setting and situational appropriateness

_____ Evaluates what is heard and offers repair or request for clarification

_____ Explains why forms are incorrect within sentences

Middle School

______ Recognizes similarities and differences in narrative and expository styles

______ Adjusts language systems for narrative and expository styles of speaking and writing

______ Uses comprehension monitoring to reflect on what is heard or read

______ Understands and uses figurative forms

______ Recognizes and uses mental activities to learn, remember, and maintain attention

Appendix 3.D
Language Development Checklist
High School and Adult Years

Articulation and Phonology

______ Articulates without error complex syllable structures in words and sentences

______ Recognizes different sounds in other languages

______ Segments new words by syllable for ease in pronunciation

______ Appreciates word similarities and differences

______ Recognizes the geographic or cultural origins of dialect

Suprasegmentals

______ Uses prosodic features to reflect mood and attitude

______ Recognizes the social prestige differences between dialects

______ Adjusts pronunciation and grammatical patterns to reflect informal and formal styles

______ Practices prosodic features in literate styles (e.g., narrative, persuasion)

______ Alters prosodic features for manipulation and sarcasm

______ Practices prosody in drama and other creative arts

Morphology and Syntax

______ Refines use of grammar and linguistic devices in speaking and writing

______ Increases understanding and use of adverbial conjuncts (e.g., *moreover, nevertheless*)

_____ Uses synonyms for greater flexibility in word choice and for cohesion between sentences

_____ Uses a variety of categorical word associations for cohesion between sentences

_____ Analyzes spoken and written language for grammatical errors

_____ Repairs grammatical errors in spoken and written language

Semantics

_____ Engages in thoughtful study and dialogue about topics

_____ Attends to subtle differences in meaning and uses precision, passion, and word economy

_____ Increases vocabulary with content area study

_____ Expands definitions of words

_____ Increases awareness of nuances in meaning conveyed by figurative forms

_____ Learns meanings of abstract and rare words

_____ Increases understanding of connectives (e.g., *because*, *during*) and double-function terms

_____ Increases understanding of words conveying psychological states

_____ Expands definition types (e.g., dictionary, operational, negation, comparison, example)

_____ Advances the use of cohesive devices

_____ Uses greater variety of explanations of metaphors

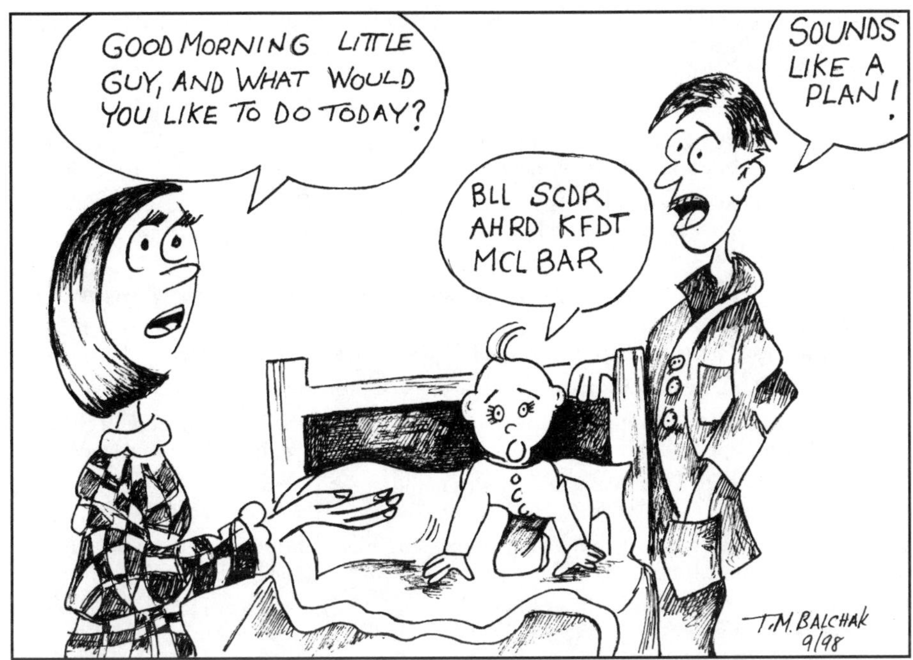

The routines established in daily life encounters with others encourage turn-taking, exploration of the environment, and the social basis for communication.

References

Ackerman, B. P. (1982). On comprehending idioms: Do children get the picture? *Journal of Experimental Child Psychology, 33*, 439–454.

Barrett, M. (1995). Early lexical development. In P. Fletcher & B. MacWhinney (Eds.), *The handbook of childhood language* (pp. 362–392). Oxford: Basil Blackwell.

Bates, E., Camaioni, L., & Volterra, V. (1975). The acquisition of performatives prior to speech. *Merrill-Palmer Quarterly, 21*, 205–216.

Beal, C. R. (1987). Repairing the message: Children's monitoring and revision skills. *Child Development, 58*, 401–408.

Beal, C. R., & Flavell, J. H. (1983). Young speakers' evaluations of their listeners' comprehension in a referential communication task. *Child Development, 54*, 148–153.

Becker, J. (1994). Sneak-shoes, sworders, and nose-beards: A case study of lexical innovation. *First Language, 14*, 195–211.

Bernthal, J. E., & Bankson, N. W. (1998). *Articulation and phonological disorders* (4th ed.). Needham Heights, MA: Allyn & Bacon.

Bradley, L., & Bryant, P. (1983). Categorizing sounds and learning to read: A causal connection. *Nature, 30*, 419–421.

Brasseur, J., & Jimenez, B. C. (1989). Performance of university students on the Fullerton subtest of idioms. *Journal of Communication Disorders, 22*, 351–359.

Brenneis, D., & Lein, L. (1977). "You fruithead": A sociolinguistic approach to children's dispute settlement. In S. Ervin-Tripp & C. Mitchell-Kernan (Eds.), *Child discourse* (pp. 245–258). New York: Academic Press.

Brown, R. (1973). *A first language: The early stages*. Cambridge, MA: Harvard University Press.

Caselli, M. C., Bates, E., Casadic, P., Fenson, J., Fenson, L., Sanderl, L., & Weir, J. (1995). A cross-linguistic study of early lexical development. *Cognitive Development, 10*, 159–199.

Clark, E. (1978). Awareness of language: Some evidence from what children say and do. In A. Sinclair, R. Jarvella, & W. Levelt (Eds.), *The child's conception of language*. New York: Springer-Verlag.

Clark, E. V. (1993). *The lexicon in acquisition*. Cambridge, England: Cambridge University Press.

Clark, E. V., & Andersen, E. S. (1979). Spontaneous repairs: Awareness in the process of acquiring language. *Papers and Reports on Child Language Development, 16*, 1–12.

Clark, H. H. (1979). Responding to indirect speech acts. *Cognitive Psychology, 11*, 430–477.

Cook-Gumperz, J. (1977). Situated instructions: Language socialization of school-aged children. In S. Ervin Tripp & C. Mitchell-Kernan (Eds.), *Child discourse*. New York: Academic Press.

Crowhurst, M. (1980). Syntactic complexity in narration and argument at three grade levels. *Canadian Journal of Education, 5*, 6–13.

Crowhurst, M., & Piche, G. L. (1979). Audience and mode of discourse effects on syntactic complexity in writing at two grade levels. *Research in the Teaching of English, 13*, 101–109.

Day, R. R. (1982). Children's attitudes toward language. In E. B. Ryan & H. Giles (Eds.), *Attitudes toward language variation* (pp. 116–131). London: Edward Arnold.

de Boysson-Bardies, B., Sagart, L., & Durand, C. (1984). Discernable differences in babbling of infants according to target language. *Journal of Child Language, 11*, 1–15.

de Villiers, J. G., & de Villiers, P. A. (1973). A cross-sectional study of the acquisition of grammatical morphemes in child speech. *Journal of Psycholinguistic Research, 2*, 267–278.

Donahue, M., & Bryan, T. (1984). Communicative skills and peer relations of learning disabled adolescents. *Topics in Language Disorders, 4*(2), 10–21.

Dore, J. (1975). Holophrases, speech acts, and language universals. *Journal of Child Language, 2*, 20–40.

Dunn, J., & Kendrick, C. (1982). The speech of two- and three-year-olds to infant siblings: "Baby talk" and the context of communications. *Journal of Child Language, 9*, 579–595.

Durkin, K. (Ed.). (1986). *Language development in the school years*. Cambridge, MA: Brookline.

Emerson, H. (1979). Children's comprehension of "because" in reversible and nonreversible sentences. *Journal of Child Language, 6*, 279–300.

Felton, R., & Brown, I. (1990). Phonological processes as predictors of specific reading skills in children at risk for reading failure. *Reading and Writing: An Interdisciplinary Journal, 2*, 39–59.

Ferguson, C. A., & Farwell, C. B. (1975). Words and sounds in early language acquisition. *Language, 51*, 439–491.

Fernald, A., & Kuhl, P. K. (1987). Acoustic determinants of infant preference for motherese speech. *Infant Behavior and Development, 10*, 279–293.

Fernald, A., & Simon, T. (1984). Expanded intonation contours in mothers' speech to newborns. *Developmental Psychology, 20*, 104–113.

Flavell, J., Speer, J., Green, F., & August, D. (1981). The development of comprehension monitoring and knowledge about communication. *Monographs of the Society for Research in Child Development, 46* (Serial No. 191).

Foster, S. H. (1986). Learning discourse topic management in the preschool years. *Journal of Child Language, 13,* 231–250.

Gardner, H. (1974). Metaphors and modalities: How children project polar adjectives onto diverse domains. *Child Development, 45,* 84–91.

Gentner, D. (1988). *Cognitive determinism: Object reference and relational reference.* Paper presented at the Boston University Child Language Conference, Boston.

Geva, E., & Ryan, E. B. (1985). Use of conjunctives in expository texts by skilled and less skilled readers. *Journal of Reading Behavior, 17,* 331–346.

Giles, H., Harrison, C., Creber, C., Smith, P. M., & Freeman, N. H. (1983). Development and contextual aspects of children's language attitudes. *Language and Communication, 3,* 141–146.

Gilmore, P. (1986). Sub-rosa literacy: Peers, play, and ownership in literacy acquisition. In B. B. Schieffelin & P. Gilmore (Eds.), *The acquisition of literacy: Ethnographic perspectives* (pp. 155–168). Norwood, NJ: Ablex.

Gleason, J. B. (1997). *The development of language* (4th ed.). Needham Heights, MA: Allyn & Bacon.

Goldfield, B. (1993). Noun bias in maternal speech to one-year olds. *Journal of Child Language, 20,* 85–99.

Golinkoff, R. M. (1986). "I beg your pardon?" The preverbal negotiation of failed messages. *Journal of Child Language, 13,* 455–476.

Grunwell, P. (1986). Aspects of phonological development in later childhood. In K. Durkin (Ed.), *Language development in the school years* (pp. 34–56). Cambridge, MA: Brookline.

Guralnick, M., & Paul-Brown, D. (1989). Peer-related communicative competence of preschool children: Development and adaptive characteristics. *Journal of Speech and Hearing Research, 32,* 930–943.

Halliday, M. (1975). *Learning how to mean: Explorations in the development of language.* New York: Arnold.

Hedrick, D. L., Prather, E. M., & Tobin, A. R. (1975). *Sequenced inventory of communicative development.* Seattle: University of Washington Press.

Hoff-Ginsberg, E. (1997). *Language development.* Pacific Grove, CA: Brooks/Cole.

Horgan, D. (1981). Learning to tell jokes: A case study of metalinguistic abilities. *Journal of Child Language, 8,* 217–227.

Hulit, L. M., & Howard, M. R. (1997). *Born to talk: An introduction to speech and language development* (2nd ed.). Needham Heights, MA: Allyn & Bacon.

Karabenick, J. D., & Miller, S. A. (1977). The effects of age, sex, and listener feedback on grade school children's referential communication. *Child Development, 48,* 678–683.

Labov, W. (1970). Stages in the acquisition of standard English. In H. Hungerford, J. Robinson, & J. Sledd (Eds.), *English linguistics* (pp. 275–302). Glenview, IL: Scott Foresman.

Larson, V. L., & McKinley, M. S. (1995). *Language disorders in older students: Preadolescents and adolescents.* Eau Claire, WI: Thinking Publications.

Leadholm, B. J., & Miller, J. F. (1992). *Language sample analysis: The Wisconsin guide.* Madison: Wisconsin Department of Public Instruction.

Leonard, L. B., Schwartz, R., Folger, M., & Wilcox, M. (1978). Some aspects of child phonology in imitative and spontaneous speech. *Journal of Child Language, 5,* 403–415.

Lepper, M. R. (1983). Social-control processes and the internalization of social values: An attributional perspective. In E. T. Higgins, D. N. Ruble, & W. W. Hartup (Eds.), *Social cognition and social development: A sociocultural perspective* (pp. 294–332). Cambridge, England: Cambridge University Press.

Lever, J. (1976). Sex differences in the games children play. *Social Problems, 23*, 478–487.

Liberman, I., & Shankweiler, D. (1985). Phonology and the problems of learning to read and write. *Remedial and Special Education, 6*, 8–17.

Local, J. (1983). How many vowels in a vowel? *Journal of Child Language, 10*, 449–453.

Lodge, D. N., & Leach, E. A. (1975). Children's acquisition of idioms in the English language. *Journal of Speech and Hearing Research, 18*, 521–529.

Lowe, R. J. (1994). *Phonology: Assessment and intervention applications in speech pathology*. Baltimore: Williams & Wilkins.

Lund, N., & Duchan, J. (1988). *Assessing children's language in naturalistic contexts*. Englewood Cliffs, NJ: Prentice-Hall.

MacLean, M., Bryant, P., & Bradley, L. (1987). Rhymes, nursery rhymes, and reading in early childhood. *Merrill-Palmer Quarterly, 33*, 255–281.

Maltz, D. N., & Borker, R. A. (1982). A cultural approach to male–female miscommunications. In J. A. Gumperz (Ed.), *Language, interaction, and social identity* (pp. 196–216). New York: Cambridge University Press.

Mann, V. (1993). Phoneme awareness and future reading ability. *Journal of Learning Disabilities, 26*, 259–269.

McNeill, D. (1966). Developmental psycholinguistics. In F. Smith & G. Miller (Eds.), *The genesis of language* (pp. 15–84). Cambridge: MIT Press.

Meacham, M. J. (1971). *Verbal Language Development Scale*. Circle Pines, MN: American Guidance Service.

Nelsen, E. A., & Rosenbaum, E. (1972). Language patterns within the youth subculture: Development of slang vocabularies. *Merrill-Palmer Quarterly, 18*, 273–285.

Nelson, K. (1973). Structure and strategy for learning to talk. *Monographs of the Society for Research on Child Development, 38*.

Nelson, K. (1985). *Making sense: The acquisition of shared meaning*. New York: Academic Press.

Nelson, N. W. (1993). *Childhood language disorders in context: Infancy through adolescence*. New York: Macmillan.

Nippold, M. A. (1998). *Later language development: The school-age and adolescent years*. Austin, TX: PRO-ED.

Nippold, M. A., & Martin, S. T. (1989). Idiom interpretation in isolation versus context: A developmental study with children and adolescents. *Journal of Speech and Hearing Research, 32*, 59–66.

Nippold, M. A., Schwarz, I. E., & Undlin, R. A. (1992). Use and understanding of adverbial conjuncts. *Journal of Speech and Hearing Research, 35*, 108–118.

Owens, R. E. (1992). *Language development: An introduction* (4th ed.). New York: Merrill.

Peevers, B. H., & Secord, P. F. (1973). Developmental changes in attribution of descriptive concepts to persons. *Journal of Personality and Social Psychology, 27*, 120–128.

Pellegrini, A. D. (1984). The development of the functions of private speech: A review of the Piaget–Vygotsky debate. In A. D. Pellegrini & T. D. Yawkey (Eds.), *The development of oral and written language in social contexts* (pp. 57–70). Norwood, NJ: Ablex.

Perfetti, C. A., Beck, I., Bell, L., & Hughes, C. (1987). Phonemic knowledge and learning to read are reciprocal: A longitudinal study of first-grade children. *Merrill-Palmer Quarterly, 33*, 283–320.

Polanski, S. (1989). Spontaneous production of figures in writing of students: Grades four, eight, twelve and third year in college. *Educational Research Quarterly*, *13*, 47–55.

Pollio, M. R., & Pollio, H. R. (1974). The development of figurative language in school children. *Journal of Psycholinguistic Research*, *3*, 185–201.

Prinz, P. M. (1983). The development of idiomatic meaning in children. *Language and Speech*, *26*, 263–272.

Reid, E. (1978). Social and stylistic variation in the speech of children: Some evidence from Edinburgh. In P. Trudgill (Ed.), *Sociolinguistic patterns in British English*. London: Edward Arnold.

Roth, F., & Spekman, N. (1984). Assessing the pragmatic abilities of children: Part I. An organizational framework and assessment parameters. Part II. Guidelines, considerations and specific evaluation procedures. *Journal of Speech and Hearing Disorders*, *51*, 8–23.

Scott, C. M. (1984). Adverbial connectivity in conversations of children 6 to 12. *Journal of Child Language*, *11*, 423–452.

Shantz, C. U. (1975). The development of social cognition. In E. M. Hetherington (Ed.), *Review of child development research* (Vol. 5, pp. 257–324). Chicago: University of Chicago Press.

Shatz, M., & Gelman, R. (1973). The development of communication skills: Modifications in the speech of young children as a function of listener. *Monographs of the Society for Research in Child Development*, *38*(Serial No. 152).

Shultz, T. R. (1974). Development and appreciation of riddles. *Child Development*, *45*, 100–105.

Sparrow, S. S., Balla, D. A., & Cicchetti, D. V. (1984). *Vineland Adaptive Behavior Scales*. Circle Pines, MN: American Guidance Service.

Stoel-Gammon, C., & Cooper, J. (1984). Patterns of early lexical and phonological development. *Journal of Child Language*, *11*, 247–271.

Storck, P. A., & Looft, W. R. (1973). Qualitative analysis of vocabulary responses from persons aged six to sixty-six plus. *Journal of Educational Psychology*, *65*, 192–197.

Strand, K. E., & Fraser, B. (1979). *The comprehension of verbal idioms by young children*. Unpublished paper, Boston University, School of Education.

Tunmer, W. E., & Cole, P. G. (1991). Learning to read: A metalinguistic act. In C. S. Simon, (Ed.), *Communication skills and classroom success* (pp. 386–402). Eau Claire, WI: Thinking Publications.

van Kleeck, A. (1987). Foreword. The metas: Implications for the language impaired. *Topics in Language Disorders*, *7*(2), vi–vii.

Weiss, C. E., Gordon, M. E., & Lillywhite, H. S. (1987). *Clinical management of articulatory and phonologic disorders* (2nd ed.). Baltimore: Williams & Wilkins.

Wimmer, H., Landerl, K., Linortner, R., & Hummer, P. (1991). The relationship of phonemic awareness to reading acquisition: More consequence than precondition but still important. *Cognition*, *40*, 219–249.

Wing, C., & Scholnick, E. (1981). Children's comprehension of pragmatic concepts expressed in "because," "although," "if," and "unless." *Journal of Child Language*, *8*, 347–365.

The Development of Written Language

Maud Kuykendall and Kathleen R. Fahey

In Chapter 3 the oral language systems were described and trends in development were discussed from infancy through adulthood. A strong foundation in oral language is critical to beginning to read and write; it provides the base on which literacy emerges and continuously supports the thinking and linguistic processes needed for literacy development. In this chapter we describe and discuss trends in the emergence of written language during the preschool and early elementary school years, and literacy for communication, learning, and enjoyment throughout formal schooling and beyond. Literacy development interests general and special education teachers and speech–language pathologists (SLPs) because of its importance to school life both as an end in itself and as a vehicle for academic achievement. As children build competence in reading and writing, they use them as avenues for independent learning, thinking, creating, and communicating. Teachers foster literacy growth in virtually every content area, classroom, and grade level. Thus, knowledge about typical trends, as well as each student's progress in literacy development, helps teachers collaborate with each other and guide student learning for successful achievement.

Literacy and Culture

Although *literacy* refers to a person's ability to participate fully in his or her community (Gee, 1990; Wallach & Butler, 1994), the term also has been widely used in a more restricted sense to refer to the acquisition of written language abilities. In this chapter the term literacy is used to remind the reader that written language is related both to oral language and to the language of the community in the broader sense. After all, reading and writing are essential to full participation in virtually all North American communities.

Maud Kuykendall is an adjunct professor at the University of Northern Colorado and a special education teacher at the Union Colony Charter School, Greeley, Colorado.

As just mentioned, although literacy is often thought of as the ability to read and write, it also encompasses a much greater realm. Langer (1987) described literacy as a way of thinking, a phenomenon of cultural activity that allows participation in the sharing of knowledge of a culture and, therefore, its goods, services, and power structures. Literacy, then, is a social process influenced by social situations and contexts (Bloome, Harris, & Ludlum, 1991).

Just as oral language develops from the interactions of people within cultures, so too does written language, and, hence, literacy. In fact, literacy development begins very early, simultaneously developing with oral language as children gain experiences with print in interaction with the environment. Written language is the focus during formal schooling, but some students come to school with a great deal of information and experience in reading and writing. They have constructed knowledge about written language simultaneously with their knowledge and abilities in oral language. Miller (1990) contended that in homes where written language exists, both oral language and written language are interwoven within the activities and values of everyday interaction. In such homes, family members are usually highly verbal, involving children in language for fun, socialization, and learning new information. These households contain many literacy artifacts (e.g., books, magazines, paper, pens) and events (e.g., bedtime stories, making grocery lists, reading the newspaper) that extend children's knowledge of the functions of written language (van Kleeck & Schuele, 1987; Wallach & Miller, 1988). The overlap of oral and written language allows children to develop oral language systems along with metalinguistic, discourse, and pragmatic knowledge of written language. As children develop greater understandings of language, their interest and knowledge about language serve as foundations for further learning. The development of written language not only extends children's knowledge about language, but has the reciprocal effect of enriching oral language development. Thus, many children come to school familiar with the oral and written discourses typically used in classrooms, which allows them to interact effectively with others and with the curriculum.

In contrast, children from homes where written language is not prevalent come to school ill prepared for the oral and written discourse of the classroom (see also Chapters 1 and 2). Further, those children from nonmainstream cultures find North American schools very different from their native language and customs (see also Chapters 5 and 6). It is no wonder that such children experience less successful achievements than their mainstream culture counterparts. The language they see and hear is new to them (Heath, 1983). This lack of familiarity with both oral and written discourse may also lead educators to erroneously conclude that language or learning problems exist.

In recent years, research has been directed to determining the relationships between family environment and emerging literacy. A wide range of types of investigations (e.g., ethnographic, adult–child interaction, and predictive and correlative studies) have shown interesting results about literacy acquisition in preschool children (van Kleeck, 1990). First, although literacy artifacts and print-related events were present in most homes, the quality and range of the artifacts varied as a function of socioeconomic status. However, poverty is not the major factor in reduced literacy preparation. Even some middle and upper class homes do not encourage literacy development. Second, literacy events that occur in homes of preschoolers are typically part of natural social interactions involving real-life activities. Even when parents teach children to read, it is not done in formal structured settings, but rather through guidance as children show interest and begin to interact with printed materials. Third, guidance and support in relating information from books to the real world through discussion has been found to be a significant factor in literacy development. Facilitative techniques in literacy development include staying on topics introduced by children (semantic contingency), structuring context to facilitate success (scaffolding), and providing highly predictable and structured contexts and routines (Snow, 1983).

Oral and Written Language Differences—A Continuum

Although oral language and written language have many similarities and indeed develop simultaneously, there are also several differences. These include physical, form and process, and situational and functional differences. Each of these is described in Table 4.1 and is further explained below.

Physical differences between oral and written language are readily apparent. The rapid and sequential production of oral language puts high demands on the speaker and the listener to keep pace with the information being communicated. Written language, on the other hand, can be produced or read without the confines of time and sequence. How many personal letters, papers for college credit, and grocery lists have been developed over days or even weeks in your own households? An advantage of written language is its permanency captured by whatever medium is used (e.g., paper, clothing, signs). We use its permanent nature to preserve and protect memories (e.g., photo albums, letters, yearbooks); reflect on thoughts, feelings, and situations through diaries and journals; and extend our understandings as we research, reflect, and write about topics (Chafe, 1985; Perera, 1984).

Table 4.1
Differences Between Oral and Written Language

Physical

Oral language exists in real time and is constrained by the capacity of individuals to process the information. It is rapid, sequential, and must be received through the hearing ability of the speaker and the listener.

Written language is free of temporal constraints and informational capacity. It is represented visually in two-dimensional space and has durability in terms of time.

Form and Process

Oral language is produced in situation-specific contexts. Its degree of formality is, therefore, highly flexible. An informal style includes simple and often incomplete sentence structures, shared vocabulary between participants, and conversational moves such as topic selection and maintenance and turn-taking. Themes and topics change frequently. More formal styles and structures are used when the situation requires them. The grammatical structure of oral language is highly redundant with many words used to convey a small amount of information. Oral language is continuous and involves the extraction of meaning as it occurs during interactions. It includes the production and perception of sounds in words and sentences accompanied by vocal characteristics, volume, rate, rhythm, and intonation changes.

Written language often incorporates formal styles, involving complete and more complex sentence structure, varied vocabulary, and correct spelling. Informal styles such as found in personal diaries or letters reflect reductions in these formal aspects. Writers develop and use phonological awareness, correspondence between phonemes and letters, word consciousness, segmentation skills, and an analytic sense about written language that is different from oral language. Writers learn the discourse structures and organizational rules for narrative and expository text. Writing is often low in redundancy and fewer words are used to convey ideas. An overall theme is necessary, and the writer must justify changes in topic. Punctuation serves to represent suprasegmentals such as intonation, pauses, and stress.

Situational and Functional

Oral language occurs most often in face-to-face interactions with verbal and nonverbal forms used together to convey and understand intentions. It is participant and situation oriented. Oral language is a principal means of communication and serves as the sole means for 40% of the world's adults who are not literate in written language (Perera, 1984). It requires turn-taking and is very important in maintaining human relationships.

(*continues*)

Table 4.1 *Continued.*

Written language is often individually constructed. It is often less personal than oral language and is explicit in both grammar and meanings. The writer has the responsibility to present intentions in clear and precise ways. The writer must specifically request feedback from readers, especially during the process of writing. Written language serves many functions. Labels inform (e.g., street signs, food names, ingredients), historical writings preserve history and acquired knowledge, writing genres extend oral forms of literature, letters maintain human relationships, and writing extends our own thinking and reasoning.

Form and process differences refer to the degree of formality of language used as reflected by grammar, vocabulary, and themes, as well as the changes speakers make in style and formality depending on the nature of situations and interactions. We are able to engage in very informal "chit-chat" as we share experiences over coffee, but can quickly modify many components, including the length and complexity of sentences, the use of specialized vocabulary, the rate and clarity of speech production, the mood of our voices, and so forth, in order to teach a class, interview a prospective teacher, or participate in an Individualized Education Plan (IEP) meeting. Additionally, the rapid and sequential attributes of oral language require us to process, integrate, and produce oral language systems in timely and coordinated ways so that meaning is derived from the utterances. Our attention, motivation, and cognitive processes must be attuned directly when we participate in oral language interactions.

Written language requires that information is provided through printed words and sentences and that thoughts and ideas are constructed and conveyed through the spellings of words, and the more conscious production of sentence structures and mechanics. It also requires knowledge and application of the styles of written discourse, such as narrative and exposition (Kamhi & Catts, 1991; Stark & Wallach, 1982; van Kleeck & Schuele, 1987; Wallach & Miller, 1988).

Situational and functional differences between oral and written language occur as purposes for communication vary. These variations allow us to use language in social contexts, to express intention and purpose appropriate to different settings, and to use language to extend thinking and reasoning. The face-to-face oral interactions we have with others require turn-taking in the exchange of information as the situation requires. Verbal and nonverbal behaviors are used to convey information. During written interactions, the exchange is not accomplished in this back-and-forth, turn-taking manner. Often, the entire message is constructed by the individual, who may or may not solicit a response from the reader in the future. The lack of face-to-face dialogue and the lack of verbal and nonverbal information require that written language be highly explicit in meaning and grammar so that intentions are clear and precise. The purposes for writing are many. Writing can serve (a) an economic function (stamps are inexpensive and most of us attempt to keep our telephone bills reasonable), (b) to label things and places in our environment (e.g., street signs, food, household products), (c) to preserve our own and society's history and acquired knowledge, (d) to extend oral forms of literature, (e) to establish and maintain human relationships, and (f) to extend our own thinking and reasoning skills (Gee, 1988; Kamhi & Catts, 1991; Perera, 1984; Westby, 1988).

In sum, oral and written language differences are numerous. Each of these differences provides challenges to young learners as they encounter them. We point out the similarities and differences to children as we guide them in their development. As they encounter new situations and purposes for the use of language, whether oral or written, the modifications in physical structure, form and process, and styles for conveying information in clear and precise ways will develop from the models and guidance that others provide.

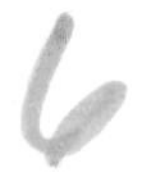

Holistic View of Written Language Development

Proponents of holistic views of language (Halliday, 1975; Piaget, 1971; Vygotsky, 1978) contend that learners actively seek information to make sense of the world. The quest for meaning, along with the social uses of language, provides sufficient impetus for development to occur. The holistic approach to written language instruction, therefore, recognizes reading and writing as social practices and places an emphasis on the reader's or writer's role to discover and create meanings through print. In school, strategies are taught to support the students' intentions to use written language in contexts that are meaningful in social and cultural situations for each student (Rhodes & Dudley-Marling, 1996). Reading and writing are learned from whole to part, as in oral language learning. That is, the goal for children (and adults) is to comprehend the whole message by deriving meaning from the words and sentences conveyed. Differences in developmental learning needs—for instance, the individual needs of children receiving special education services—are not treated as deficits in holistic literacy instruction. Rather, instruction remains focused on providing meaningful learning opportunities by meeting children at their own specific levels of understanding.

Consequently, literacy skills taught in holistic instruction develop with explicit support and direction based on each student's needs. Assessment and instruction is interwoven during classroom interactions so that teachers analyze each student's efforts and products in order to adjust instruction appropriately. Rhodes and Dudley-Marling (1996) addressed several aspects of reading and writing that can be assessed and taught within a holistic philosophy. Table 4.2 lists aspects based on each student's previous experiences and instruction in reading and writing. Past experiences influence memories, attitudes, and beliefs about reading; the role of reading in the student's social interactions; and the student's ease and comfort in modifying effort and rate depending on the purpose he or she has for reading or writing. Assessment and instruction should also be directed to each student's current understandings of

Table 4.2
Aspects of Reading and Writing To Assess and Teach

Previous Literacy Experience and Instruction

Role of past experiences and instruction in reading and writing

Attitudes and interest toward reading and writing

Beliefs about how reading and writing develop

Flexibility in adjusting effort and rate to suit situational purpose (e.g., homework assignments, pleasure reading, writing a personal letter)

Role of literacy to enhance social interactions and thinking processes

Current Literacy Development

Use reading and writing to construct meaning

Process words and other text features (e.g., punctuation, italics, quotations) effectively for comprehending text

Use writing conventions to convey intentions to readers

Use composition strategies to achieve clear organization and appeal to the intended audience

Understand and use procedures to gain access to information (e.g., library, Internet)

Note. Adapted from *Readers and Writers with a Difference: A Wholistic Approach to Teaching Struggling Readers and Writers* (2nd ed.), by L. K. Rhodes and C. D. Dudley-Marling, 1996, Portsmouth, NJ: Heinemann.

text, including: (a) meanings of vocabulary- and sentence-level comprehension, (b) use of text features and conventions, (c) use of discourse strategies, and (d) use of procedures to gain access to reading and writing opportunities.

Predictable routines in the assessment and instruction of reading and writing enhance the effect of holistic instruction (Rhodes & Dudley-Marling, 1996). Routines are especially beneficial for emergent readers or for those students who struggle with reading. The benefits of routines for students include (a) expectations in how time is spent, how they should behave, and what assistance will be provided; (b) mutual support from student peers; and (c) avenues of participation, practice, and independence.

Teachers benefit from routines, too. By scheduling predictable activities, teachers increase opportunities to assess and instruct students. They can individualize instruction, coordinate and share routines between classrooms and resource environments, and build routines into all of the academic areas.

A model of literacy development based on a holistic view has been offered by K. Goodman (1986). This perspective regards literacy development within an integrated environment with oral language. He wrote,

> Learning to read and write is a matter of learning to comprehend written language. It involves learning to apply the psycholinguistic strategies already learned in listening, with orthographic rather than phonological input. We learn to read and write, as we learn to speak and listen, from whole to part, not from part to whole. . . . Only when we can comprehend the whole are we fully able to see how the parts relate to it. Kids who can read are usually good at learning phonics, because they can put phonic relationships into the context of making sense from print. (p. 84)

The first phase in K. Goodman's (1986) model, *preschool literacy,* includes building awareness of print through the environment and experiences with literary artifacts. This phase allows for expansions of children's sense of narratives, expositions, and the style and form of written language. The second phase, *primary level literacy*, includes the development of print knowledge and productive reading. This phase involves the development of reading fluency and comprehension strategies. *Developmental literacy*, the third phase, broadens and refines interests and efficiency in reading and writing skills. It allows for continued development of confidence and supports growth of learning through written language (Hoffman, 1990).

In that the primary goal of reading and writing instruction in the elementary grades and beyond is comprehension of meaningful and useful information, an integrated, holistic approach is superior to more skills-based approaches, because it encourages a focus on meaning with direct support provided for decoding and meaning-making. Students active in learning use all modes of language in direct response to the opportunities that present themselves in the context of purposeful communication.

This chapter addresses the development of reading and writing according to an integrated and holistic philosophy. The phases of reading outlined by K. Goodman (1986) do not precisely conform to age ranges; however, for ease in discussing development, preschool, elementary and middle, and secondary grades will serve as a guide to the typical developmental changes that occur.

In addition, general and special education teachers and SLPs should understand that students who have language problems or language differences develop reading and writing in the same ways that children without such problems do. The development may be somewhat slower and students may struggle with one of more aspects, such as comprehension, decoding, or fluency, yet each child will continue to advance in this process given ample time, instruction, guidance, and encouragement.

9 Dyslexia

Students with severe reading and writing problems, called *dyslexia*, need intensive and explicit instruction in reading and writing, with particular attention to the development of phonological coding and phonemic awareness. (See Chapter 3 for information on development and Chapter 12 for interventions.) There is not one universally accepted definition of dyslexia; each group with a vested interest in the problem supports a slightly different definition that meets its own needs (Jordan, 1996). The term derives from Greek. The prefix *dys* refers to something that is different and the stem *lexicos* is literally "pertaining to words." Therefore, dyslexia is a term that refers to someone who is having difficulty with language, specifically written language. Many educationists are uncomfortable using the term dyslexia, which seems medical, and prefer instead more educational terms such as *poor readers*, *individuals with severe reading impairment*, and the like. These latter terms encourage some consideration of poor instruction or sociocultural differences and not merely some dysfunction in the child. Although the manifestation that gets a person labeled as dyslexic is difficulty with reading and writing, difficulties with language in general are certainly involved (Vellutino, 1979). For our purposes, the definition advocated by the World Federation of Neurology is useful (Critcheley, 1970):

> *Specific developmental dyslexia* is a disorder manifested by difficulty learning to read despite conventional instruction, adequate intelligence, and

> adequate sociocultural opportunity. It is dependent upon fundamental cognitive disabilities which are frequently of constitutional origin. (p. 6)

Simply stated, the child must have a neurological deficit, usually assumed rather than documented (Spafford & Grosser, 1996), that is pretty much limited to reading and does not extend too far into other areas of cognitive functioning (Stanovich, 1988). In the early years, the problem may indeed be restricted to reading and writing, but the impact of a reading disability becomes increasingly severe as the student ages. The reason, as Stanovich (1986) explained, is that the failure to learn to decode words leads to other problems—problems with reading comprehension, vocabulary, syntactic development, and even general knowledge acquisition. He labeled this phenomenon "the Matthew effect," a reference to the Bible verses in which the rich get richer and the poor get poorer; that is, those who can read and write develop language competencies more easily, whereas those who have difficulties lag more and more behind over time.

In their review of the literature, Clark and Uhry (1995) pointed out that the research substantiates a significant relationship between early language processing problems and later reading problems. Follow-up studies of children with language impairment show that 90% of them have difficulty learning to read. On the other hand, as Clark and Uhry also noted, not all children ultimately diagnosed with dyslexia have had histories of oral language problems—only about a half of them score below the screening cutoff as 4-year-olds.

A strong relationship exists between dyslexia and the perception of speech sounds, which Stanovich (1986) called the "phonological core deficit." Brady, Poggie, and Rapala (1989), for example, found in their word repetition studies that the participants with dyslexia had difficulty remembering sounds and encoding them into phonological information. Likewise, Tallal and Stark (1982) detected that these participants had difficulties perceiving and analyzing speech sounds rapidly. When students cannot discriminate between phonemes in spoken words, they lose the ability to correlate sounds with graphemes. Catts (1986) studied the relationship between speech *production* and phonological deficits in children with reading disorders and, once again, found that the students with dyslexia had problems. Bradley and Bryant (1983) found difficulties in the categorization of sounds. Finally, Snowling and Hulme (1989) showed that phonological awareness develops prior to reading, but that it is also aided by experience with reading (i.e., there is a reciprocal relationship between them).

Dyslexia, then, is a disorder specific to written language, probably based on a more fundamental problem associated with phonological processing. As students get older, the disorder seems less and less specific, because more and more aspects of their functioning are affected. Many people with dyslexia have difficulties that continue throughout their lifetimes. Spelling difficulties, for example, usually persist.

Reading Development in Preschool

DEBBIE (3 YEARS OLD): Mommy, whatcha doing?

MOMMY: I'm reading a book about gardening.

DEBBIE: Why you do that?

MOMMY: Because I want to learn about growing vegetables so we can have a garden this summer.

DEBBIE: Mommy, I better read it too so I can help you with the garden.

This short exchange demonstrates children's awareness of and interest in reading. Youngsters are curious about such items as newspapers and books, letters from friends and family, street signs, and being able to select their favorite toy from the box design at the store. They observe the uses of oral language and reading in their homes and neighborhoods. Indeed, both oral language and reading are learned in the context of daily interactions with other language users.

By around 3 years of age, children have developed many of the foundation abilities of oral language and writing and can use them to interact with people in their environments. They refine these abilities, which continue to build in complexity throughout the preschool years and beyond. As oral language develops, children use it to help them cope with the complicated demands of acquiring reading and writing. Their interest and knowledge about oral language serves as a foundation for further learning. The acquisition of reading and writing not only extends children's knowledge by equipping them with another avenue of communication, but has the reciprocal effect of enriching oral language development.

Reading Aloud and Story Retelling: Important Routines

Reading before bedtime or at other times during the day is an early and important social activity that occurs in literate households. This routine can provide emotional support and security, as well as linguistic information, to youngsters. It is one of the most significant activities parents can do to influence reading development (Anderson, Hiebert, Scott, & Wilkinson, 1985; Wells, 1985).

Because children *observe and participate in* these story reading interactions, reading becomes a natural part of family life. When adults read to children, they both note and give their children practice with important characteristics about story structure. In fact, children as young as 18 months have been observed to page through books and babble as though they are reading (Sulzby & Teale, 1984). On average, children handle books and become aware of the top, bottom, front, and back by age 3. They follow with their eyes or fingers in the left to right direction of the written words, especially when another child or adult reader provides these cues (Y. Goodman, 1986).

Two- to 4-year-old children tell stories aloud or "read" them from familiar storybooks to familiar adults. This *pretend reading* is an important development in the acquisition of literacy. During the story retelling, even 2- and 3-year-olds modify the structure and content of the stories to be like the written stories. For example, familiar characters may be introduced and children may fictionalize themselves in stories. They use formal openings (e.g., "Once upon a time"), closings (e.g., "and they lived happily ever after"), and even wordings and styles that reflect written text structure (e.g., "so it came to be known around the land") (Applebee, 1978; Sulzby, 1986). They also respond to written product logos, dictate and reread language experience stories, and pretend to read stories and letters (Harste, Woodward, & Burke, 1984).

Children who are read to hear the story grammars common to their native culture and develop the ability to generate their own personal stories or to retell stories in the same organized way (van Kleeck, 1990). Parents usually respond to the slightest reaction from their children about books by using interactive scaffolding techniques to create two-sided interactions. For example, a child may show great interest in the hats that the cat wears in a Dr. Seuss story. The following exchange may occur as the child points to the different hats:

PARENT: Yes, look at all the different hats. They are big and little.

CHILD: This one's big, this one's big. Here is a little one.

PARENT: This one looks like your baseball cap, doesn't it.

CHILD: My baseball cap, the green one?

PARENT: Yes, you like to go to Matt's baseball games with Daddy.

CHILD: I go to baseball with Daddy today?

Eventually, children use words and phrases to become more independent in emergent book reading. Sulzby and Teale (1984) described book reading situations as a weaving between oral and written interactions over time. The interactions families engage in about reading result in "literacy socialization." Consequently, children from high-print homes often enter school having book awareness and book reading routines; knowing how to respond to questions; being able to recite the alphabet; recognizing letters; and being able to do some sight word reading and rudimentary writing (Kamhi & Catts, 1989).

Metalinguistics: Phonological Awareness

An area that has gained much attention in emergent reading is the development and role of metalinguistics. In particular, phonological awareness is central to children's development of written language. Children's awareness of sounds in words, words' resemblances to other words, and the manipulations that can be done to change meaning, allows them to participate in social routines in play with other children (e.g., rhymes, songs, chants, jokes). Phonological awareness is a strong predictor of reading development, and research has shown that this relationship is reciprocal (Wagner, Torgeson, & Rashotte, 1994). That is, phonological awareness becomes more explicit and highly developed as experience with written language increases. Good readers demonstrate the ability to deliberately reflect on and manipulate the structural features of language and treat the language system itself as an object of thought (Tunmer & Cole, 1991). Poor readers have deficiencies in their knowledge and awareness of oral language or may have differences in their general phonological processing abilities (Flood & Menjuk, 1983; Stanovich & Siegal, 1994; Wagner et al., 1994).

Preschoolers begin to recognize, analyze, and reflect about sounds in words. They make corrections and manipulate sounds in words during spontaneous speech, creative sound play, and rhyming games. Such reasoning, which occurs gradually (Karmiloff-Smith, 1986), requires the ability to segment oral language. For example, 3-year-olds demonstrate the ability to segment sentences based on meanings, understanding that the main ideas of a sentence are "the parts" of the sentence, and exhibit the ability to segment sentences into words. Segmentation of words into syllables and individual sounds emerges much later, usually as children complete their fourth year (Ehri, 1975; Liberman, Shankweiler, Fisher, & Carter, 1974), but it is not unusual for children as late as 6 or 7 to be working on syllable and sound segmentation. Three- and 4-year-olds usually recognize a relationship between letters and sounds. Note that these areas of metalinguistic awareness can develop without explicit instruction in some children, especially among those from high-print households; however, youngsters without such experiences often need explicit instruction and plenty of practice time in kindergarten and the early elementary grades. Further, children who have difficulty developing awareness of phonological and other language segments will have difficulties in learning to read (Adams, 1990; Bradley & Bryant, 1983; Tunmer, Herriman, & Nesdale, 1988).

As oral language development continues through the preschool years, much knowledge is accrued about the nature of reading. Table 4.3 is a summary

Table 4.3
Preschoolers' Knowledge of Oral and Written Language

Page through books and babble as though reading
Page through books and use words and phrases as though reading
Name pictures
Name printed alphabet
Produce rhymes and alliterations
Divide sentences into main ideas
Divide sentences into words
Segment words into syllables
Begin to segment words into phonemes
Handle books and orient to the top and bottom
Recognize letters that vary from conventional forms
Realize that print is meaningful and is used for several functions
Recognize different uses and ways that printed language occurs (e.g., newspapers, books, lists)
Respond to global organizational structures of stories (e.g., openings, closings)
Be aware of relationships between letters and sounds
Recognize written product logos
Pretend to read
Dictate and reread language experience stories
Repair errors in spontaneous speech
Creatively engage in sound play
Recognize, analyze, and reflect about sounds in words
Understand that meanings in print are independent of the immediate social context

of preschoolers' knowledge and abilities that are acquired across oral language, early reading, and the interactions between them (e.g., phonological awareness and the meanings and functions of print). It is fair to say that these expressions of language interact continuously and it is, therefore, somewhat artificial to separate the two areas of knowledge.

In summary, the preschool period is an important time for significant attainments in reading. Generally, formal instruction in reading has not yet occurred. Still, many children have developed emergent reading abilities through home and preschool activities. One of the most important attainments is phonological awareness. Beyond the preschool years, reading development takes on a more prominent focus with intentional instruction provided in elementary school.

Reading Development in Elementary School

The rich oral and written literacy base that many children have when they begin school allows teachers to guide students in more advanced reading activities. Elementary classrooms are often print-rich and have areas designated for blackboard instruction, tasks for which students are responsible (e.g., calendar, distributing materials, collecting materials), computer time, library time, and so on. This environment creates an atmosphere in which literacy is part of daily interactions with other students. Students typically immerse themselves in their classrooms, enjoying the expanded options they have to explore with other students the materials and activities available. However, we cannot assume that chronological age or grade in school corresponds to a particular individual's literacy level. Those students who lack exposure to preschool literacy activities in their homes prior to entering school require additional time as well as direct experience with printed materials and oral language activities. We must remember that while some youngsters enter kindergarten just after turning 5, others are more mature 5-year-olds, and still others are 6 years old. These varied ages and experiences due to culture, time in preschool, developmental ability, and interest and motivation result in a wide variety of starting points for classroom learning. Early elementary teachers and SLPs who provide holistic, language-based experiences in reading engage in activities that promote and support the development of primary reading. These activities include listening and reading comprehension strategies and metalinguistics and decoding strategies.

Listening and Reading Comprehension

During the early elementary school years, students are asked to focus on listening for characters and events in orally read stories, and making predictions about what comes next in stories that have familiar structures. Additionally, students are exposed to teacher models about the purposes of reading and the social rules of the classroom. For instance, at 5 years old, Carrie was able to read stories containing lengthy paragraphs (5 to 7 sentences) and full pages of print. Imagine the shock when at age 6½ she arrived at school and was given books loaded with pictures and only a few lines of print on each page. At home, she proceeded to "read" the story aloud to her family by alerting everyone to the pictures, reading the few sentences, and turning the book toward all so that the picture was seen again. Carrie provided a vivid demonstration of the circle time "read-to-the-class" style that one sees in early grades. Although her reading level was beyond this style, she put some importance on this new teacherlike reading behavior of the classroom. She had learned a style of language typical for instruction in the early grades.

Comprehension of oral and written texts involves transactions between the reader and the text, with interpretations influenced by factors such as linguistic and conceptual level, social and cultural attitudes, and personality. Children's comprehension of text must be viewed with these areas in mind, especially considering the purposes each child has as he or she engages in deriving meaning from text (Fish, 1980; Iser, 1978; Langer, 1987).

A person's ability to take in and comprehend oral and written language can vary from shallow to deep processing, depending on the relationships being drawn between new information and information previously stored in memory (Craik & Lockhart, 1972). In regard to reading comprehension, one level involves *understanding the literal meanings of words and sentences*. It includes the understanding of the vocabulary and the relationships between the words and sentences (i.e., semantics). A second level is called *inspectual reading*. This is the level engaged when the purpose of the reader is to understand the text within a short amount of time, involving the ability to scan for information in a systematic fashion. The *analytic level* involves active seeking of deep understandings of text. The fourth level involves *comparative reading*, in which the reader must use all the previously described levels to understand meanings, inspect and analyze topics, then use the information to compare the ideas presented in multiple sources. Knowledge about these levels of comprehension can help teachers determine strengths or difficulties particular children may have and can facilitate instruction for advancing comprehension. Note that a particular child's comprehension can depend on the nature of the material and the interest and motivation that child has in reading any particular piece.

Refer to Table 4.4 for examples of the types of questions at each level that children might answer after reading a story about a school basketball game.

Metalinguistics and Decoding Strategies

Teachers often give attention to metalinguistic development through oral and written activities such as rhyming, alliteration, segmentation of sentences, and segmentation of words by syllables and by phonemes. These and other activities tune children into the segments of oral language and the manipulations that can occur in words to change meaning. Recall that many children have prior experience with oral and written words and sound awareness activities. Classroom activities often serve to provide more practice for some and new experiences for others. Directed, and perhaps more structured, activities make the metalinguistic knowledge more explicit by increasing attention to and awareness of language. Some techniques used to heighten awareness include using redundancy in examples and practice activities, linking oral language with its written form, and focusing on changes in meaning through sound manipulations in words, word order, or word changes in sentences.

Participation in metalinguistic activities promotes awareness of language units which, in turn, increases students' ability to decode during reading. As students develop the ability to decode rapidly and automatically, they tend to improve in comprehension of what they read. Traditional skill-based phonics approaches emphasize decoding activities as prerequisite to reading and writing. Students engage in activities such as (a) reciting the alphabet, (b) recognizing and naming letters, (c) sounding out letters in single words, (d) finding words beginning or ending with particular sounds, and (e) determining which words contain certain vowel sounds (Adams, 1990). Students learn to look carefully at written words and make judgments about their similarities and differences. Kamhi and Catts (1991) described two problems that readers of English face with this approach. The first problem is that the sounds of speech are abstract and do not correspond to discrete letter sounds. In connected speech, the segments (sounds, syllables, words) blend together so that individual segments are often not heard. The second problem is that sounds can vary depending on the other sounds around them. Such variations interfere with constructing the phoneme–grapheme correspondences that are required in decoding through phonics. Perhaps the most frustrating problem for teachers and their students is the problem of irregularities in the orthographic spellings of words and the variations created by upper- and lowercase print, script, and typed words. However, when language is predictable, explicit instruction in decoding for reading and

Table 4.4
Types of Questions To Probe Reading Comprehension

Level 1—Elementary: Literal meanings of words and sentences

What does it mean to dribble the ball?

What did Alison do after she made the basket?

What was the score at the end of the game?

Describe the crowd's reaction when Alison was getting ready for the shot.

Level 2—Inspectual: Systematic skimming for information

Where did the basketball game take place?

Why was this particular game so important to each team?

How did the score change as the game continued in the second quarter?

What event led to the tension displayed by the crowd?

How did the game end?

Level 3—Analytic: Active seeking of deep understandings

In the second paragraph the team was described as watchful, nervous, and high-strung. Why did the author create this image?

Do you see the use of flashback in the episode? What are the advantages of using this technique here?

Think about a similar experience that you have had. How did you feel?

Rewrite the ending to this story to change the outcome.

Level 4—Comparative: Inspect and analyze to compare and construct information

As we study drama through writing, how does this story compare to the one about the fishing expedition?

What specific devices did this author use to build the dramatic tone of the story?

How would the story be different if the author eliminated these devices?

encoding for spelling can provide students with regular patterns that are useful, if they are taught from a whole-to-part-to-whole perspective.

In integrated, holistic approaches, phonics activities are incorporated *simultaneously* during connected and meaningful written language experiences. For example, reading high-interest stories, using written language to solve a problem, or writing procedures about how the classroom hamster will survive during the Thanksgiving holiday provide opportunities for phonics instruction within rich language contexts. K. Goodman (1993) defined phonics as "the set of complex relationships between phonology (i.e., the sound system of an oral language) and orthography (i.e., the system of spellings and punctuation of written language)" (p. 8). This relationship is broader than "sound–symbol relationship" or "letter–sound correspondence" that is often used in the literature and in discussions about phonics. Liberman and Shankweiler (1991) clarified these expressions by discussing the importance of teaching the relationship between the word's phonology and the visual shapes of a word. That is, the phoneme patterns of the word must be related to the letters used to represent it. This task is not simply making the relationships between visual and auditory images, but rather involves making the linguistic connections from both apparent. Decoding written language includes using the visual and auditory information to represent units of language. As mentioned earlier, phonological awareness has been shown to be highly correlated and predictive of future reading success (Blachman, 1983; Bradley & Bryant, 1983; Fox & Routh, 1980; Vellutino & Scanlon, 1985). While phonological awareness is important, the alphabetic principle is not accomplished effectively only by sounding out words. Rather, readers must develop the ability to group the consonant and vowel sounds into pronounceable units that convey meaning (Liberman & Shankweiler, 1991).

As students develop decoding strategies for single words, they also learn to use their knowledge of the regularities of spoken syntax and semantics to assist them in decoding. This knowledge provides students with multiple strategies for decoding print easily and effectively. Comprehension is facilitated when students recognize individual words and, more important, when they relate the words within the context of sentences and the sentences within paragraphs. Competent readers use prediction, monitor comprehension, and correct errors more readily than poor readers (Perfetti, Goldman, & Hogaboam, 1979; Stanovich, 1982). Difficulty with comprehension monitoring can suggest that a student's ability to think about and reflect on the cognitive processes needed to understand text is not well developed.

In summary, holistic classrooms provide environments rich in literacy opportunities. Teachers and SLPs observe each child in authentic reading and writing and provide support in making sense from print. Children become effective readers and writers by spending a great deal of time reading and writing (Allington, 1993; Gee, 1994; Weaver, 1994). Students with difficulties might also require direct and explicit instruction (Adams, 1990).

Reading Development in Middle and High Schools

The middle and high school years are characterized by continued use of reading and writing in all content areas. Skillful readers can maintain silent reading rates of 300 words per minute, perceiving whole words and whole phrases very quickly and with little effort, while focusing attention on meaning (Adams, 1990). Students engage in reading at literal, inspectual, and analytic levels during these years (Kamhi, 1997). They show their comprehension of texts through written summaries or outlines, oral reports, answering questions on teacher-made tests, or applying the information in related projects.

Often during these years (especially around Grade 4) nonreaders or slow readers show a decline in their ability to succeed in the academic content areas. Reading fluency is often hampered by a strategy of sounding out text word by word or by failure to use syntactic and semantic cues to achieve word recognition (Rhodes & Dudley-Marling, 1996). The slow pace and the difficulty constructing meaning make it difficult for students to keep abreast of information they are required to know. In these grades, teachers expect students to read textbooks independently in order to comprehend science, social studies, or math. In addition to reading fluency and comprehension difficulties, content area textbooks present material in a structure different from what some students are used to. These books organize information through headings and subheadings, visual aids such as graphs or charts, boxes embedded in the text that elaborate a topic, the use of italics and bold to emphasize concepts, and study questions before or after the chapter. All students benefit from an introduction to and instruction in using this structure to aid comprehension (Slater & Graves, 1989). Some students require more direct and more frequent instruction so that the organization of texts becomes clear and useful for comprehension.

During high school, more complex thought and reasoning abilities position the reader to use analytic and comparative comprehension strategies (Kamhi, 1997). Such strategies can facilitate the student's ability to retain information and to study information for performance-based demonstrations, such as tests and projects. Competent students engage in several activities, including (a) text scanning exercises, (b) implicit self-questioning, (c) examination of text structures, (d) elaboration of texts, (e) drawing inferences, (f) finding the main ideas and supporting points (and also outlining), (g) summarizing text in their own words, (h) using several sources to research topics, and (i) relating information verbally or in written reports (Tunmer & Cole, 1991). Most students are able independently to access information from the library, the Internet, newspapers, and other sources. They read to fulfill a variety of needs and purposes in school, at home, and in jobs.

Poor readers in high school struggle to keep up with the content areas and have difficulty employing both analytic and comparative strategies. Unfortunately, reading instruction is seldom provided in most high schools. Students try to use the decoding and comprehension strategies they have already acquired, but because they are ineffective, many give up and sometimes even drop out of school. Poor grades, low mathematics and reading scores, failing of one or more grades, failing to see the relevance of education to life, and having verbal and language deficiencies are among the 21 symptoms associated with dropping out of school (Larson & McKinley, 1995).

In sum, the development of reading spans many years, from preschool through high school and continues into adulthood. The development of metalinguistic knowledge, comprehension, and decoding during the preschool and early elementary years allows students to engage in reading for learning across the curriculum. Most students learn to read with ease, but about 20% struggle to acquire written language.

Learning To Write

Children learn to write through acts of discovery. Shortly after birth, they begin such discoveries through the myriad of social interactions that families have with written language. Y. Goodman (personal communication, June 1996) noted that families and other caregivers engage in countless interactions involving literacy. Parents read, write, talk, listen, and think in the company of their children. Youngsters see others read and write for a variety of purposes and they participate, actively or passively, in pastimes and rituals that vary widely in complexity and function. For example, they observe others reading the daily paper and watch as lists are made, notes are written, and recipes are followed. They may watch others work on computers, connect to the Internet, and send and receive e-mail. Sometimes they participate in religious activities that involve reading and writing. In this way, young children are involved in literacy traditions that are unique to each family and social setting, but are constrained by the larger aspects of the culture into which the child is born (Vygotsky, 1978).

When children are read to, they learn about a written form of language that can present and explain things without the use of oral speech. Eventually, when surrounded by meaningful print and encouraged to produce their own, they learn to write. Most children follow similar discovery paths (Temple, Nathan, Temple, & Burris, 1993), yet they evolve their own strategies—such as prediction, confirmation, and integration strategies—to learn about how print works for writing, as they do with reading (Y. Goodman & Burke, 1980; Rhodes & Dudley-Marling, 1996). They discover *rules* about how language works initially in learning to talk, and then coincidentally with learning to read and write. To make meaning out of their worlds, children form tentative concepts about how to *do* language. They gradually revise their attempts until they approach conventional correctness through an ongoing process of trial and error. This process does not occur in isolation but, as mentioned earlier, through social interactions within the cultural and historical context of a particular community of language users.

As with learning to talk, children, through their own efforts, take the majority of the responsibility for learning how to write (Cambourne, 1988). For young children, usage of correct forms in writing does not result from direct teaching, but through gradual conceptual learning controlled by the children themselves (Temple et al., 1988). Parents, caregivers, and preschool teachers, in addition to models of literacy, become environmental engineers to ensure that children are surrounded by meaningful print and opportunities to engage in learning at their own rate and level. For young children with special needs or a shortfall of early literacy experiences, parents and others may need to provide additional sustained interventions.

General and special educators and SLPs recognize that children receiving special education services follow the same developmental pathway in learning to write as other children. These children usually differ from other learners in the amount and type of facilitation needed to facilitate growth in written language. Although they pass through the same levels that every child experiences, such as scribbling and forming letters, they may develop writing skills and strategies more slowly or not at all. Teachers and SLPs must be alert to each child's level of writing development, making sure that instruction matches the learning needs. Writing development may suffer because instructional strategies are not appropriate for the level of development a child has achieved (Kuykendall, 1997). In addition, educators and SLPs should not expect high levels of writing competence from students experiencing reading difficulties.

Writing development involves an interaction between cognitive processes and the educational and cultural contexts of children's environments. It is also a highly integrated process involving linguistic, cognitive, and motor skills.

Y. Goodman (1992) referred to this conglomerate of contexts and abilities as aspects of complex literacy events that impact, influence, and constrain each piece of writing that children produce. She defined three broad categories that interact in each literacy event: the writer, the written text, and the literacy community. Throughout our lives, we learn to write by continually interacting with oral and written text and by interacting in our literacy communities. To understand writing development, it is essential to consider these complex influences that affect each learner's writing process.

Writing research, as well as what writers report about their composing processes, indicates that writers of all ages engage in a complex, nonlinear process when they write. Calkins (1994) and Graves (1983) compared the writing process to a *craft*. Graves noted that "a craft is a process of shaping material toward an end" (p. 6). Writing is a process of shaping text toward an end. Therefore, as with any craft, writing takes time to perfect and is learned, in part, in apprenticeship with more knowledgeable writers, just as oral language is learned by interacting with other language users. Time is crucial for writers to engage in the recursive nature of writing. Writers of all ages engage in an iterative process of selecting, composing, and reading what they have written (Graves, 1983).

In summary, children learn to write through their own efforts in discovering how writing works. Their efforts are situated within social and collaborative contexts beginning with the family into which they are born. Through gradual conceptual learning, children control and construct their own understandings about writing and the purposes that writing serves. Additionally, learning to write is an interactive venture involving cognitive, educational, and cultural constraints. Therefore, writing is a multifaceted, recursive process. *All* children experience learning to write as a process and learn to write in ways that are similar, whether or not they have special education labels. Vygotsky (1978) reminded us that, historically and culturally, we humans harbor negative perceptions toward those we label as *disabled*. Educators and SLPs must hold the expectation that learning to read and write is essential in the lives of each student by responding to each student's needs with appropriate teaching strategies.

Writer, Text, and Literacy Community at the Preschool Level

Preschool students engage in what Scott (1991) described as *emergent writing*. This early writing bears little resemblance to more mature writing. Importantly, however, it is a process of expressing thoughts through written symbols and, therefore, is an important beginning toward becoming literate. When children scribble or write several letters and ascribe meaning to them, they are actively involved in the process of writing even though they have not yet learned the alphabet. By using marks or a few letters to communicate, children are showing that they understand the function of writing (Siu-Runyan, 1992). Gradually, they may switch or combine writing systems, such as using scribbling, pictures, or invented spellings, depending on the situation or setting (Sulzby, 1986). This flexibility shows that children call upon their repertoire of knowledge to engage in writing for different purposes.

At around 18 months, children begin to experiment with pencils or crayons to produce and to respond to scribbles on paper (Gibson & Levin, 1975; Henderson, 1981). Sometimes they use less desirable surfaces, including walls, furniture, and even themselves! Children gradually combine scribbles with lines that intersect or close the scribble. The scribbles then take on linear and repetitive qualities (Fields, 1989), which develop into letterlike creations and conventional forms. In all, children's active participation in writing may include some or all of the following developmental forms of writing: (a) scribble writing, (b) scribbling plus some letters or letterlike characters, (c) a combination of letters and numbers, (d) copying environmental print, and (e) writing by repeating well-learned units.

As mentioned earlier, children adopt rules as strategies for creating early writings. One rule is the use of a letter (i.e., grapheme) or a symbol (e.g., picture, symbol) to represent a word (e.g., T = bird). The selection of the letter is arbitrary, but it is used to differentiate one word from another (Ferreiro, 1984). Another rule is to use a combination of three or more letters to represent a word (e.g., xyt = bird). Ferreiro and Teberosky (1982) refer to this as the *minimum number principle*. Eventually, children develop an awareness of sounds in words and begin to represent these in their invented readings and writings of words (e.g., brd = bird). The development of this *alphabetic principle* is considered to be an important characteristic in the development of reading and writing.

Young children learn that letters are objects with names (Ferreiro, 1984) and that letter combinations (words) can be used as substitutes for other objects. Prior to the acquisition of the alphabetic principle, children do not understand that letters represent the sound patterns of words (Dyson, 1986). Writing is for the sake of activity rather than for creation (Calkins, 1994). With the development of the alphabetic principle (when written symbols designate speech sounds), young children begin to appreciate that the number of letters or the sounds of syllables distinguish objects. They begin to write messages to others, label objects in the environment, and produce longer texts for personal or social reasons. In terms of text structure, the most common genres during this time are the *book* genre and the *draw and write* genre. The book genre often contains a title in capital letters, numbered pages, and left-to-right and top-to-bottom orientation (Himley, 1986). The draw and write genre has the drawing at the top of the page and the text at the bottom.

In summary, preschool children need plenty of opportunities to practice their emerging writing (Taylor & Walls, 1990). Classrooms are designed to surround the children with useful, meaningful print—their own as well as others. Opportunities for writing for real purposes and real audiences occur daily. Children are encouraged to build on their current understandings of how print works. Reading to children continues to be an extremely important way for children to learn about writing. Additionally, children learn about letters and letter sounds through repetitive readings and through their own texts. In keeping with a holistic approach, they learn about grapheme–phoneme connections within the context of learning to write and read.

Writer, Text, and Literacy Community at Elementary School

Writing instruction is often a part of elementary curricula; however, historically, reading instruction has dominated most language arts programs. Recently, extensive research conducted at elementary, secondary, and college levels is changing the way we view writing development, and hence writing instruction, by supporting a holistic approach to learning (Maxwell & Meisser, 1997). In classrooms that apply a holistic philosophy, reading and writing are taught in an integrated fashion along with speaking and listening (Shanklin, 1991). In addition, the writing process movement that emerged during the 1970s and 1980s emphasizes writing as a problem-solving activity that evolves from authentic activities in social situations and experiences. In these classrooms, teachers provide mini-lessons to guide the development of text writing. Students write on topics of choice across many half-hour or full-hour sessions, so that various processes can be developed and practiced. Individual conferencing, library work, and gaining input of other students are encouraged. The holistic approach to the development of writing creates many more opportunities to explore and develop purposeful writing than when writing is controlled and produced by students for the teacher. Shanklin (1991) outlined and described the 10 principles shared by holistic and writing process movements. These are listed in Table 4.5.

The length of writings and the types of genres written by students in the elementary grades change with age and experience. The book and the draw and write texts mentioned earlier are produced in the early grades, followed by

Table 4.5
Ten Principles Shared by Holistic Language and Writing Process Movements

1. Role of prediction
2. Importance of prior knowledge
3. Integrated use of cueing systems
4. Function before form
5. Risk-taking and gradual approximation
6. Self-correction and revision
7. Role of writing in reading and reading in writing
8. Ongoing assessment
9. Peer interaction
10. Concept of continued development

Note. Adapted from "Whole Language and Writing Process: One Movement or Two?" by N. L. Shanklin, 1991, *Topics in Language Disorders, 11*(3), pp. 45–57.

recount and fictional narratives. As described in Chapter 2, a recount is a series of events based on personal experience. These narratives include a setting, the series of events related by temporal words such as "and then," and the closing. A fictional narrative, as indicated in Chapter 2, is similar; however, the story is created from the imagination or based on real-life experiences and often a problem is presented that requires a solution. Other types of genres, including opinion essays, expository texts, persuasive writing, and narratives, develop during the elementary years (Pellegrini, Galda, & Rubin, 1984; Scott, 1991). These genres require experience in reading as well as writing, since they are styles that appear in books used as texts in the classrooms or those obtained from libraries or bookstores.

By the end of first grade, children typically can use the alphabetic principle to match speech and print to produce stable wording, print words as units with space between, and combine morphemes with constant spellings to form new units of meaning (Dobson, 1988). Consequently, children in elementary school spend much time learning to produce sentence structure. Sentences increase in length and complexity from third to sixth grade, with students using more subordinating clausal structures. Students also replace the informal oral forms of speaking with the structured formal language used in writing (Scott, 1991). Punctuation changes occur in school-age writers to reflect their growing sophistication with syntactic knowledge. An example of a letter written and typed by a 7-year-old shows the emergence of several aspects of writing.

dear Aunt kathy,

I Am having A great summer. how about you? how do you and molly, like your new house? dose it feel like home yet? how are Uncle Tome, Aunt Natalie, Ali, & matthew, School is starting soon I Am going to be in 2nd grade. how are you and molly? how do molly and pepper get along? In my swimming lessons I started in level 2 and ended in level 4. at my Indian princess meeting which was at my grandpas farm this is what I did: I did A lot of swimming little of jumping off the dock A little Eating and A little riding on the trailer we put the innertubes in the trailer. PS. Hope to hear from you soon!

Teachers expect that spelling will become more conventional during the elementary school years. Students develop further orthographic knowledge and learn strategies to spell unknown words. Rhodes and Dudley-Marling (1996) discussed a continuum of spelling abilities where each phase is not discrete and a particular student may cross stages depending on the spelling demands of tasks. Figure 4.1 shows this continuum. The *prephonetic* speller uses letters or letterlike symbols, numbers, or other forms to represent words. Children in the *phonemic* phase progress from representing the first and last letters of words to being able to represent all or most of the sounds within words. Students use a letter naming strategy until they incorporate some visual features of the orthography into spellings. At this point they become *transitional* spellers. During this phase, students learn that not all sounds are represented by single letters and that some words have letters that do not represent sounds. Transitional spellers engage in the application of rules along with the visual features of words to deal with these irregularities. The final stage of spelling is the *correct* phase. Students regularly spell words correctly by employing the visual features of spelling with phonemic knowledge. Of course, it takes time, experience, and practice to reach a level of spelling proficiency. Even very skilled spellers

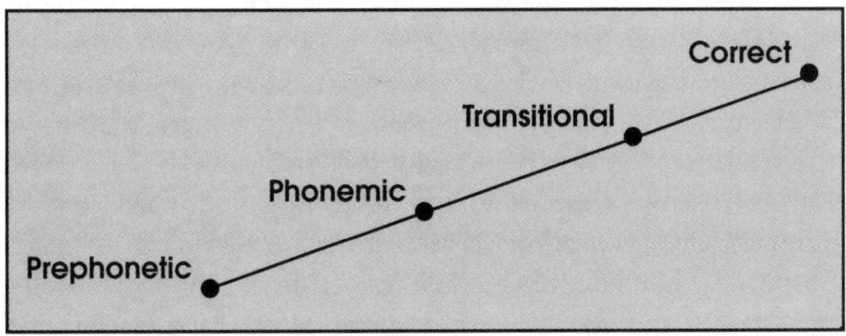

Figure 4.1. Continuum of spelling development.

depend on dictionaries and spell checks in word processing programs during writing.

Teachers also expect students to acquire handwriting abilities. Changes in student handwriting between the ages of 5 and 13 years reflect qualitative and quantitative developments. For example, they change the way the pen is held, the kinds of strokes made, the patterns of the strokes, and the speed of writing (Martlew, 1986). Most students have the motivation to develop legible handwriting, since it is useful for allowing audiences to read what has been written. Handwriting exercises should be done as a part of meaningful tasks, such as copying compositions for publication with attention to letter formation (Rhodes & Dudley-Marling, 1996). One instructional aid that is useful in the classroom to help students with handwriting is a list of guide words. By referring often to the list, students learn the correct spellings of commonly misspelled words. Other useful materials include dictionaries and other reference materials. Postural or motor difficulties can be overcome with position changes, guided instruction, and practice (Graves, 1983; Rhodes & Dudley-Marling, 1996).

In this age of computers, keyboarding skills can and should be a part of writing programs. Word processing can facilitate children's quantity and speed of writing and decrease anxiety caused by spelling errors, or dissatisfaction with or embarrassment regarding penmanship. Software programs also help students organize stories or reports and create many different forms of writing, such as brochures, newsletters, and so forth (Cunningham & Allington, 1994; Katzer & Crnkovich, 1991; Routman, 1991). "In our experience, children who have regular access to computers for processing are more willing to write, write more, revise more, and feel more confident in their writing" (Cunningham & Allington, 1994, pp. 121–122).

Research on elementary children's use of process in writing shows that they begin to plan during writing between the ages of 10 and 14 years. Ten-year-olds, when given specific planning instruction, produced written sentences. They did not change them for use within the text. Fourteen-year-olds first wrote notes containing ideas, then expanded the notes into complete ideas within texts (Bereiter & Scardamalia, 1987). In holistic language classrooms, teachers encourage students to pay more attention to process. For example, the process of planning involves "forming intentions," which includes activities such as (a) choosing topics; (b) determining the audience; (c) finding out, selecting, and ordering information; and (d) using appropriate forms. Teachers can use modeling and scaffolding techniques to help students engage in these planning aspects. They encourage students "to make their own decisions on what to write about, and how to set their own research questions, thus enabling them to be independent writers" (Bereiter & Scardamalia, 1987, p. 32).

Graves (1983) described writing development for children during the primary and intermediate grades in terms of the problems children must solve. Children in the first and second grades seek solutions that involve spelling so that their readers can understand their messages. They also focus on the motor-aesthetic aspects of their writing, which involve their handwriting and the visual qualities of their work. During the resolution of these issues, children begin to focus on the conventions of writing—capitalization and punctuation. During the third grade and beyond, children involve themselves in many aspects of literacy that require the integration of the other language processes of listening, thinking, speaking, and reading with writing. There is a shift in focus from learning to write to writing to learn. They concern themselves with topic information, resolving problems about topic choice and topic content. Lastly, they attack problems concerning the revision of their writing, struggling with issues about information—what to add and what to take out. Writing, by the end of the intermediate grades for most children, becomes a tool for thinking (Zemelman & Daniels, 1988).

It is important to stress that *children receiving special education services do not differ from their peers in the process of writing development*. They encounter the same set of problems in the same order. Kuykendall (1997) found that one intermediate student labeled as learning disabled did not differ in writing from three other students who were struggling with writing. (The only difference was in his classroom behavior.) All four students exhibited similar patterns of errors, as well as similar developmental levels of writing. Although they, in turn, did not differ significantly from their peers in their writing development, their writing experiences and products fell toward the lower end of the classroom developmental writing continuum. This finding supports the belief that writing instruction, opportunities to write, and expectations should be high for every student, allowing and encouraging each to make progress in writing development.

Writer, Text, and Literacy Community in Middle and High Schools

Students entering middle and secondary schools face many changes in writing instruction. They also face dramatic changes in their own lives. Zemelman and Daniels (1988) pointed out that, whereas the elementary writing curriculum often involves expressive and narrative activities, secondary school programs concentrate on the more formal and expository forms of writing—reports, explanations, arguments, essays, research writing, term papers—that may be less appealing and less stimulating to students (see Chapter 2). In addition, students are developing in many ways during adolescence and, therefore, may be reluctant to expose their thoughts and feelings during speaking or writing in ways that might make them vulnerable to adults.

Additionally, it should be noted that a holistic approach to writing and the departmentalized approach of most traditional secondary settings are incompatible. The extensive research on how students learn supports holistic principles in teaching writing (as well as in other learning). Maxwell and Meisser (1997), for example, pointed out that we have experienced a paradigm shift in our understanding of teaching and learning: from behaviorist to holistic (see also Reid & Kuykendall, 1996). When given the opportunity, students actively engage and participate in their own learning. They set their own goals, develop criteria for evaluating their work, and choose products for evaluation. Teachers understand that students are the center of teaching and learning and recognize that they themselves are co-learners and writers. The emphasis of learning is on meaning-making within learning contexts.

In a holistic learning environment, writing development for students at the secondary level continues to be supported as an interactive language process in conjunction with the other language processes of thinking, listening, speaking, and reading. Writing is integrated into the curriculum in balance with these other language processes. Students are encouraged to engage actively in writing for real and varied purposes across content areas and for the purposes emerging in their own lives. Lastly, writing is viewed as a communicative act with a genuine purpose, for an intended audience, and within a meaningful context (Maxwell & Meisser, 1997).

Whether encountering traditional or holistic approaches in secondary settings, students continue to experience reading for understanding. They read new information in order to engage in writing activities that require demonstration of the knowledge acquired, such as homework, test-taking, and discussions. Students also write summaries from single texts or use several sources to construct their own expositions. This integration of information and the ability to construct written products develop slowly over time with experience and guidance from teachers and other writers.

Note-taking, another highly integrative activity, becomes a critical component of writing at the secondary level. Oral language instruction through lectures, movies, presentations by students, and directions places many cognitive demands on students. Students have to be able to listen intently, understand the language being used, remember it, and paraphrase it. They have to write it down quickly and organize it while simultaneously attending to new information. This ability to engage in deep processing (Craik & Lockhart, 1972) is important for abstracting critical meanings.

Writing development at the secondary level also includes the development of categorization skills for abstracting important points from larger units of oral or written texts (Williams, 1988). Five summarization rules have been found to develop from fifth grade to college level: (1) deleting unimportant information, (2) deleting redundant information, (3) substituting category names for lists, (4) selecting a topic sentence, and (5) inventing a topic sentence (Nelson, 1993).

An example of a letter from a girl in the eighth grade (the same girl who wrote the previous letter in the second grade) shows the remarkable development from the early elementary grades to middle school.

> Aunt Kathy—
>
> So how is all in Colorado? Everthing is okey doky here. I don't need a cast which a HUGE relief. I don't even have a split. It just is wraped up in some gauze that he will probably take off tomorrow. He will also cut the ends of the stiches off and I can finally get it wet. Of coure that's what were HOPING will happen. Also I have been walking since last Sun. In a post-op shoe. Tomorrow hopefully he will say I can were a tennis shoe because this thing is sooo ungly and I am definitlay not starting a fashion trend. He said no running, jumping or playing for about 4 weeks. It's still a little sore but I really have no trouble walking. Our first cheerleading competion is on Oct. 24 or something like that and dance starts this week so I really hope it hurrys up and heals. I know, I know. I won't rush it. I would rather have it heal than mess it up again. So I'll lay low until I am sure it's better, but it's such a pain!!!!! Hope to hear from you soon.

When students reach high school, they refine previously learned abilities and apply their knowledge in a variety of ways. Comprehension and production demands are greater at the high school level than at the middle school level. Students must integrate larger and more complex amounts of incoming information and then formulate and produce information across several different modes. For example, students listen to lectures and read from textbooks, highlighting or taking notes about main ideas in the material. They are asked to formulate and write expository texts, such as book reports or essays, and then present them or discuss them orally (Larson & McKinley, 1995). Teachers can support the development of these abilities through modeling and scaffolding techniques. A key-word strategy can be used to frame cues for students to help them recognize different kinds of expository structures (Westby, 1991). Table 4.6 provides a guide to the key words often found within text structures (Larson & McKinley, 1995). Other techniques include the use of bridging questions and mediation strategies (Larson & McKinley, 1995).

During these years, high school students develop their writing to have an effect on the reader. The readers' perspectives are kept in mind as the writer

Table 4.6
Key Words for Different Expository Text Structures

Text Structure	Key Words
Comparing and Contrasting	same, different, however, but, on the contrary, similar, dissimilar, yet, still, common, alike, rather than, instead of, compare, contrast
Problem and Solution	one problem, the problem is, the issues are, a solution(s) is (are)
Cause and Effect	if, then, because, reason, affected, influenced, resulted in, therefore, since, thus, hence, consequently, cause, caused, effect, net effect, result, consequence
Chronological Sequence (episodic sequence)	first, second, third, after that, antecedent, before that, preceding, next, last, in order, subsequent, proceeding, finally, eventually, gradually
Order of Importance (hierarchical)	first, second, third, most, least, all, none, some, always, never, more, less, ____________+er, ____________+est, frequent, infrequent
Category (topical cluster or list)	group, set, for instance, another, an illustration of, such as, an example of, like, category, class
Physical Location	here, there, left, right, above, below, north, south, east, west, around, on top, under, bottom, front, back, forward, backward, side
Description	defined as, called, labeled, refers to, is someone who, is something that, means, can be interpreted as, describe, procedure, how to
Matrix	interpret, intersection, come together, overlap, influenced by, simultaneously, at the same time, converge

Note. From *Language Disorders in Older Students: Preadolescents and Adolescents* (p. 194), by V. L. Larson and M. S. McKinley, 1995, Eau Claire, WI: Thinking Publications. Copyright 1995 by Thinking Publications. Reprinted with permission.

presents information in expository or persuasive forms (Bereiter, 1980; Scott, 1991). Additionally, writers use feedback by reading their own writing, revising it, and developing personal styles and standards (Bereiter, 1980). Unfortunately, the writing required of high school students is often restricted to demonstrating knowledge to teachers by using informational summaries or analyses (Applebee, 1984; Britton, Burgess, Martin, McLeod, & Rosen, 1975).

The ability to consider the reader's point of view is an important aspect in planning, generating, and revising writing. As discussed earlier, planning was not a strong component that young and middle teens demonstrate in their writing, and revision was often only at the level of sentence structure (Hayes & Flower, 1980, 1987). High school seniors show the use of think-aloud strategies to plan text organization and to consider the forms of language used. More proficient adult writers revise to consider the global perspective of the text.

Summary

Learning to write is a continual act of discovery for children and adolescents. As early as 18 months of age, children experiment with writing. Soon they discover that writing serves a function. It provides another way to communicate other than talking. Preschool children draw, scribble, and eventually form letters. They learn that letters represent sounds and make up their own spellings to represent words. Over time, and given ample opportunities to write with demonstrations and feedback on their writing, children learn how spelling communicates their messages. In kindergarten, a holistic approach to writing instruction continues to support writing development by providing daily writing opportunities in meaningful ways. General and special educators applying a holistic approach recognize that children follow the same developmental pathway in their writing development regardless of special education labeling.

In elementary school, children continue to learn to write in the primary grades, gradually shifting their focus to use writing to learn new information. Students concern themselves with resolving issues surrounding spelling, handwriting, and the conventions of capitalization and punctuation in the primary grades. Once these issues are dealt with, if writing development is proceeding smoothly, children work on topic choice and content. Finally, they tackle issues of revision—what to leave in and what to take out.

In middle and high school, students encounter more complex writing instruction and writing challenges, such as essays, reports, and note-taking. At the same time, they experience their own adolescence, a period of self-definition that may complicate their attitude toward writing instruction, and hence their willingness to write. Throughout students' writing development, writing as presented in a holistic approach remains integrated with reading, speaking, thinking, and listening—the other language processes. Writing is recognized as an iterative, nonlinear process that is controlled by the learner, who, in turn, is influenced by social, educational, and cultural factors. Lastly, writers of all ages follow the same recursive process in writing: selecting, composing, reading, editing, and revising what they have written.

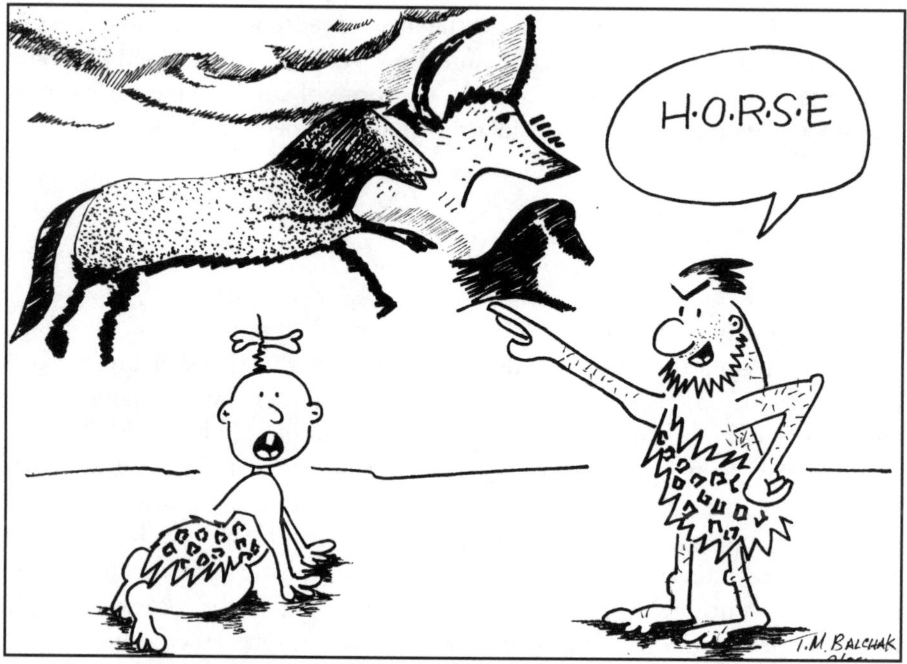

Just as oral language develops from the interactions of people within cultures, so too does written language, and hence, literacy. In fact, literacy development begins very early, simultaneously developing with oral language as children gain experiences with print in interaction with the environment.

References

Adams, M. J. (1990). *Beginning to read: Thinking and learning about print—A summary*. Austin, TX: Center for the Study of Reading.

Allington, R. L. (1993). Literacy for all children: Michael doesn't go down the hall anymore. *Reading Teacher, 46*, 602–606.

Anderson, R. C., Hiebert, E. H., Scott, J. A., & Wilkinson, I. A. G. (1985). *Becoming a nation of readers*. Champaign, IL: University of Illinois, Center for the Study of Reading.

Applebee, A. N. (1978). *The child's concept of story*. Chicago: University of Chicago Press.

Applebee, A. N. (1984). Writing and reasoning. *Review of educational research, 54*, 577–596.

Bereiter, C. (1980). Development in writing. In L. W. Gregg & E. R. Steinberg (Eds.), *Cognitive processes in writing*. Hillsdale, NJ: Erlbaum.

Bereiter, C., & Scardamalia, M. (1987). *The psychology of written composition*. Hillsdale, NJ: Erlbaum.

Blachman, B. (1983). Are we assessing the linguistic factors critical in early reading? *Annals of Dyslexia, 33*, 91–109.

Bloome, D., Harris, O. L., & Ludlum, D. E. (1991). Reading and writing as sociocultural activities: Politics and pedagogy in the classroom. *Topics in Language Disorders, 11*(3), 14–27.

Bradley, L., & Bryant, P. E. (1983). Categorizing sounds and learning to read—A causal connection. *Nature, 301*, 419–421.

Brady, S., Poggie, E., & Rapala, M. (1989). Speech repetition abilities in children who differ in reading skill. *Language and Speech, 32*, 109–122.

Britton, J., Burgess, T., Martin, N., McLeod, A., & Rosen, H. (1975). *The development of writing abilities* (pp. 11–18). London: Macmillan.

Calkins, L. M. (1994). *The art of teaching writing*. Portsmouth, NH: Heinemann.

Cambourne, B. (1988). *The whole story: Natural learning and the acquisition of literacy in the classroom*. Auckland, New Zealand: Scholastic.

Catts, H. (1986). Speech production/phonological deficits in reading disordered children. *Journal of Learning Disabilities, 19*, 504–508.

Chafe, W. (1985). Linguistic differences produced by differences between speaking and writing. In D. R. Olson, N. Torrance, & S. Hildyard (Eds.), *Literacy, language, and learning*. New York: Cambridge University Press.

Clark, D., & Uhry, J. (1995). *Dyslexia: Theory and practice of remedial instruction*. Baltimore: York Press.

Craik, F., & Lockhart, R. (1972). CHARM is not enough: Comments on Eich's model of cued recall. *Psychological Review, 93*, 360–364.

Critcheley, M. (1970). *The dyslexic child*. Springfield, IL: Thomas.

Cunningham, P. M., & Allington, R. L. (1994). *Classrooms that work: They can all read and write*. New York: Harper Collins.

Dobson, L. (1988). *Connections in learning to write and read: A study of children's development through kindergarten and grade one*. (Tech. Rep. No. 418). Champaign, IL: University of Illinois, Center for the Study of Reading.

Dyson, A. (1986). Children's early interpretations of writing: Expanding research perspectives. In D. Yaden & S. Templeton (Eds.), *Metalinguistic awareness and beginning literacy* (pp. 201–218). Portsmouth, NH: Heinemann.

Ehri, L. (1975). Word consciousness in readers and prereaders. *Journal of Educational Psychology, 67,* 204–212.

Ferreiro, E. (1984). The underlying logic of literacy development. In H. Goelman, A. Oberg, & F. Smith (Eds.), *Awakening to literacy*. Exeter, NH: Heinemann Educational Books.

Ferreiro, E., & Teberosky, A. (1982). *Literacy before schooling*. Exeter, NH: Heinemann Educational Books.

Fields, M. (1989). *Literacy begins at birth*. Tucson, AZ: Fisher Books.

Fish, S. (1980). *Is there a text in this class?* Cambridge, MA: Harvard University Press.

Fox, B., & Routh, D. K. (1980). Phonetic analysis and severe reading disability in children. *Journal of Psycholinguistic Research, 9,* 115–119.

Gee, J. (1988, June). *Perceptions on literacy: Cultural and social diversity*. Workshop presented at Emerson College Language Learning Disabilities Institute, Boston.

Gee, J. P. (1990). *Social linguistics and literacies: Ideology in discourses*. New York: Falmer Press.

Gee, J. (1994). First language acquisition as a guide for theories of learning and pedagogy. *Linguistics in Education, 6,* 331–354.

Gibson, E. J., & Levin, H. (1975). *The psychology of reading*. Cambridge, MA: MIT Press.

Goodman, K. (1986). *What's whole in whole language?* Portsmouth, NH: Heinemann.

Goodman, K. (1993). *Phonics phacts: A common-sense look at the most controversial issue affecting today's classrooms!* Portsmouth, NJ: Heinemann.

Goodman, Y. (1986). Children coming to know literacy. In W. Teale & E. Sulzby (Eds.), *Emergent literacy*. Norwood, NJ: Ablex.

Goodman, Y. M. (1992). The writing process: The making of meaning. In Y. M. Goodman & S. Wilde (Eds.), *Literacy events in a community of young writers* (pp. 1–16). New York: Teachers College Press.

Goodman, Y. M., & Burke, C. L. (1980). *Reading strategies: Focusing on comprehension*. New York: Holt, Rinehart & Winston.

Graves, D. H. (1983). *Writing: Teachers and children at work*. Portsmouth, NH: Heinemann.

Halliday, M. (1975). *Learning how to mean: Explorations in the development of language*. New York: Arnold.

Harste, J., Woodward, V., & Burke, C. (1984). *Language stories and literacy lessons*. Portsmouth, NH: Heinemann Educational Books.

Hayes, J. R., & Flower, L. S. (1980). Identifying the organization of writing processes. In L. Gregg & E. Steinberg (Eds.), *Cognitive processes in writing*. Hillsdale, NJ: Erlbaum.

Hayes, J. R., & Flower, L. S. (1987). On the structure of the writing process. *Topics in Language Disorders, 7*(4), 19–30.

Heath, S. (1983). *Ways with words: Language, life, and work in communities and classrooms*. New York: Cambridge University Press.

Henderson, E. H. (1981). *Learning to read and spell: The child's knowledge of words*. DeKalb: Northern Illinois University Press.

Himley, M. (1986). Genre as generative: One perspective on one child's early writing growth. In M. Nystrand (Ed.), *The structure of written communication* (pp. 137–158). New York: Academic Press.

Hoffman, L. P. (1990). The development of literacy in a school-based program. *Topics in Language Disorders, 10*(2), 81–92.

Iser, W. (1978). *The act of reading: A theory of aesthetic response*. Baltimore: Johns Hopkins University Press.

Jordan, D. (1996). *Overcoming dyslexia in children, adolescents, and adults* (2nd ed.). Austin, TX: PRO-ED.

Kamhi, A. G. (1997). Three perspectives on comprehension: Implications for assessing and treating comprehension problems. *Topics in Language Disorders, 17*(3), 62–74.

Kamhi, A. G., & Catts, H. W. (Eds.). (1989). *Reading disabilities: A developmental language perspective*. Boston: College Hill/Little, Brown.

Kamhi, A. G., & Catts, H. W. (1991). *Reading disabilities: A developmental language perspective*. Needham Heights, MA: Allyn & Bacon.

Karmiloff-Smith, A. (1986). Some fundamental aspects of language development after age 5. In P. Fletcher & M. Garman (Eds.), *Language acquisition: Studies in first language development* (pp. 455–474). Cambridge, England: Cambridge University Press.

Katzer, S., & Crnkovich, C. (1991). *From scribblers to scribes: Young writers' use of the computer*. Englewood, CO: Teacher's Idea Press.

Kuykendall, M. (1997). *A collaborative classroom ethnography of a fourth–fifth grade community of writers, including students with and without the label of learning disabilities*. Unpublished dissertation, University of Northen Colorado, Greeley.

Langer, J. A. (1987). A sociocognitive perspective on literacy. In J. A. Langer (Ed.), *Language, literacy, and culture: Issues of society and schooling*. Norwood, NJ: Ablex.

Larson, V. L., & McKinley, M. S. (1995). *Language disorders in older students: Preadolescents and adolescents*. Eau Claire, WI: Thinking Publications.

Liberman, I., & Shankweiler, D. (1991). Phonology and beginning reading: A tutorial. In L. Reiben & C. Perfetti (Eds.), *Learning to read: Basic research and its implications* (pp. 3–18). Hillsdale, NJ: Erlbaum.

Liberman, I., Shankweiler, D., Fisher, F., & Carter, B. (1974). Explicit syllable and phoneme segmentation in the young child. *Journal of Experimental Child Psychology, 18*, 201–212.

Martlew, M. (1986). The development of written language. In K. Durkin (Ed.), *Language development in the school years*. Cambridge, MA: Brookline Books.

Maxwell, R. J., & Meisser, M. J. (1997). *Teaching English in middle and secondary schools* (pp. 117–138). Upper Saddle River, NJ: Prentice-Hall.

Miller, L. (1990). The roles of language and learning in the development of literacy. *Topics in Language Disorders, 10*(2), 1–24.

Nelson, N. (1993). *Childhood language disorders in context: Infancy through adolescence*. New York: Merrill.

Pellegrini, A., Galda, L., & Rubin, D. (1984). Context in text: The development of oral and written language in two genres. *Child Development, 55*, 1549–1555.

Perera, K. (1984). *Children's writing and reading: Analysing classroom language*. Oxford: Blackwell.

Perfetti, C., Goldman, S., & Hogaboam, T. (1979). Reading skills and the identification of words in discourse context. *Memory & Cognition, 7*, 273–282.

Piaget, J. (1971). *Psychology and epistemology*. New York: Grossman.

Reid, D. K., & Kuykendall, M. (1996). Literacy: A tale of different belief systems. In D. K. Reid, W. P. Hresko, & H. L. Swanson (Eds.), *Cognitive approaches to learning disabilities* (3rd ed., pp. 497–544). Austin, TX: PRO-ED.

Rhodes, L. K., & Dudley-Marling, C. D. (1996). *Readers and writers with a difference: A wholistic approach to teaching struggling readers and writers* (2nd ed.). Portsmouth, NJ: Heinemann.

Routman, R. (1991). *Invitations: Changing as teachers and learners K–12*. Portsmouth, NH: Heinemann.

Scott, C. M. (1991). Learning to write: Context, form, and process. In A. G. Kamhi & H. W. Catts (Eds.), *Reading disabilities: A developmental language perspective* (pp. 261–302). Boston, MA: Allyn & Bacon.

Shanklin, N. L. (1991). Whole language and writing process: One movement or two? *Topics in Language Disorders, 11*(3), 45–57.

Siu-Runyan, Y. (1992). An ingenious approach to emergent literacy. *The Colorado Communicator, 15*(3), 4–7.

Slater, W. H., & Graves, M. F. (1989). Research on expository text: Implications for teachers. In K. D. Muth (Ed.), *Children's comprehension of text* (pp. 140–166).

Snow, C. (1983). Literacy and language: Relationships during the preschool years. *Harvard Educational Review, 53*(2), 165–189.

Snowling, M. J., & Hulme, C. (1989). A longitudinal case study of developmental phonological dyslexia. *Cognitive Neuropsychology, 6*, 379–401.

Spafford, C., & Grosser, G. (1996). *Dyslexia: Research and resource guide*. Needham Heights, MA: Allyn & Bacon.

Stanovich, K. (1982). Individual differences in the cognitive processes of reading: II. Text-level processes. *Journal of Learning Disabilities, 15*, 549–554.

Stanovich, K. (1986). Matthew effect in reading: Some consequences of individual differences in the acquisition of literacy. *Reading Research Quarterly, 21*, 360–407.

Stanovich, K. (1988). The right and wrong places to look for the cognitive locus of reading disability. *Annals of Dyslexia, 38*, 154–177.

Stanovich, K. E., & Siegal, L. S. (1994). Phonotype performance profile of children with reading disabilities: A regression-based test of the phonological-core variable-difference model. *Journal of Education Psychology, 86*(6), 350–357.

Stark, J., & Wallach, G. P. (1982). The path to a concept of language learning disabilities. In G. P. Wallach & K. G. Butler (Eds.), *Language disorders and learning disabilities*. Rockville, MD: Aspen.

Sulzby, E. (1986). Writing and reading: Signs of oral and written language organization in the young child. In W. Teale & E. Sulzby (Eds.), *Emergent literacy: Writing and reading* (pp. 50–89). Norwood, NJ: Ablex.

Sulzby, E., & Teale, W. H. (1984). *Young children's storybook reading: Hispanic and Anglo families and children* (Interim report to the Spencer Foundation). Evanston, IL: Northwestern University.

Tallal, P., & Stark, R. (1982). Perceptual/motor profiles of reading impaired children with or without concomitant oral language deficits. *Annals of Dyslexia, 32*, 163–176.

Taylor, D., & Walls, L. (1990). Educating parents about their children's early literacy development. *The Reading Teacher, 44*(1), 72–74.

Temple, C. A., Nathan, R. G., Temple, F., & Burris, N. A. (1993). *The beginnings of writing*. Needham Heights, MA: Allyn & Bacon.

Tunmer, W. E., & Cole, P. G. (1991). Learning to read: A metalinguistic act. In C. S. Simon (Ed.), *Communication skills and classroom success* (pp. 386–402). Eau Claire, WI: Thinking Publications.

Tunmer, W., Herriman, C., & Nesdale, A. (1988). Metalinguistic abilities and reading. *Reading Research Quarterly, 23*, 135–158.

van Kleeck, A. (1990). Emergent literacy: Learning about print before learning to read. *Topics in Language Disorders, 10*(2), 25–45.

van Kleeck, A., & Schuele, C. (1987). Precursors to literacy: Normal development. *Topics in Language Disorders, 7*, 13–31.

Vellutino, F. (1979). *Dyslexia: Theory and research*. Cambridge, MA: MIT Press.

Vellutino, F. R., & Scanlon, D. M. (1985). Verbal memory in poor and normal readers: Developmental differences in the use of linguistic codes. In J. Kavanagh & D. Gray (Eds.), *Biobehavioral measures of dyslexia* (pp. 177–214). Parkton, MD: York Press.

Vygotsky, L. S. (1978). *Mind in society: The development of higher psychological processes*. Cambridge: MA: Harvard University Press.

Wagner, R. K., Torgeson, J. K., & Rashotte, C. A. (1994). Development of reading-related phonological processing abilities: New evidence of bi-directional causality from a latent variable longitudinal study. *Developmental Psychology, 30*, 73–87.

Wallach, G. P., & Butler, K. G. (1994). Creating communication, literacy, and academic success. In G. P. Wallach & K. G. Butler (Eds.), *Language learning disabilities in school-age children and adolescents: Some principles and applications*. Needham Heights, MA: Allyn & Bacon.

Wallach, G. P., & Miller, L. (1988). *Language intervention and academic success*. Boston: College Hill/Little, Brown.

Weaver, C. (1994). *Reading process and practice: From socio-psycholinguistics to whole language* (2nd ed.). Portsmouth, NH: Heinemann.

Wells, G. (1985). Preschool literacy-related activities and success in school. In D. Olson, N. Torrance, & A. Hildyard (Eds.), *Literacy, language, and learning: The nature and consequences of reading and writing* (pp. 229–255). New York: Cambridge University Press.

Westby, C. (1988, October). *Oral language and reading connections*. Paper presented at American Speech-Language-Hearing Association Weekend Workshop, Denver, CO.

Westby, C. (1991). Learning to talk—Talking to learn: Oral-literate language differences. In C. S. Simon (Ed.), *Communication skills and classroom success: Assessment and therapy methodologies for language and learning disabled students* (pp. 334–357). Eau Clare, WI: Thinking Publications.

Williams, J. P. (1988). Identifying main ideas: A basic aspect of reading comprehension. *Topics in Language Disorders*, 8(3), 1–13.

Zemelman, S., & Daniels, H. (1988). *A community of writers: Teaching writing in the junior and senior high school*. Portsmouth, NH: Heinemann.

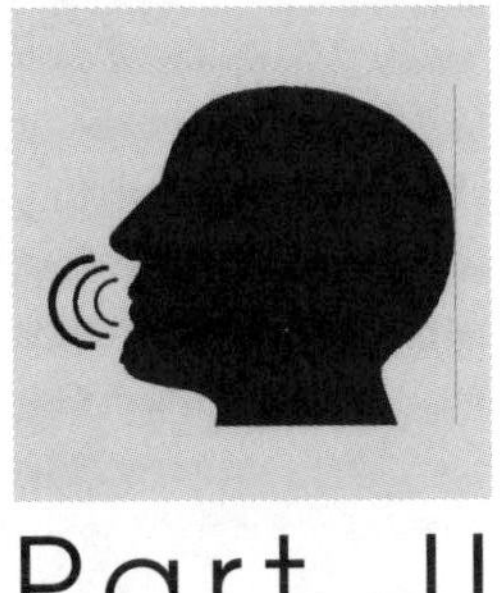

Part II

Language Differences

Language Acquisition and Usage: Multicultural and Multilinguistic Perspectives

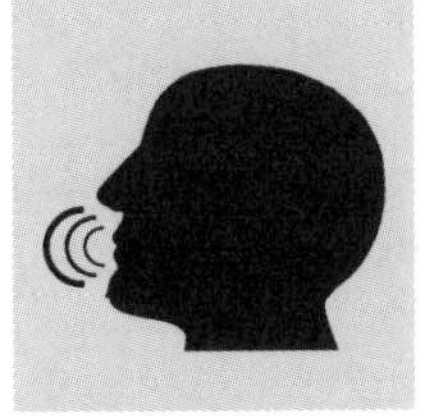

Chapter 5

J. M. Lagrander and D. Kim Reid

The traditional school curriculum reflects the European American, middle and upper middle class (i.e., the mainstream) culture and norms that have been derived from our nation's European heritage. This traditional *Eurocentric curriculum* is based on the 18th- and 19th-century European standards and values that have shaped our canon (i.e., the criteria by which we judge beauty, excellence, etc.) and privileged European American males. As a result and as noted in earlier chapters, the educational system welcomes the typical learning and behavior of middle class students who speak Standard American English (SAE), while frequently alienating those students from other social and linguistic cultures and subcultures (Cheng, 1996; Hillis, 1996). In short, in the typical classroom, educators portray—and in the process teach, privilege, and maintain—a limited view of the world. Students who are nonwhite, members of a lower socioeconomic class, or even female may thus be marginalized. Race and class segregation and the gender inequalities of the larger society, therefore, confound instruction in schools.

Teaching for Diversity

U.S. society is becoming increasingly diverse and students who attend U.S. schools represent this diversity. In 1990 the Bureau of the Census reported that one third of all school children were members of a nonmainstream group. It is projected that by the year 2000, more than 40% of school-age children will be

J. M. Lagrander is an educational specialist and part-time teacher for homebound students in the Boulder Valley Public Schools. She is also a doctoral student in the Division of Special Education at the University of Northern Colorado, Greeley.

nonmainstream group members. Currently, in 33 of the largest school districts in the nation, students from nonmainstream families already represent a majority (Lara, 1994). Further, the census data show that almost half the Hispanic and Asian American respondents indicated that English was not the primary language used in the home. To better serve these students, educationists must learn to value diversity (and bilingualism) and work to integrate all students into the educational community.

Language both shapes and mirrors the values and beliefs of a culture. Therefore, the language that a student brings to school is intrinsically connected with family, community, and individual identity (Gee, 1990). One's culture provides the foundation that determines the way an individual experiences and participates in society. Culture defines for each group a lifestyle and language that are its own. Too often, however, because of the hegemony (i.e., dominance not by laws, but by common acceptance) of the Eurocentric curriculum, schools fail to reflect and accept the diversity and multiple world views that are actually represented within classrooms and, as a result, fail to validate and appreciate the richness of our nation's myriad cultural traditions.

No culture is inherently better than another. Still, we tend to view different cultures through the lens of the dominant one, which we presume to be best. As a consequence, educators often assume students who are culturally or linguistically different from the mainstream culture will exhibit deficient academic achievement related to both language and behavior. Delpit (1995) addressed this assumption:

> When a significant difference exists between the students' culture and the school's culture, teachers [and speech–language pathologists (SLPs)] can easily misread students' aptitudes, intent, or abilities as a result of the difference in styles of language use and interactional patterns. . . . when such cultural differences exist, teachers [and SLPs] may utilize styles of instruction and/or discipline that are at odds with community norms. (p. 167)

Many of the difficulties that minority-language students experience in mainstream classrooms can be attributed to the devaluing of their culture by their teachers and other educationists (Darder, 1991; Macedo, 1994). Forced to choose between family and school, between the familiar and the unknown, too often language minority students or those from poor families, families of color or of nonmainstream ethnicities, perceive themselves as outsiders and are at risk of feeling as if they do not belong anywhere. Honoring cultural and linguistic differences goes a long way toward stemming students' feelings of alienation. Consequently, *effective* teachers and SLPs communicate a clear assumption that the language and culture each nonmainstream learner brings into the classroom is both appropriate and deserving of respect.

Whether students enter formal schooling able to speak, read, or write in English or in another language, they do not begin as blank slates. Children learn to communicate in a manner determined by the accepted norms within the communities in which they are raised. Building on the linguistic foundation that students bring with them to school is certainly more efficacious than starting from scratch. Despite the political debates around bilingual education, there is a body of research that indicates that students learning a second language achieve optimally when literacy instruction proceeds from their primary language (e.g., Bialystok, 1991; Collier, 1989, 1995; Cummins, 1979, 1981, 1991; Fishman, 1987; E. Garcia, 1994; Genesee, 1987, 1994; Hakuta, 1986; Krashen & Biber, 1988; McCollum & Walker, 1990; Reyes, 1987; Skutnabb-Kangas, 1981). In addition, Cummins (1979, 1981) proposed that learning that occurs in a student's native language more easily transfers to a second language, because knowledge is already grounded in the language and schema in which it was originally comprehended. Second language learning is thus greatly facilitated when a native language foundation is well developed.

However, advocacy for native-language instruction does not presuppose that students should not learn to communicate effectively in SAE. English is, after all, the primary language spoken in the majority of our classrooms, as well as the principal discourse in this country. At this point in our history, learning to speak, read, and write in the dominant language is necessary if these students are to succeed in the adult world. The goal, however, should be to *teach* students to become competent in mainstream society *without* making them feel inadequate and taking away their cultural roots.

Language and Dialectal Variations Associated with Race

Dialects are variations in the standard language rule system of a particular linguistic group. People from a specific geographic region of a country, for example, will speak in a different dialect from those of other regions. These *dialectal differences* are often related to racial, ethnic, socioeconomic, situational or contextual, peer-group influenced, and first- or second-language learning factors (Owens, 1992). Sometimes, as is the case with Ebonics (also sometimes called Black English or Black Vernacular English), what many in the popular culture view as a dialect is considered by linguists to be a separate language

(American Society of Linguists, cited in "Linguists Find the Debate over 'Ebonics' Uninformed," 1997), and the arguments about the appropriateness of its initial use and acceptance in schools, then, become political rather than linguistic.

Most dialects spoken in this country are variants of SAE (i.e., they share a common set of grammatical rules with SAE), the form of English used in textbooks and formal communication. English speakers, however, rarely use SAE in informal conversation (Edwards, 1991). Owens (1992) pointed out that at least 10 regional dialects have been identified in the United States. The primary racial and ethnic languages and dialects found in this country are what are known as Ebonics and Hispanic English (see Chapter 6 for their characteristics). Geographic and socioeconomic factors have influenced and continue to influence both. Other ethnic dialects include Hawaiian Creole or Islands English, Appalachian English, and those of the various Native American and Asian communities.

Although some languages or dialects generally have higher status among some listeners (again for political reasons), all languages and dialects are actually valid rule systems within a particular social context and merely reflect differences (Owens, 1992), not disorders or lower level forms of language.

> Any deficit view of linguistic behavior is incorrect—no language, or language variety, has been shown to be more accurate, logical or capable of expression than another. Rather, it should be realized that different language communities develop speech patterns that differ in their modes of expression, vocabulary and pronunciation. There is also the possibility that different groups assign different functions to language. (Edwards, 1991, p. 73)

To consider a language or dialect inferior to another is to view the speakers and their culture also as inferior. As Delpit (1995) asserted, "Children have a right to their own language, their own culture" (p. 37). Teachers and SLPs, therefore, need to invite all students' voices into the learning discourse.

African American Voices

Ebonics is the linguistic system used by most working-class African Americans, primarily in urban centers and the rural south (Owens, 1992). Although much of the American populace thinks of Black Vernacular English or Black English (i.e., Ebonics) as just plain bad English (probably because it evolved from the languages of slaves), linguists defend it as a legitimate communication method

(Gollnick & Chinn, 1994) and argue that Ebonics fulfills the criteria for embodying an intact rule system. It is, therefore, not an aberrant form of English (Dillard, 1973; Fairchild & Edwards-Evans, 1990; Labov, 1973; Owens, 1992). Ebonics is its own language.

A 1997 article in *Newsweek* affirmed that a small body of research indicates that African American students learn to use SAE optimally when it is compared explicitly to their native language, Ebonics. African American students taught using a technique called "contrastive analysis," in which texts contrasted Ebonics with SAE, transposed fewer Ebonics constructions into their SAE writing, as compared to those who learned SAE in isolation (Leland & Joseph, 1997). Allowing students to translate their primary language into SAE rather than punctuating language instruction with continual correction is also affirming of the linguistic diversity of African American speakers and writers. Delpit's (1995) research illustrates that constant correction of a student's language- or dialect-influenced pronunciation and grammar during reading instruction inhibits fluency and comprehension, and in some cases engenders resentment toward both the task and the teacher (or other educationist).

Educators and SLPs need to realize that what might look like a language deficit in nonmainstream students when seen through the lens of middle class—that is, SAE—expectations, is often merely a language or dialectal difference. We must also realize that differences do not end with language usage per se: Cultural styles also vary and they carry over into interactions with teachers and SLPs. Studies have shown, for example, that African Americans benefit from more direct and explicit instruction in oral and written language than many European American students (Delpit, 1988; Macías, 1989; Reyes, 1991; Siddle, 1986). Further, Heath (1982) found that questions to elicit information for exhibition (i.e., questions for which the questioner already knows the answer) were not generally used in the homes of African Americans, although they are used extensively in early schooling. Thus, for example, when an African American student replies to a question with "I don't know," the student may be indicating discomfort or lack of familiarity with the question type, dislike for working in isolation, or a need for further instruction (G. Garcia, 1992). Those who engage such students in instructional activities need to be aware that there are several alternative interpretations of the students' behavior and to distinguish among them.

Storytelling and writing also differ in African American culture. As noted in Chapter 1, Michaels (1981) found that, contrary to the expected, SAE mode of following a theme centering on a single topic, African American students tended to tell stories about associated topics with no overall theme—a preference also shared by African American adults. Because they differ so radically from Eurocentric, SAE classroom norms, teachers and SLPs may have difficulty validating both Ebonics usage and African American forms of storytelling and writing; many simply consider them to be inadequate. Educators and SLPs need to recognize, however, that difference does not necessarily translate into deficiency and disadvantage. With immersion into mainstream language or culture and metacognitively based instruction that explicitly compares the language children bring to school with that expected in the classroom (i.e., SAE), students can be both appreciated for who they are and helped to cross the linguistic boundaries that will enable them to be successful in school and, later, in society (Gee, 1990).

Hispanic American Voices

Both *Latino* and *Hispanic American* are umbrella terms under which we cluster several subgroups of Americans of Spanish origin. Although these terms are convenient, they should not obscure the fact that these groups differ in racial or ethnic ancestry and cultures. The largest of these subgroups consist of Mexican Americans, Puerto Ricans, Cuban Americans, and people from Central or South America. A variety of Spanish dialects are spoken by Latinos, who together are the largest ethnic population in the United States, which is the fifth largest Spanish-speaking country in the world (Kayser, 1993). Spanish often affects students' understanding and production of English and interacts with the English dialect spoken in the surrounding community. Additionally, Latino speakers often use vocabulary words that are of Spanish origin (Owens, 1992).

Students who speak both Spanish and English are bilingual. Most bilingual students develop a primary language in the home and a second language in school or other community setting. Until the age of 3, second-language learning mirrors the sequence of development of initial language acquisition (Owens, 1992). However, students who learn a second language later and, therefore, already possess a rule-governed linguistic system are better able to understand and learn a second language when literacy instruction proceeds from their primary language. Rather than attempting to change minority-language students to conform to extant classroom expectations, instruction should thus be based on the language abilities that students already possess. In this way, educators and SLPs honor the student's voice and employ best practices, as indicated by the already listed research findings. As Bruner (1983) noted, "Learning is most often figuring out how to use what you already know in order to go beyond what you currently think" (p. 183).

Bilingual education consists of the pairing of two languages as a strategy for instruction. The objective is not merely to teach English as a second language, but also to instruct children in the language with which they are already familiar and reinforce this knowledge through the use of English (Baca & Cervantes, 1989). Bilingual education, then, is different from learning a second language through standard English as a Second Language (ESL) approaches in which all instruction is given in English. Collier (1995) found that students who are taught English primarily through ESL methods take 7 to 10 years or more to reach age- and grade-level norms of native English-speaking students. Students who have had the benefit of 2 to 3 years of first-language learning in their home country before emigrating to the United States, however, typically take only 5 to 7 years to reach native English-speaking proficiency when taught by the same ESL techniques (Collier, 1989; Cummins, 1981). Therefore, the *most significant predictor* of achievement in second-language learning is the amount of prior formal schooling students receive in their primary language. Bilingual education, which encourages second-language learning by means of the knowledge and abilities a student already possesses, is, therefore, the most effective practice to pursue with language-minority students. "Bilingual education still represents the best and most effective program for most students for whom English is a second language" (Nieto, 1992, p. 166). The controversy that surrounds bilingual education is, then, a political, not linguistic or educational, one.

According to Nieto (1992), there are several interpretations of bilingual education. The most common approach found in the United States is probably the *transitional bilingual model*, in which students receive content-area instruction in their native language, while learning English as a second language. This approach is a means of transitioning from the language most commonly used in the home to the mainstream language of schooling. Thus, there is usually a limit of 3 years before students are required to exit this program.

The *maintenance or developmental model*, on the other hand, has no set limit on the time students can be in the program. The rationale is that children will be more successful when literacy in a native language is utilized as a foundation for continued learning and, hence, students also become functionally bilingual (i.e., they continue to acquire competence in their native tongue as well as master English).

The *two-way bilingual model* integrates students whose native language is English with those for whom English is a second language. The goal for both groups is to develop bilingualism through learning content in their native language while being introduced to a new language.

Finally, in the *immersion bilingual model*, students are immersed in learning a second language for 1 to 2 years before their native language is introduced as the mode of instruction. By the fifth or sixth year of schooling, an equivalent amount of instruction in both languages or most instruction in the secondary language may be occurring.

In addition to being effective in teaching students content-area knowledge in their native language and English as a secondary language, bilingual education motivates students to stay in school rather than drop out (Paulston, 1980). Bilingual education, with its emphasis on acknowledging native language and culture, provides a more meaningful and enjoyable school experience for the Hispanic American student than traditional ESL practices, which are not designed to value and build on the student's prior linguistic knowledge and experience.

In a survey of the kinds of services for students with limited English proficiency that SLPs were delivering in schools, Roseberry-McKibbin and Eicholtz (1994) found that the majority of the clients were Hispanic Americans, 90% of whom did not speak a second language (i.e., English) fluently enough to receive services in that language, which may account at least in part for the poor showing of ESL instruction. Of the SLPs responding to the survey, 76% had not had prior coursework or classes teaching them how to address services for language-diverse students. Consequently, the "experts" often need to learn as they go. The problems that SLPs encounter most frequently relate to a lack of appropriate assessment practices and instruments and their inability to speak the languages of the students they serve. The American Speech-Language-Hearing Association (ASHA) has tried to respond to this situation with two initiatives: Multicultural Agenda 2000 and the establishment of an Office of Multicultural Affairs (Quinn et al., 1996).

With Latino as well as African American students, however, it is not only language usage per se that varies. Different cultural communities interact with and socialize their children to use language in many ways that vary from European American, middle class norms (Boggs, 1985; Damico & Damico, 1993; Heath, 1983; Philips, 1983; Schieffelin, 1979). The dominant culture in the United States values individuality and extroversion. Hispanic culture, on the other hand, places a higher value on community and introversion (Poplin, 1992). Further, Delgado-Gaitan (1987) found that Mexican immigrant children were more familiar with cooperating and negotiating with others in their environment than in competing, although competition is valued by the Eurocentric educational system that is based on rank-ordering through testing and grading.

Further, Hispanic American students often enter school without print experiences comparable to those of their middle class peers (Ruiz, 1989). Again, cultural differences play an important role. For example, Latino parents may not consider knowledge of letters, numbers, and colors as relevant for their children to learn as respect for and courtesy toward others (Slobin, 1983). Latino parents also do not generally see themselves as teachers. They demonstrate predominantly nonverbal interactions with infants (Garcia Coll, 1990) and emphasize observation and independence in the learning process (Valdes, 1986). Additionally, Latinos are taught to hold authority figures in high regard, thus according status to teachers and other educationists that promotes relying on them for more direct intervention than might normally be offered in classrooms catering to European American, middle and upper middle class students (Delgado-Gaitan, 1987; Macías, 1989). The cultural expectations of the public school system and the diametrically opposed guiding principles of the home lead to conflicts in values for large numbers of Latino students.

These conflicts pervade the curriculum. Poplin (1992) pointed out, for example, that Spanish writers tend to embellish their compositions with adjectives, which is typical of that culture's preferred speaking style. Teachers and SLPs may be critical of this writing style, viewing it as too flowery and rambling. Educationists always need to keep in mind that when students' values go unacknowledged, unappreciated, or even criticized, schools will fail to engage these students meaningfully in the learning process.

Asian American Voices

People from myriad Asian cultures live in this country. Although each culture is distinctive, they possess some commonalities. As with Hispanic cultures, however, one should use caution in generalizing about Asian cultures as a group, because generalizing can lead to stereotyping and erroneous conclusions. Asian American students are usually regarded as good students, because they are generally quiet and well mannered in the classroom and have attained the highest educational level of any immigrant group (Lott & Felt, 1991). However, as Delpit (1995) pointed out, this stereotype can easily lead teachers to overlook their academic needs:

> There is a widespread belief that Asian-American children are the "perfect" students, and that they will do well regardless of the academic setting in which they are placed. This stereotype has led to a negative backlash in which the academic needs of the majority of Asian-American students are overlooked. (p. 170)

Asians are generally viewed as formal by Western standards and this formality is reflected in their languages (Kepler, Royse, & Kepler, 1996). The Asian writing style reflects circularity and indirectness, traits also found in Asian oral language, and this indirectness is often misinterpreted as their lacking the ability to express themselves (Poplin, 1989). Teachers may also interpret Asian students' perceived passive participation style in the classroom as indicative of intellectual dullness (Miyanaga, 1991). However, this propensity for quiet attention has been shaped by an Asian educational system that discourages the asking of questions by students who may well consider themselves to be active rather than passive learners (Takada & Hanahan, 1995). Further, because the sound of Asian languages is more modulated, enthusiasm and excitement expressed by English speakers can be misinterpreted by Asians as anger (Kepler et al., 1996).

Both Japanese and Chinese cultures value group-oriented norms (Masahiko, 1994). A sense of community, collaboration, and interaction with others is esteemed (Delpit, 1995) over the individualism that prevails in the Eurocentric curriculum. Such differences in values between cultures may cause academic difficulty for Asian students.

A major difference between Japanese and English languages is syntax. English depends on word order for structure, whereas word order in Japanese is more flexible, with the exception that the verb always falls in the final position (Takada & Hanahan, 1995). Additionally, in conversations between Japanese individuals, the status of the speakers influences word choice (Kepler et al., 1996). Hence, Japanese students learning English as a second language have to contend with more rigid structural variations in ordering words and the status of the person who is being addressed. Sometimes these simultaneous concerns lead to confusion and miscommunication. Another potential communication difficulty for students of Japanese culture is the differing norms regarding eye contact. In Western cultures, for example, eye contact is expected between students and their teachers, but it is considered a sign of disrespect in Japanese society.

The communicative style of Japanese speakers is considered to be "intuitive" and "indirect" when compared to the style of the dominant culture in this country (Clancy, 1986, p. 213). For example, a direct "no" in answer to a question is generally avoided (so as to avoid conflict); as a result, "yes" answers can also be vague. Also, a pause in conversation is an integral part of Japanese discourse; it serves the function of allowing time for reflection (Kepler et al., 1996). Particularly in the IRE (Initiate–Respond–Evaluate) model of instruction, however, where rapid responses are required, reflective Japanese students may be at a disadvantage. Teachers need to adapt classroom participatory frameworks to accommodate these students. In conversation, educationists and peers need to learn to wait this silence out before responding, rather than assume that the conversation has ended.

The Chinese language consists of a uniform written system, with several dialects and subdialects. Although similar words are graphically represented by the same character, speakers of differing Chinese dialects are usually unable to understand each other (Cheng, 1995). Chinese is a tonal language, in which variations in pitch signal differences in meaning, but the pitch remains unchanged at the end of sentences. In English raising or lowering pitch at the end of a sentence can change it from a declaration to a question. Obviously, this can cause misunderstanding across cultural lines (Kepler et al., 1996).

As in Japanese culture, Chinese students are discouraged from interrupting the teacher to ask questions. However, there are distinct differences between expectations found in Chinese and Japanese educational systems. The former are "more performance oriented," whereas the latter are "more reflective" (Stigler & Perry, 1988, p. 40). Thus, educators and SLPs should take note of these differences and adjust instructional methods accordingly.

Other Asian cultures, such as Vietnamese and Hmong, also have similar characteristics as well as distinct differences. Like Japanese, Korean culture is also concerned with status. In this case, age establishes rank, so it is not unusual for a Korean student to ask an adult, "How old are you?" which would seem to be an impertinent question by United States standards (Kepler et al., 1996). Teachers should not mistake this as a penchant for rudeness, but rather consider it as clarification of the standing of those engaged in conversation.

The overall message for educators is to use caution when making assumptions based on mainstream norms and values regarding ethnically and linguistically diverse students. Behavior that may seem to conflict with traditional school standards may very well be typical and acceptable in specific cultures. If schools are to engage all students fully in the educational process, intrinsic cultural variations must be acknowledged and accepted, at least initially.

Native American Voices

Currently, in the United States, there are about 2 million North Americans of indigenous ancestry; of this number, approximately one third live on reservations (Hess, Markson, & Stein, 1995). A similar situation exists in Canada. Although knowledge and tradition vary among Native American nations, most share a common world view and collective experience. However, as with African American, Latino, and Asian cultures, commonalities should not be used to portray Native Americans as a nondiverse population.

The indigenous people of North America spoke between 250 and 300 different languages when the Europeans first arrived (Crawford, 1995). Because of past assimilationist policies, approximately 30% of tribal proficiency in ancestral language has either disappeared altogether or is retained currently only among the oldest generation (Leap, 1995). Early on, missionary schools, not generally affirmative of native cultural values, were located on or near reservations to educate Native American youth. As we are finding today with speakers of other languages or dialects, the missionaries reported that their attempts to promote literacy among Native Americans were more successful when they used their native languages as the basis for teaching them (Reyhmer, 1992).

The federal government decided that in order to hasten assimilation of Native Americans into the dominant culture, native youth needed to be removed physically from indigenous cultural influences by being sent to boarding schools where they were expected to speak English and emulate white, European culture. Promoting assimilation into the mainstream society (rather than education per se) was the goal of these boarding schools (Hess et al., 1995). Government officials presumed that stripping native languages from Native Americans would hasten their assimilation. A statement by the Commissioner of Indian Affairs in 1887 reflects this premise: "If we expect to infuse into the rising generation the leaven of American citizenship, we must remove the stumbling blocks of hereditary customs and manners, and of these language is one of the most important elements" (cited in D. Adams, 1988, p. 8). Ironically, the majority of Native Americans were not even granted citizenship until 1924. Nevertheless, between 1889 and 1930, most Native American youth learned to speak English through the boarding school experience (Ovando & Gourd, 1996).

In the 1950s the focus shifted from boarding schools to local, state-administered public schools, but the goal of assimilation remained essentially the same (Saravia-Shore & Arvizu, 1992). Once children began attending schools that employed English as the language of instruction, native languages eroded more rapidly and literacy achievement levels in English also dropped. The Cherokees, for example, had a literacy rate of 90% in their native language (McDonald, 1989) and high levels of English literacy (Medicine, 1979) during the 1850s. After the takeover of schools by the federal government, however, literacy levels in both Cherokee and English dropped dramatically (Medicine, 1979). This loss of literacy, particularly the loss of the native language—the primary means for oral communication—has had profound effects on Native American communities, where there are high rates of poverty, unemployment, alcoholism, and substance abuse. Retention of language is imperative for cultural survival—when the connection between language and community is broken, a culture is lost.

A 1988 Bureau of Indian Affairs (BIA) status report found that 90% of all Native Americans attended public schools; the remainder were enrolled in BIA and private schools. Most schools have been unresponsive to tribal concerns and needs regarding education. The dropout rate for Native American students was 45% in 1980, and family illiteracy continues to hinder youth from mastering basic educational skills (Saravia-Shore & Arvizu, 1992). Further, school dropout rates among Native Americans tend to be higher in urban schools than in schools located on reservations (National Coalition of Advocates for Students, 1985).

Although there is no substantial support for the recognition of a single Native American–English dialect, there is evidence that the dialects of English spoken by Native Americans differ enough from the SAE used in schools to cause learning difficulties for the speakers (Jasper, 1980; Kwachta, 1981; Leap, 1977). Native American students have been found to have an incidence of communicative disorders 5 to 15 times higher than those in the general population when assessment is based on SAE speech and language tests (McCardle & Walton, 1995). However, this high percentage does not necessarily represent an accurate measure of communication disability among students in this population, but rather probably to a very large extent reflects language differences.[1] In observing Native American speakers, Leap (1995) found that "sentence word order and pronunciation patterns often reflect constraints which parallel features from the speaker's tribal (or ancestral) language" (p. 1).

Additionally, Native American narrative structure is far removed from the typical story grammar structure taught and expected in the Eurocentric classroom (Highwater, 1981). For example, Worth and Adair (1972) observed that Navajos devoted more attention to details about the background and setting than to the plot of the story. According to Highwater, Native Americans do not generally view events, which are the basis of most SAE stories, as involving succession and causality. To mainstream educators, these narratives may not appear to be adequate in terms of content, because structure and organization follow a more oral tradition in which ideas differ markedly from narratives based on the Western world view.

Tharp (1989) observed that Native American students usually take longer to respond in the traditional classroom, because most indigenous cultures tend to value deliberate thought. Once again, we see that IRE models of instruction (see Chapter 1) put these students at a disadvantage. Further, Philips (1972, 1983) found that Native American students did not willingly respond when solicited by teachers to answer questions in front of a group. Participation increased, however, when students were given the opportunity to interact on a one-to-one basis with the teacher or in self-directed small groups—that is, participation styles that parallel interactions on the reservation.

Native American students tend to learn best in a holistic manner, rather than in the analytical mode fostered in the majority of Eurocentric classrooms

---

[1]Because of limited health care, Native Americans have a high incidence of chronic otitis media. This condition also is likely to contribute to language difficulties. It alone, however, cannot explain the very high overestimation of language disorders among this population (Harris, 1993).

(Ovando & Gourd, 1996). In addition, like African and Mexican Americans, Native American students tend to learn best in highly social settings (Ramirez & Castañeda, 1974). Cooperative learning environments capitalize on these preferred learning styles and are compatible with many of the values of Native Americans, including cooperation, a sense of community, and sharing (Nieto, 1992).

Revitalization of Native American languages and cultures has increased in the past few years. The Native American Languages Act (Public Law 101-524), enacted in 1992, provides for the preservation of indigenous languages. Despite past efforts to extinguish native languages, ancestral languages continue to be the primary language used in the home and community in many Native American tribes until students begin to attend Head Start programs or other schools where English is introduced. As for Hispanic Americans, bilingual education programs are effective purveyors of literacy for Native Americans (Rosier & Holm, 1980; Tharp, Dalton, & Yamauchi, 1994). Demonstration schools have been established on reservations to promote bilingualism and biculturalism, as well as knowledge and abilities valued by Native American communities. As a result, English literacy competency and reading scores have improved for students attending such schools, concurrent with increased native language proficiency (Dick & McCarty, 1994). This success once again demonstrates the validity of the premise that academic learning and English proficiency are enhanced through the use of native language as a foundation on which to build literacy instruction.

Another educational practice that benefits Native American learners is a culturally relevant curriculum that encourages students to speak, read, and write about their own cultural experiences. An example of a culturally relevant activity is employing indigenous creation myths and poetry as a means of improving reading skills and increasing literature appreciation (Saravia-Shore & Arvizu, 1992). Above all else, educators must be sensitive to inaccurate and biased historical textbook accounts of Native Americans (often portrayed as savages attacking the homesteads of European American settlers), which hinder educational progress by causing Native American students to become further disengaged from the Eurocentric.

Summary

The cultural knowledge and values that African American, Hispanic American, Asian American, and Native American students bring to mainstream educational programs often conflict with those of the school and with the ways teachers and SLPs interpret and mediate learning and cognition. Consequently, as a nation we lose an important opportunity to learn and enjoy the potential benefits of our wonderfully rich and diverse cultural legacy. To honor, appreciate, and (in the bargain) maintain diversity while building community, educators and SLPs need to become first aware, then understanding, and finally inviting of the behavioral and linguistic traditions that students bring to the classroom, while teaching them the language and culture of schools (i.e., helping them to become bicultural and bilingual). Additionally, relating instruction to students' specific cultures, particularly as they are instantiated in language, is one means of fostering optimal learning for all students. As Reyes (1992) wrote, a "one size fits all" approach does not work. Further, when faced with language differences that can be somewhat intimidating and with what might appear to be unresponsive students, teachers should not assume that these differences denote inferior abilities (Owens, 1992). They simply represent different ways of meaning-making. Literacy programming should always promote sensitivity for the language, values, and norms of other cultures.

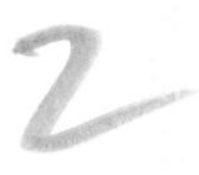

The Impact of Socioeconomic Class

A *social class* is a group of people associated by common economic factors, values, and practices (Nieto, 1992). Although there are discrete class divisions in the United States, vocabulary signifying social class strata is largely absent from public discourse; one rarely hears social class referred to in ordinary conversation or in the media (Mantsios, 1995). Despite our reluctance as a society to acknowledge class divisions overtly, we cannot escape the recognition that variations in socioeconomic status have a powerful impact on the education of children. "Education is strongly influenced by societal factors such as race, class, and the sociocultural context in which it occurs" (Hillis, 1996, p. 115).

According to the Department of Commerce (Bureau of the Census, 1993), 15% of the people living in the United States were living below the U.S. government's official poverty line (calculated in 1992 at $7,143 for an individual and $14,335 for a family of four). Of these, about 3 million were homeless people and 25% were children under the age of 6. Additionally, over 42% of households earned less than $25,000 in 1990 (Bureau of the Census, 1992). Poverty is most likely to be a condition of children, the aged, minorities, women, people who are illiterate, and full-time workers employed in the lowest paying jobs (Gollnick & Chinn, 1994).

As we know from government statistics, the vast majority of poor people do not choose to live in poverty. Rather, they are casualties of a social system they often do not understand well and whose opportunities favor more mainstream groups (Kozol, 1995). It is not surprising, then, that African Americans, Hispanic Americans, and Native Americans are the most economically deprived ethnic groups in this country (Gollnick & Chinn, 1994).[2] According to the 1992 Census Bureau, African American families' median income is 58% that of European Americans and Hispanic families' is 63%. Further, a disproportionate number of people of color live in poverty: while 11% of the white population fall below the federal poverty level, 32% of the African American and 38% of the Hispanic American populations do so (Bureau of the Census, 1992). The poverty rate on reservations is generally between 45% and 58% (Bureau of the Census, 1988) and life expectancy is the lowest of all ethnic groups in the United States (Hess et al., 1995). A number of factors perpetuate this disparity. One of the most important is educational level: Because U.S. public schools are generally so inhospitable to students of color, these students drop out in greater numbers and are thus more likely to be either employed in lower paying jobs or unemployed (Gollnick & Chinn, 1994).

Performance in school (Mantsios, 1995; Persell, 1993) and level of school completed (Bowles & Gintis, 1976; National Coalition, 1985) have been strongly correlated with social class. Mantsios found that class position is probably the single greatest factor in determining future educational success. In a 1978 study by the Carnegie Council of Children, de Lone examined the test scores of over half a million students who took college entrance examinations. Consistent with previous studies (e.g., Sewell, 1971), he found that a relationship exists between social class and *Scholastic Aptitude Test* (SAT) scores and concluded, "the higher the student's social class, the higher the probability that he or she will get higher grades" (p. 19). This pattern continues to persist. Table 5.1 depicts the correlation between social class and SAT scores in 1996.

Poverty, in particular, has been consistently associated with low academic achievement (Allington & Cunningham, 1996; Cooley, 1993; Gadsden & Wagner, 1995). Parents who live in poverty may not have access to the resources that more financially stable families may possess, such as books, school supplies, and other tools needed to promote literacy. Additionally, economically oppressed parents may, out of necessity, be more concerned and involved with basic survival than their children's education, at least in traditionally expected ways (Allington & Cunningham, 1996; Nieto, 1992). However, despite these possible explanations, no specific factor can be blamed

---

[2]Remember that Asians are the most highly educated immigrant group in the United States and that, when educated Cubans settled in Miami, they established a community that flourished. African, Hispanic, and Native Americans have not had the benefit of highly literate family backgrounds.

Table 5.1
Average Combined *Scholastic Aptitude Test* (SAT) Scores by Income (on a 400 to 1,600 scale)

Family Income	Median SAT Score
More than $100,000	1,129
$80,000 to $100,000	1,085
$70,000 to $80,000	1,064
$60,000 to $70,000	1,049
$50,000 to $60,000	1,034
$40,000 to $50,000	1,016
$30,000 to $40,000	992
$20,000 to $30,000	964
$10,000 to $20,000	920
Less than $10,000	873

Note. From *College-Bound Seniors: 1996 Profile of SAT and Achievement Test Takers,* by College Entrance Examination Board, 1996, Princeton, NJ: Author. Copyright 1996 by College Entrance Examination Board. Reprinted with permission.

for lack of academic achievement. Indeed, and most important for our purposes, Nieto (1992) pointed out that teacher perception of a student's social class has also been shown to be a significant factor in school failure for these students.

Furthermore, Anyon (1980) and Cheng (1996) have described attitudes among educationists that both imitate and perpetuate the social class stratification in society. The practical outcome of such attitudes is that they lead to messages, both subtle and blatant, that may influence student achievement. One example is the widespread belief that poor or working class students are less capable than their middle class peers. "It is important to understand that as teachers [and SLPs], all the decisions we make, no matter how neutral they seem, may impact in unconscious but fundamental ways on the lives and experiences of our students" (Nieto, 1992, p. 219). Hence, the expectations of teachers and SLPs, albeit both unintentional and unintentionally communicated, can have a profound effect on the way students view themselves.

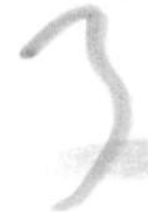

Multiculturalism and Special Education

It has long been known that ethnicity and social class are related to the issue of exceptionality; students from nonmainsteam and poor families have traditionally been overrepresented in special education placements. Significant numbers of African, Hispanic, and Native American students, many of lower socioeconomic status, are labeled as developmentally delayed, learning disabled, or emotionally disturbed. Dunn pointed out as early as 1968 that 60% to 80% of the students labeled as having mental retardation were nonmainstream children from low socioeconomic backgrounds. Mercer (1973) later documented the disproportionate numbers of both Mexican and African Americans in programs for students with mental retardation in a California school district. He found that although Hispanics represented only 11% of the total school population, over 45% were placed in classes for the developmentally delayed, while African Americans were overrepresented in the same placements at a rate 3 times greater than their overall representation in the school population. Further, although Caucasians comprised 81% of the school population, only about 32% were receiving special education for mental retardation.

Through their analysis of the 1978 to 1984 U.S. Office of Civil Rights Surveys of elementary and secondary schools, Chinn and Hughes (1987) concluded that African Americans continued to be overrepresented in classes for students with mild and moderate developmental delays and serious emotional disturbance. Indeed, twice the percentage of African Americans found in the general school population were labeled as having mild developmental delays. Similarly, Native Americans were overrepresented in classes for students with moderate developmental delays and learning disabilities. Additionally, Latinos, African Americans, and Native Americans were all significantly underrepresented in gifted and talented programs. Unfortunately, these trends persisted in the 1986, 1988, and 1990 Office of Civil Rights Surveys (Office of Civil Rights, 1988, 1990, 1992) and continue today. Table 5.2 depicts the breakdown of blacks, whites, and Hispanics in special education placements, based on the 1990 Civil Rights Survey results.

Although true exceptionalities certainly exist among nonmainstream students, the disproportionate numbers enrolled in special education suggest that *difference rather than disability* may well be a causal factor in referrals, a factor that represents one way that disabilities are socially constructed. There is no syndrome from which many of these students suffer. Indeed, it was suggested nearly two decades ago that attitudes toward culturally and linguistically diverse students affect referral for special education services (High & Udall, 1983). The majority of teachers and SLPs in this country are from European

Table 5.2
Breakdown by Race of Special Education Students (in percent)

Special Education Category	Black	White	Hispanic
Retarded	26	11	18
Learning disabled	43	51	55
Emotionally disturbed	8	8	4
Speech impaired	23	30	23

Note. Derived from *1990 Elementary and Secondary Schools Civil Rights Survey,* by Office of Civil Rights, 1992, Washington, DC: U.S. Department of Education.

American, middle class backgrounds with inherent values and norms that may be incompatible with those of nonmainstream and lower socioeconomic class students. When teachers *perceive* students as exhibiting social, learning, and linguistic deficits, they are likely to refer them to special education (Chinn & Harris, 1990; Edwards, 1991). That is why it is so important for teachers and SLPs to be aware that what often look like disabilities are really language or dialectal differences.

The assessment process also has been implicated as a reason for the disproportionate placement of students from nonmainstream groups in special education. Qualification for special education services are partially based on standardized test scores. Standardized tests are, however, for the most part biased against culturally and linguistically different populations (Gardner, 1995; Gollnick & Chinn, 1994; Perkins, 1995; Samuda & Lewis, 1992), because they are standardized in ways that reflect racial and socioeconomic distributions in the society at large. Hence, through their use of averages to calculate norms, they always favor the most numerous group in the United States, the white middle class. Furthermore, assessments conducted in English with minority-language students will not yield accurate results. Nor will test items normed on predominantly white, middle class samples elicit "correct" responses from nonmainstream students. Educators and SLPs, therefore, need to monitor test results to determine whether they are consistent with what they observe in the classroom and whether they indicate a real disability or merely an ethnic difference (i.e., a characteristic that is not considered a disadvantage in the student's home community).

Lack of acceptance in the home community is the key test for a language disorder. The language and learning disabilities label is commonly given to linguistically different students, especially students with dialectal (as opposed to language) differences, because we professionals have not been as careful as we should be about examining the social and cultural factors found in a student's speech community (Taylor, Payne, & Anderson, 1987). Furthermore, assessment in the student's native language is essential to revealing a true communication disorder (Kayser, 1993). Still, as noted earlier, we do not often have appropriate tests or the skill to administer them. It is incumbent that SLPs and school psychologists differentiate between true pathology and language or dialectal variation. ASHA (1983) addressed linguistic differences thus:

> An essential step towards making accurate assessments in communicative disorders is to distinguish between those aspects of linguistic variation that represent the diversity of the English language from those that represent speech, language, and hearing disorders. The speech–language pathologist must have certain competencies to distinguish between dialectical differences and communicative disorders. These competencies include knowledge of the particular dialect as a rule-governed linguistic system, knowledge of the phonological and grammatical features of the dialect, and knowledge of nondiscriminatory testing procedures. Once the difference–disorder distinctions have been made, it is the role of the speech–language pathologist to treat only those features or characteristics that are true errors and not those attributable to the dialect. (pp. 23–25)

Hence, teachers, SLPs, and other specialists should begin with the premise that all students are members of a community who share a common communication norm and then determine what the student needs to know to communicate appropriately within this community. Taylor et al. (1987) suggested that, to ensure optimal understanding of tasks and a successful evaluation, children should be observed in a variety of settings that embody familiar objects and activities: "Less structured conversational activities elicit more language than structured activities and picture-describing tasks" (p. 421). Family members and significant people in the student's cultural environment can provide the necessary information regarding communicative norms (Taylor et al., 1987).

Additionally, research on language acquisition has yielded relevant information regarding nonstandard English norms. Stockman (1986), for example, found that the acquisitional patterns of children who acquire Ebonics prior to 3 years of age are similar to those of children who acquire SAE. Hence, a disorder may be present when young children fail to exhibit these expected language behaviors. However, between the ages of 3 and 7, children acquiring Ebonics demonstrate different patterning and specific grammatical rules. Therefore, these norms suggest that older children acquiring Ebonics who fail to evidence SAE forms are more likely to be exhibiting a different language or

Table 5.3
Basic Assumptions of Multicultural Education

1. The diagnostic and therapeutic process needs to be family centered.
2. Communication and language are always culturally based.
3. Every person belongs to some culture.
4. The client and family direct the intervention process.
5. The clinical process is a social occasion.
6. Intervention must be culturally sensitive.
7. Intervention should focus and build on the child's strengths.
8. All children have the potential to make substantial gains.
9. Intervention should include strategies to support the development of natural speech and literacy skills.

Note. From *Building Bridges: Multicultural Preschool Project, Assistive Technology,* by the American Speech-Language-Hearing Association, no date, Rockville, MD: Author. Reprinted with permission.

dialect rather than a disorder. Table 5.3 delineates some basic assumptions that teachers, SLPs, and other specialists should presume in diagnosing and serving language minority students.

The danger in misdiagnosing a communication difference as a disability lies in further confusing students when they observe the speech and language patterns of others in their community, as this suggests that they need to become different and, thus, alienated from others in their speaking circle (Taylor et al., 1987). The goal should always be to preserve students' native dialects while teaching them SAE.

Implications for Educators and Speech–Language Pathologists

What do educators and SLPs do, then, to create classroom climates in which the knowledge, languages, and experiences that students bring to school with them are respected and honored? How does one develop a multicultural perspective where differences are affirmed rather than negated? Foremost, it should be assumed that all children come to school with previously learned strategies which, although different from the mainstream, are nonetheless just as valid. "To be inclusive of all learners, teaching practices, literacy instruction in particular, must begin with the explicit premise that each learner brings a valid language and culture to the instructional context" (Reyes, 1992, p. 443).

Further, we should endeavor to gather knowledge of students' lives outside the classroom—it is as simple as asking or interviewing them or their parents—in order to ascertain their strengths, and to introduce new skills and concepts in contexts with which students are already familiar. "Knowledge about culture is but one tool that educators may use when devising solutions for a school's difficulty in educating diverse children" (Delpit, 1995, p. 167). A multicultural perspective, therefore, goes beyond merely celebrating the diversity in students, but rather acknowledges and builds on the strengths and abilities of all students and incorporates this knowledge into the curriculum. Indeed, connecting the curriculum and reading and writing tasks with students' personal experiences has been shown to support greater progress and increased investment in school and learning (Au & Jordan, 1981; Barnitz, 1986; Flores, Rueda, & Porter, 1986; Steffensen, Joag-dev, & Anderson, 1979; Willig & Swedo, 1987).

Generally, as noted in Chapter 4, skills-oriented approaches that focus on isolated, decontextualized parts, such as typical readiness activities, are less effective in encouraging language acquisition than are approaches that emphasize meaningful context and connectedness for the student (Delpit, 1995). Engaging students fully in the learning process necessitates using activities and techniques that are familiar and generate interest and enthusiasm (see Appendix 5.A for suggestions). Of utmost importance, however, is recognizing the student's potential and promoting high expectations for success. "When teachers do not understand the potential of the students they teach, they will underteach them no matter what the methodology" (Delpit, 1995, p. 175).

Also, cooperative learning has been shown to (a) build successfully on the interactional styles of some cultural groups (Slavin, 1983) and (b) encourage trusting relationships in the classroom (Oakes, 1985). In cooperative learning, small heterogeneous groups of students work together for collective reward (Gollnick & Chinn, 1994). Hence, the focus is on interacting, negotiating, and cooperating with others, a format similar to the socialization principles found in many ethnic communities. In fact, the concept of cooperative learning came about through observing how Native and Mexican American students interacted with each other as a result of cultural socialization (Poplin, 1992). Additionally, Collier (1995) found that interactive classes, problem-based discovery, and thematic learning promote language acquisition:

> In our current research, we have found that classes in school that are highly interactive, emphasizing student problem-solving and discovery learning through thematic experiences across the curriculum are likely to provide the kind of social setting for natural language acquisition to take place, simultaneously with academic and cognitive development. (p. 7)

Another technique that fosters both oral and written language acquisition is negotiating linguistic forms and meaning among peers (Ellis, 1985; Enright & McCloskey, 1988; Freeman & Freeman, 1992; Goodman & Wilde, 1992; Swain, 1985; Wong Fillmore, 1991). An example of this method is analyzing rap songs to discover inherent patterns and using rules for creating new rap songs based on these patterns. Such a technique can become a base for teachers to explain the structure of grammar and to make comparisons across languages or be used as an actual writing assignment for a real audience (Delpit, 1988).

Reading to children is the single most important predictor of achievement among independent readers (M. Adams, 1990). Reading to children not only models the process of reading, but also fosters the growth of vocabulary and syntax. The language of books is different from that of speech and television (two other primary sources of exposure to language) and is also more interactive. Reading several texts per day, therefore, appears to be one of the best strategies to promote literacy. Use of predictable texts, repeated readings of stories, and writing language experience stories are all excellent ways to enhance classroom support for children acquiring English as a second language (Rigg, 1989).

Students literate in a native language other than English need to continue reading and writing in their native language while learning English (Cummins, 1994). Foreign language books, films, and computer software should be available in classrooms and school libraries to promote literacy acquisition. An additional benefit of providing foreign language materials in schools is that it helps nonmainstream as well as other students develop a better understanding of the cultures of their classmates. Parents of second-language learners can be recruited as volunteers to read books to children in their native language. Many favorite big books are available in Spanish and multiple-language editions; the English and other-language editions can thus be contrasted. Fairy and folktales are a good source of reading material, as they often touch on universal themes. Poetry also mirrors one's culture and presents big, important thoughts in a few words.

Student-made bilingual dictionaries are an inexpensive tool for incorporating non-English speaking students into the classroom (Allington & Cunningham, 1996). These can be put together by both English and non-English speaking children who are literate in their first language. Vocabulary should be drawn from the core curriculum, with sections for different subjects, such as social studies, science, and math, as well as a general vocabulary section. Dictionaries can be updated, via computer, as needed, and copies can be sent home with students to further support language learning. Parents who are bilingual can be asked to help in proofreading final copies.

"Language buddies" are another way to support non-English speaking students (Allington & Cunningham, 1996). Children pair up with older students with English language proficiency who help with homework, reading, and writing in a quiet, comfortable space provided for these activities. Additionally, students with the same first language should be placed in the same classroom so that they can support each others' learning.

Students with non-English language proficiency can also serve as tutors for English-speaking children interested in learning a second language. An after-school program can be set up to facilitate tutoring. The staff can consist of students, parents, people from the community, or staff members who speak the language to be learned. English speakers can thus learn the rudiments of another language while non-English speakers have an opportunity to practice a second language.

Telecommunications is another option for promoting literacy. For example, Vasquez (1993) discussed an after-school program for Latino children called "La Clase Magíca." Using computer software, Spanish-speaking students participate in a role-playing activity and later write letters and progress reports, via a telecommunications network, to other students in schools also involved in the activity. Another telecommunications program is the "Scholastic Place Network" of American Online, which links second-language learners to other speakers, readers, and writers of their native language.

An approach linked more directly to classroom instruction is the *Cognitive Academic Language Learning Approach* (CALLA), which supports students learning English as a second language in the regular classroom by targeting high-priority content from the grade-level core curriculum (Chamot & O'Malley, 1994). The premise is that all language learners succeed best when instructional activities are meaningful and authentic. Hence, CALLA uses natural language involving the regular curriculum, rather than drill and practice of isolated speech components. Learning is supported concurrently with developing language proficiency (Allington & Cunningham, 1996).

> If ESL students are to catch up academically with their native English-speaking peers, their cognitive growth and mastery of academic content must continue while English is being learned. Thus the teaching of English as a second language should be integrated with the teaching of other academic content. . . . All content teachers must recognize themselves also as teachers of language. (Cummins, 1994, p. 56)

Currently, a wide range of children from homes where SAE is not the primary language attend schools in which the Eurocentric curriculum is the norm. Because the population of students in our schools is becoming increasingly diverse, SLPs and teachers need to become even more responsible for enhancing educational support for learners who are acquiring English proficiency. Collectively, we need to rise to the challenge of better serving these children by valuing their diversity (rather than thinking of them as students who do not fit the mold), fostering literacy in a multitude of languages, and promoting the successful integration of *all* students in the educational community. To do otherwise is to sustain an educational system that benefits primarily the mainstream few.

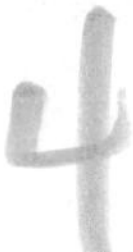

Gender Issues

No discussion of attitudes and prejudices that affect educational outcomes would be complete without a discussion of gender-based expectations, which often have a negative impact on both males and females. Nevertheless, the Eurocentric curriculum has tended to privilege males, while silencing females. Until recently, education, for example, was the only institution in which those who entered with an advantage—that is, girls—exited doing less well than their male counterparts—and that after 12 years of instruction and "nurturance" (Sadker & Sadker, 1994). According to a report aired on National Public Radio on October 14, 1998, however, the National Association for University Women's newest study on gender equity in schools indicates that great strides have been made in recent years toward the use of nonsexist language in educational settings and in female students' achieving educational parity. According to their report, the one difficulty for female students that may still remain, although there is some controversy about this issue, is whether female students use technology in the same ways as males. As teachers and SLPs, we must acknowledge that language practices have played and continue to play a key role in what happens to girls and women throughout schooling. As Moore (1995) pointed out in his essay on racism in the English language, "Language not only develops in conjunction with a society's historical, economic, and political evolution; it also reflects that society's attitudes and thinking. Language not only *expresses* ideas and concepts but actually *shapes* thought" (p. 376).

Through concerted efforts to change the climate for females, according to the National Association of University Women study, the society has both changed and been changed by our attention to sexist language and its relation to privilege. As Bosmajian (1995) pointed out, we had become used to making women invisible in our everyday references to humankind and to the professions; to having women identified in the media in ways that would be ludicrous if they were applied to descriptions of men (and vice versa); and to using words typically associated with helplessness and immaturity to refer to women (e.g., *baby, doll, girl, lady*). This language, then, both passed on societal conceptions of what women and men should be like and shaped the behavior and expectations of the male and female students we taught and the ways in which we taught them. Furthermore, there have been numerous popular and scholarly books that suggest that women have been socialized to use language differently from men and, although the findings are still controversial and their authors careful to say that the language is "different" and not inferior, they have often been interpreted as casting women in an inferior light when compared to the male standard or when described from the male point of view. Finally, some language-based stereotypes still influence what happens in schools, particularly with respect to how girls are treated within curricular settings.

Language About Women

In the English language, the generic form of most terms related to groups, roles, and professions (e.g., *mankind, chairman, doctor, senator*) is masculine (the National Association of University Women study is silent on such issues). For that reason, we also use the masculine pronouns *he* and *him* when we speak of non-specified persons or use the term to refer to all persons, both male and female. In every case, we make women invisible and, as Hernandez remarked in 1971, through such language usage "in all areas that count, we discount women" (p. 6).

Attempts to correct such omissions have often led to cumbersome and even ludicrous constructions, such as *Madam Chairman* or *person hours* and, for that reason, many people have been reluctant to construct alternatives to the masculine form. Furthermore, many men and women argue that we *understand* the term *mankind* or *doctor*, for example, to mean both sexes, so we need not change the phrasing. The consequence of resisting linguistic change is that the visions women and girls may have about the range of possibilities for their own lives are limited. They cannot be judges or senators, but must always be labeled as the outsider, the female judge, the female senator. It is good to know that these problems no longer hamper girls in school, but they are still very much a part of the larger society.

Because of our assumption that the agent is male unless otherwise noted, awkward and insidious references to women often appear in the media. Bosmajian (1995, p. 390) listed several examples from newspaper headlines—"Grandmother Wins Nobel Prize," "Blonde Hijacks Airliner," and "Housewife To Run for Congress"—all of which would be thought to contain superfluous, and even ludicrous, information if the agents were males. We simply cannot imagine the headline that announces "Grandfather Wins Nobel Prize."

In addition, women are often introduced in terms of their husbands, rather than as professionals in their own right. In January 1998, the host of the television show "Jeopardy" introduced three celebrity panelists. When he introduced the two men, there was no reference to their wives, but he introduced the woman, a highly accomplished and renowned reporter, as the wife of the chairman of the Federal Reserve Board.

Even more demeaning in many instances is the penchant of the media to use the language and perspective of men when reporting about women. A major New York newspaper, for example, described a Supreme Court nominee as having a "bathing beauty figure"—a comment that in its comparable masculine form (e.g., body builder's, or perhaps, athlete's figure) would have been considered completely irrelevant.

Teachers and SLPs must be aware of the subtle and not-so-subtle messages that these language forms send to female students about what the expectations are for them in life and teach students—both males and females—to analyze and reflect on such messages. Males, of course, are also harmed by the perpetuation of gender-biased stereotypes, particularly males who deviate from the image of the individualistic, athletic, go-getter. The focus here is on women, however, because it is they who are most affected by issues of language usage.

Furthermore, now that we have apparently made significant gains, teachers and SLPs need to continue to instruct students to use nonsexist language, particularly when writing. Although constructions that make women visible are often cumbersome, one can usually avoid the use of such sexist expressions as "the executive, he," by using the plural form "executives, they" or in the case of a female executive, "the executive, she" (American Psychological Association, 1994).

Language of Women

In 1975 Lakoff published a book that both established a new line of research—studies of how women's language usage differed from that of men—and prompted assertiveness training programs that were designed to help women overcome their more deferential language behaviors and, therefore, succeed better in the corporate world. Since that time, a controversy has raged about whether women's language is, in fact, different from that of men, how it differs, and whether those differences should be considered as deficiencies.

One of the best known sociolinguists who studies and defends the idea that women use language differently from men is Tannen (1986, 1990, 1993, 1994, 1997). She argues that women and men grow up primarily in same-sex groups, so communication between men and women is essentially cross-cultural and often leads to misunderstanding and confusion. She posits that women are more comfortable using language in private settings and that this language can be characterized as "rapport-talk." That is, it is used to establish connections and negotiate relationships. Men's language, on the other hand, is used to establish independence and to negotiate and maintain their status in our society's hierarchical social order. Although Tannen is careful to note that the language patterns of the two sexes are simply different, she does acknowledge that it is but a short step from people's translating *different* into *worse*. Because men are dominant in our society, they serve as the standard and it is consequently women who are usually encouraged to change, to become more like men.

Tannen argues, furthermore, that despite the possible dangers, it is important to recognize the differences, because recognizing them helps people to understand that the differences are often cultural, rather than personal (e.g., "Men tend not to talk much at home"—that is, engage in private talk—versus "My *husband* doesn't talk much at home") and they also work to expose stereotypes. For example, it is commonly believed that females talk more than males. This belief is so pervasive that teachers who viewed a film in which boys did three times as much talking as girls perceived and reported that the girls had done most of the talking (Sadker & Sadker, 1995). Such beliefs are likely implicated in the earlier finding that teachers call more often on boys and use follow-up questions and the like that support reasoning and enable boys to talk longer (Sadker & Sadker, 1994). It probably feels to teachers as if boys need more encouragement to talk, since they believe that girls just naturally do most of the talking.

Similarly, LaFrance and Henley (1997) have argued that well-documented differences between men and women exist in nonverbal behavior, with women being both more sensitive and more expressive nonverbally. They argue that these differences are "attributable to power inequities rather than personality differences" (p. 105). LaFrance and Henley believe that women become better at nonverbal communication because it is safer. It enables them to demonstrate compliance with the social order (i.e., to show that their subordinate status is intact). It is after all, the authors argue, wise of the less powerful to monitor behaviors among those who are in power.

Aries (1997) has reviewed the objections to Tannen's hypothesis that men and women use language differently, and Hall and Haberstadt (1997) have raised similar arguments against the subordination hypothesis proposed by LaFrance and Henley (1997). Primary among the objections is that we cannot essentialize women (i.e., pretend that there is an "essential" woman and therefore talk about women as a group, rather than respect the individual differences among them; Butler, 1990): Some women may use language differently or be superior in nonverbal communication and others not. Furthermore, in both cases, although the results of studies are consistently *statistically* different, the actual size of the effects tends to be small and nonsupporting examples abundant. Language usage is not a trait that is a stable characteristic. Rather, language usage is a process that is culturally sensitive (see, e.g., Philips, Steele, & Tanz, 1987), dynamic, and flexible. It changes with circumstances, needs, and partners. Consequently, it is probably more appropriate to locate usage in the *interaction* between the conversants, rather than attribute specific characteristics to a particular person, who may use language quite differently in a new situation. For example, a teacher may dominate a conversation with a learner during a social studies lesson and respond altogether differently just a few minutes later when the student is guiding the teacher through the use of an unfamiliar computer program.

In conclusion, there is some indication that women as a group might be more concerned with issues of rapport, while men are more individualistic. Similarly, it may be the case that women are more sensitive and expressive nonverbally. What is important, however, is that both women and men have the capacity to develop a wide range of preferences, styles, and competencies in communication. It is the obligation of teachers and SLPs to make certain that their female students develop as broad and useful a range of competencies as their male counterparts and that male students be given the freedom to explore their natures without similar restrictions. Furthermore, it is incumbent upon teachers and SLPs to help students understand how language is used to play out and conserve societal expectations and stereotypes. It is likely that whatever differences do exist are the results of socialization (as the new National Association of University Women's study bears out) rather than immutable characteristics of women and men. What we want to work toward in a demo-cratic culture is the freedom to be who and what we are with no more regard for gender than for eye color.

Language and the Curriculum

Chapman (1997) provided some idea how important gender issues are in schooling in the opening words of her text on equitable education for girls and boys:

> Who am I? and What can I become? are questions of great urgency for children and adolescents. Their own lives and the society of the future will be affected by their answers. The ideas they absorb from those around them about being male or female will be of decisive importance in the answers they are able to construct. (p. i)

Furthermore, language is a central factor in influencing aspirations and supporting or impeding their realization. Consequently, language differences have serious educational implications, especially when race, socioeconomic status, and gender are all confounded as in the case of poor African American women (hooks, 1994).

Whether or not differences in communication styles between females and males actually exist, they are perceived to exist and, as a result, certain language patterns have become female or male associated. *Female-associated language* (a) is supportive of other speakers, usually through the use of nonverbal cues and short, uninterrupting comments, such as "Mmmmm" and "Right"; (b) uses questioning intonation frequently and therefore appears deferential and uncertain; and (c) involves considerable self-disclosure. *Male-associated language*, on the other hand, is characterized by (a) friendly arguing that often reaches the status of a bonding ritual; (b) verbal posturing in an impersonal and somewhat abstract style that focuses on contents and yields little self-disclosure; and (c) tends toward monologues that assert dominance and leave little time for listening to others. Of course, either style may be used by women or men in any given situation and most people probably move back and forth between them, depending on the situation. However, the perceptions that women should behave one way and men another are so pervasive that these perceived style differences may continue to have a subtle impact on schooling.

In her review of the literature on the impact of gender-associated language in classrooms, Chapman (1997) concluded that female-associated speakers are at a disadvantage. While girls are being taught, however subtly, to adopt female-associated language patterns and are judged by their ability to do so (see Carli, 1990), the evidence suggests that both female and male teachers prefer classroom comments that are made in the assertive male-associated style. Female-associated speakers, whether they be males or females, are less convincing and are interrupted more often by both teachers and peers. Not only do they not finish what they want to say, but they stay out of the conversation once interrupted. This lack of participation may then be reflected in grades or affect levels of achievement.

There are also some difficulties associated with male-associated language usage, but they are typically less detrimental. Boys are much more likely to call out in class than girls, but teachers are also more likely to let boys (than girls) get away with not raising their hands. Male-associated language behaviors, however, may be interpreted as challenges to authority or may prohibit speakers from listening to and learning from others. Furthermore, males who believe that they must conform to male-associated expectations are just as limited and constrained in the range of behaviors they allow themselves to engage in as are females who are limited by female-associated constraints.

Finally, differences in expectations can lead to miscommunications and even hurt feelings, when students who must collaborate in classrooms are unaware of the differences in communication patterns that are expected of female and male students. Another source of miscommunication can be differences in expectations for nonverbal communications. Eye contact is a case in point. In mainstream culture, looking at other people while listening to them talk is generally perceived as less powerful, while looking at a person to whom one is talking is interpreted as a sign of having higher status. As a result, teachers generally expect students who are listening to them to maintain eye contact. Yet, as we mentioned earlier, eye contact in some cultures is considered rude and looking down a sign of respect. The evidence suggests that white females are most likely to maintain eye contact, while African American males are least likely (Chapman, 1997). Teachers must be aware of such propensities, so that they do not equate the maintenance of eye contact as a sign of attentiveness or of interest.

In sum, although the recent study by the National Association of University Women reveals positive findings, the variables studied were about the use of sexist language in its most obvious form, the presence of females in science courses, the achievement levels as specified in grades, the numbers of women going on to college and other forms of advanced training, and so forth. They did not include some of the more subtle forms of sexism described in much of the recent scientific literature. Consequently, although we should find comfort in the fact that things are getting better for our female students, we should be aware that the job of monitoring our language usage and language expectations is not yet done.

Conclusion

Race, class, and gender are all associated with variations in language patterns, dialects, and nonverbal communications that have consequences for schooling. In fact, females, people from nonmainstream cultures, and the poor often experience very similar life situations and events (Chafe, 1995). Teachers, SLPs, and other specialists must be aware of these variations in communication patterns and styles, so as to interpret them in ways that support the enhancement of individual potential and reduce the incidence of the stereotyping and miscategorization that lead to the overrepresentation of nonmainstream students in special education and the possible undervaluing and consequent underdevelopment of females. As SLPs and teachers, we must learn to invite all voices into the classroom and to accept the language and associated styles that students bring to school. We can then help the students make direct comparisons between their speech and writing patterns and those of the SAE that we must teach them for ideological purposes (Gee, 1990).

Furthermore, we must teach our students about cultural and language differences, about prejudice and hierarchy, and the impact they are likely to have on their lives (Banks, 1996; Friere, 1998; hooks, 1994; Macedo, 1994). We must help them understand the political nature of the educational enterprise and help them to succeed within it while inviting them to have an impact upon it. We cannot rely on the banking system of education in which teachers "impart" knowledge of the Eurocentric curriculum to students. Students must become agents and collaborators in their own learning (hooks, 1994). If we cannot as a nation accommodate our race-, class-, and gender-based diversity within education, our society's primary instrument of acculturation, and promote the talents of all citizens, how will we as a nation fare in this increasingly competitive world?

Appendix 5.A
Annotated Bibliography of Selected Resources

Ada, F. A., Harris, V. J., & Hopkins, L. B. (1993). *A chorus of cultures: Developing literacy through multicultural poetry*. Carmel, CA: Hampton-Brown Books.

An anthology of hundreds of multicultural poems, songs, sayings, and folklore, with techniques for infusing multiculturalism into the classroom through the use of poetry. Included are scores of multicultural themes and whole-language activity ideas to develop literacy and extend concepts across the curriculum by the authors, who are themselves teachers. Additional professional resources for promoting multiculturalism are provided.

Bigelow, B., Christensen, L., Karp, S., Miner, B., & Peterson, B. (Eds.). (1994). *Rethinking our classrooms: Teaching for equity and justice*. Milwaukee, WI: Rethinking Schools.

A collection of creative teaching ideas to promote values of community, justice, and equality. Included are articles, poems, reproducible student handouts, lesson plans, teaching tips, role plays, and activities to help develop critical skills. A related teaching guide and available resources, including books, videos, periodicals, and organizations, are also included.

Kepler, P., Royse, B. S., & Kepler, J. (1996). *Themes for multicultural understandings: Windows to the world*. Glenview, IL: Good Year Books.

A book of resources for Grades 4 through 8 that goes beyond multicultural awareness to focus on the attitudes and skills needed to interact successfully across cultural lines. Each chapter emphasizes a theme common to all cultures, such as language, time, work, and leisure, and shows how cultures differ in their interpretation and expression of some aspect of life. Included are a wide array of interesting instructional strategies and activities. Interspersed throughout are quotations, proverbs, new words, and "Did You Know" facts about beliefs and behaviors in other cultures. Professional resources are provided at the end of each chapter.

Sierra, J. (1992). *The onyx multicultural folktale series: Cinderella*. Phoenix, CA: Oryx Press.

Consists of 24 variants of the Cinderella fairytale told in English, representing a broad range of cultures, geographical areas, and styles. Included are notes on the tales from ancient Egypt, China, France, Germany, England, Ireland, Portugal, Norway, Finland, Iceland, Republic of Georgia, Russia, Iraq, South

Africa (Zulu), India, Native America (Micmac, Zuni), United States (Appalachia), Japan, the Philippines, and Vietnam. Also included are suggested related activities, a bibliography of Cinderella picture books, guide to variants in collections, and recommended further readings. Sierra has also coauthored *Multicultural Folktales* available through the same publisher.

Materiales
Papier-Mâché
DIRECTIONS
1. Tear the Newspaper
2. Begin To PAPER-Mâché
• Place The 1/4 liter container face down.
Pasta de trigo
Papier Mâché
Dirección de la actividad
1. Romper el papel
2. Empezar a hacer papier-mâché
• Coloquen los recipientes de 1/4 litro boca abajo
FLOUR
H2O
T.M. BALCHAK 9/98

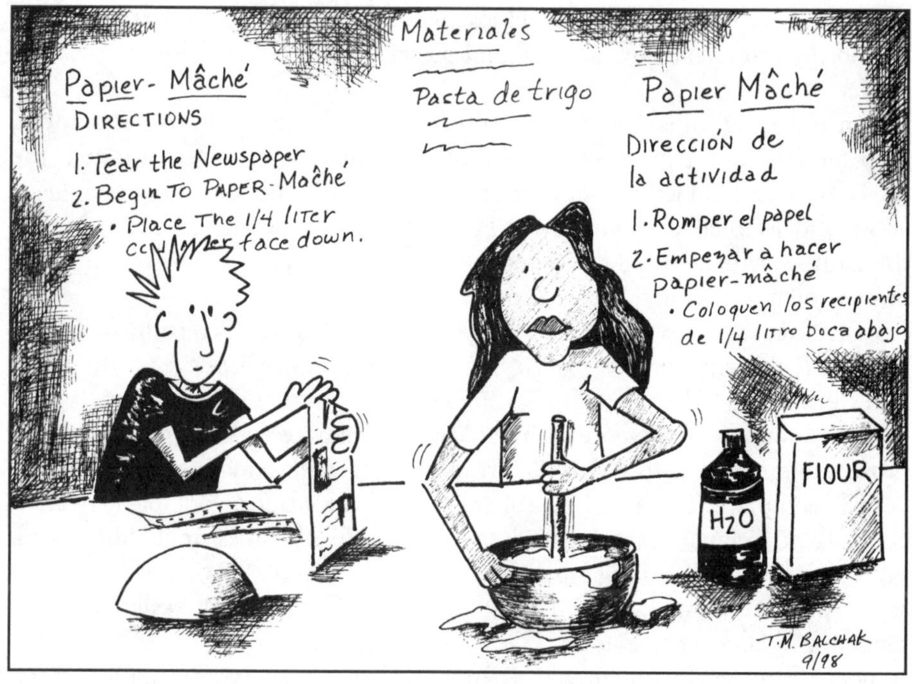

To better serve students, educationists must learn to value diversity (and bilingualism) and work to integrate all students into the educational community.

References

Adams, D. W. (1988). Fundamental considerations: The deep meaning of Native American schooling, 1880–1900. *Harvard Educational Review, 58*(1), 1–28.

Adams, M. J. (1990). *Beginning to read: Thinking and learning about print*. Champaign: University of Illinois at Urbana-Champaign, Center for the Study of Reading, The Reading Research and Education Center.

Allington, R. L., & Cunningham, P. M. (1996). *Schools that work: Where all children read and write*. New York: HarperCollins.

American Psychological Association. (1994). *Publication manual of the American Psychological Association* (4th ed.). Washington, DC: Author.

American Speech-Language-Hearing Association. (1983). Position of the American Speech-Language-Hearing Association on social dialects. *Asha, 25*, 23–25.

American Speech-Language-Hearing Association. (no date). *Building bridges: Multicultural preschool project, assistive technology*. Rockville, MD: Author.

Anyon, J. (1980). Social class and the hidden curriculum at work. *Journal of Education, 162*(1), 67–92.

Aries, E. (1997). Women and men talking: Are they worlds apart? In M. R. Walsh (Ed.), *Women, men, and gender* (pp. 91–100). Rensselaer, NY: Hamilton.

Au, K., & Jordan, C. (1981). Teaching reading to Hawaiian children: Finding a culturally appropriate solution. In H. T. Trueba, G. P. Guthrie, & K. H. Au (Eds.), *Culture in the bilingual classroom: Studies in classroom ethnography* (pp. 139–152). Rowley, MA: Newbury House.

Baca, L. M., & Cervantes, H. T. (1989). *The bilingual special education interface*. New York: Merrill/Macmillan.

Banks, J. A. (1996). *Multicultural education: Transformative knowledge and action: Historical and contemporary perspectives*. New York: Teachers College Press.

Barnitz, J. G. (1986). Towards understanding the effects of cross-cultural schemata and discourse structure on second language reading comprehension. *Journal of Reading Behavior, 18*, 95–113.

Bialystok, E. (Ed.). (1991). *Language processing in bilingual children*. Cambridge, England: Cambridge University Press.

Boggs, S. T. (1985). *Speaking, relating and learning: A study of Hawaiian children at home and at school*. Norwood, NJ: Ablex.

Bosmajian, H. (1995). The language of sexism. In P. S. Rothenberg (Ed.), *Race, class, and gender in the United States: An integrated study* (pp. 386–392). New York: St. Martin's Press.

Bowles, S., & Gintis, S. (1976). *Schooling in capitalist America: Educational reform and the contradictions of economic life*. New York: Basic Books.

Bruner, J. (1983). *In search of mind: Essays in autobiography*. New York: Harper and Row.

Bureau of the Census. (1988). *Statistical Abstract of the United States, 1988* (108th ed.). Washington, DC: Government Printing Office.

Bureau of the Census. (1990). *Statistical Abstract of the United States, 1990* (110th ed.). Washington, DC: Government Printing Office.

Bureau of the Census. (1992). *Statistical Abstract of the United States, 1992* (112th ed.). Washington, DC: Government Printing Office.

Bureau of the Census. (1993). *Poverty in the United States: 1992* (series P-60, no. 185). Washington, DC: U.S. Department of Commerce.

Butler, J. P. (1990). *Gender trouble*. London: Routledge.

Carli, L. L. (1990). Gender language and influence. *Journal of Personality and Social Psychology, 59*, 941–951.

Chafe, W. (1995). Sex and race: The analogy of social control. In P. S. Rothenberg (Ed.), *Race, class, and gender in the United States: An integrated study* (pp. 417–431). New York: St. Martin's Press.

Chapman, A. (1997). *A great balancing act: Equitable education for girls and boys*. Boston: National Association of Independent Schools.

Chamot, A. U., & O'Malley, J. M. (1994). *The CALLA handbook: How to implement the Cognitive Academic Language Learning Approach*. Reading, MA: Addison-Wesley.

Cheng, L. L. (1995, December). *Chinese influenced English*. Paper presented at the American Speech-Language-Hearing Association Conference, Orlando, FL.

Cheng, L. L. (1996). Enhancing communication: Toward optimal language learning for Limited English Proficient students. *Language, Speech, and Hearing in the Schools, 27*, 347–354.

Chinn, P. C., & Harris, K. C. (1990). Variables affecting the disproportionate placement of ethnic minority children in special education programs. *Multicultural Leader, 3*(1), 1–3.

Chinn, P. C., & Hughes, S. (1987). Representation of minority students in special education classes. *Remedial and Special Education*, 8(4), 41–46.

Clancy, P. M. (1986). The acquisition of communicative style in Japanese. In B. B. Schieffelin & E. Ochs (Eds.), *Language socialization across cultures* (pp. 213–250). New York: Cambridge University Press.

College Entrance Examination Board. (1996). *College-bound seniors: 1996 profile of SAT and achievement test takers*. Princeton, NJ: Author.

Collier, V. P. (1989). How long? A synthesis of research on academic achievement in second language. *TESOL Quarterly, 23*, 509–531.

Collier, V. P. (1995). Acquiring a second language for school. *Directions in Language and Education, 1*(4), 1–11.

Cooley, W. (1993). The difficulty of the educational task: Implications for comparing student achievement in states, school districts, and schools. *ERS Spectrum, 11*, 27–31.

Crawford, J. (1995). Endangered Native American languages: What is to be done, and why? *Bilingual Research Journal, 19*(1), 17–38.

Cummins, J. (1979). Linguistic interdependence and the educational development of bilingual children. *Review of Educational Research*, 49, 222–251.

Cummins, J. (1981). The role of primary language development in promoting educational success for language minority students. In *Schooling and language minority students: A theoretical framework* (pp. 3–49). Sacramento: California Department of Education.

Cummins, J. (1991). Interdependence of first- and second-language proficiency in bilingual children. In E. Bialystok (Ed.), *Language processing in bilingual children* (pp. 70–89). Cambridge, England: Cambridge University Press.

Cummins, J. (1994). The acquisition of English as a second language. In K. Spangenberg-Urbschat & R. Pritchard (Eds.), *Kids come in all languages: Reading instruction for ESL students* (pp. 36–63). Newark, DE: International Reading Association.

Damico, J. S., & Damico, S. K. (1993). Language and social skills from a diversity perspective: Considerations for the speech language pathologist. *Language, Speech, and Hearing in the Schools, 24*, 236–243.

Darder, A. (1991). *Culture and power in the classroom: A critical foundation for bicultural education*. Westport, CT: Bergin & Garvey.

de Lone, R. (1978). *Small futures*. New York: Harcourt Brace Jovanovich.

Delgado-Gaitan, C. (1987). Traditions and transitions in the learning process of Mexican children: An ethnographic view. In G. Spindler & L. Spindler (Eds.), *Interpretive ethnography of education: At home and abroad* (pp. 173–187). Hillsdale, NJ: Erlbaum.

Delpit, L. (1988). The silenced dialogue: Power and pedagogy in educating other people's children. *Harvard Educational Review, 58*(3), 280–298.

Delpit, L. (1995). *Other people's children: Cultural conflict in the classroom*. New York: The New Press.

Dick, G. S., & McCarty, T. L. (1994). Navajo language maintenance and development: Possibilities for community-controlled schools. *Journal of Navajo Education, 11*(3), 15–20.

Dillard, J. L. (1973). *Black English*. New York: Vintage.

Dunn, L. (1968). Special education for the mildly retarded: Is much of it justifiable? *Exceptional Children, 7*, 5–24.

Edwards, J. (1991). *Language and disadvantage: Studies in disorders of communication* (2nd ed.). London: Whurr Publishers.

Ellis, R. (1985). *Understanding second language acquisition*. Oxford: Oxford University Press.

Enright, D. S., & McCloskey, M. L. (1988). *Integrating English: Developing English language and literacy in the multicultural classroom*. Reading, MA: Addison-Wesley.

Fairchild, H. H., & Edwards-Evans, S. (1990). African American dialects and schooling: A review. In A. M. Padilla, H. H. Fairchild, & C. M. Valadez (Eds.), *Bilingual education, issues and strategies* (pp. 96–116). Newberry Park, CA: Sage.

Fishman, J. (1987). *English only: Its ghosts, myths, and dangers*. Keynote address at the Conference of the California Association for Bilingual Education, Anaheim.

Flores, B., Rueda, R., & Porter, B. (1986). Examining the assumptions and instructional practices related to the acquisition of literacy with bilingual special education students. In A. Willig & H. Greenberg (Eds.), *Bilingualism and learning disabilities* (pp. 149–165). New York: American Library.

Freeman, Y. S., & Freeman, D. E. (1992). *Whole language for second language learners*. Portsmouth, NH: Heinemann.

Friere, P. (1998). *Teachers as cultural workers: Letters to those who dare teach*. Boulder, CO: Westview Press.

Gadsden, V. L., & Wagner, D. A. (Eds.). (1995). *Literacy among African-American youth: Issues in learning, teaching, and schooling*. Cresskill, NJ: Hampton Press.

Garcia, G. E. (1992). Ethnography and classroom communication: Taking an "emic" perspective. *Topics in Language Disorders, 12*(3), 54–66.

Garcia, E. (1994). *Understanding and meeting the challenge of student cultural diversity*. Boston: Houghton Mifflin.

Garcia Coll, C. T. (1990). Developmental outcome of minority infants: A process-oriented look into our beginnings. *Child Development, 61*, 270–289.

Gardner, H. (1995). Scholarly brinkmanship. In R. Jacoby & N. Glauberman (Eds.), *The bell curve debate: History, documents, opinions* (pp. 61–72). New York: Times Books.

Gee, J. (1990). *Social linguistics and literacies: Ideology in discourses*. New York: Farmer.

Genesee, F. (1987). *Learning through two languages: Studies of immersion and bilingual education*. Cambridge, MA: Newbury House.

Genesee, F. (Ed.). (1994). *Educating second language children: The whole child, the whole curriculum, the whole community*. Cambridge, England: Cambridge University Press.

Gollnick, D. M., & Chinn, P. C. (1994). *Multicultural education in a pluralistic society* (4th ed.). New York: Merrill/Macmillan.

Goodman, Y. M., & Wilde, S. (Eds.). (1992). *Literacy events in a community of young writers*. New York: Teachers College Press.

Hakuta, K. (1986). *Mirror of language: The debate on bilingualism*. New York: Basic Books.

Hall, J. A., & Haberstadt, A. G. (1997). Subordination and nonverbal sensitivity: A hypothesis in search of support. In M. R. Walsh (Ed.), *Women, men, and gender* (pp. 120–133). Rensselaer, NY: Hamilton.

Harris, G. A. (1993). American Indian cultures: A lesson in diversity. In D. Battle (Ed.), *Communication disorders in multicultural populations* (pp. 81–82). Boston: Andover Medical.

Heath, S. B. (1982). Questioning at home and at school: A comparative study. In G. Spindler (Ed.), *Doing the ethnography of schooling: Educational anthropology in action* (pp. 96–101). New York: Holt, Rinehart, & Winston.

Heath, S. B. (1983). *Ways with words: Language, life, and work in communities and classrooms*. New York: Cambridge University Press.

Hernandez, A. (1971, January 1). The preening of America. *Star-News* (Pasadena, CA), p. 10.

Hess, B. B., Markson, E. W., & Stein, P. J. (1995). Racial and ethnic minorities: An overview. In P. S. Rothenberg (Ed.), *Race, class, and gender: An integrated study* (3rd ed., pp. 176–188). New York: St. Martin's Press.

High, M. H., & Udall, A. I. (1983). Teacher ratings of students in relation to ethnicity of student and school ethnic balance. *Journal of Education and the Gifted, 6*, 154–166.

Highwater, J. (1981). *The primal mind: Vision and reality in Indian America*. New York: Harper & Row.

Hillis, M. R. (1996). Allison Davis and the study of race, social class, and schooling. In J. A. Banks (Ed.), *Multicultural education, transformative knowledge, and action: Historical and contemporary perspectives* (pp. 115–129). New York: Teachers College Press.

hooks, b. (1994). *Teaching to transgress: Education as the practice of freedom*. New York: Routledge.

Jasper, S. P. (1980). *Selected grammatical characteristics of Mojave English*. Unpublished doctoral dissertation, University of Arizona, Tucson.

Kayser, H. G. (1993). Hispanic cultures. In D. E. Battle (Ed.), *Communication disorders in multicultural populations* (pp. 114–157). Boston: Andover Medical.

Kepler, P., Royse, B. S., & Kepler, J. (1996). *Windows to the world: Themes for cross-cultural understanding*. Glenview, IL: Good Year/Scott Foresman.

Kozol, J. (1995). *Amazing grace: The lives of children and the conscience of a nation*. New York: Crown.

Krashen, S., & Biber, D. (1988). *On course: Bilingual education's success in California*. Sacramento: California Association for Bilingual Education.

Kwachta, P. (1981). *The acquisition of English by Choctaw speaking children*. Unpublished doctoral dissertation, University of Florida, Gainesville.

Labov, W. (1973). The logic of nonstandard English. In N. Keddie (Ed.), *Tinker, tailor . . . The myth of cultural deprivation*. Harmondsworth, England: Penguin.

LaFrance, M., & Henley, N. M. (1997). On oppressing hypotheses: Or, differences in nonverbal sensitivity revisited. In M. R. Walsh (Ed.), *Women, men, and gender* (pp. 104–119). Rensselaer, NY: Hamilton.

Lakoff, R. (1975). *Language and woman's place*. New York: Harper and Row.

Lara, J. (1994). Demographic overview: Changes in student enrollment in American schools. In K. Spangenberg-Urbschat & R. Pritchard (Eds.), *Kids come in all languages: Reading instruction for ESL students* (pp. 9–21). Newark, DE: International Reading Association.

Leap, W. L. (Ed.). (1977). *Studies in Southwestern Indian English.* San Antonio: Trinity University Press.

Leap, W. L. (1995, December). *American Indian English.* Paper presented at the American Speech and Hearing Association Conference, Orlando, FL.

Leland, J., & Joseph, N. (1997, January 13). Hooked on Ebonics. *Newsweek, 129,* 78–79.

Linguists find the debate over "Ebonics" uninformed. (1997, January 17). *Chronicle of Higher Education,* pp. A16–A17.

Lott, J. T., & Felt, J. C. (1991). Studying the pan-Asian community. *Population Today, 19*(2), 6–8.

Macedo, D. P. (1994). *Literacies of power: What Americans are not allowed to know.* Boulder, CO: Westview Press.

Macías, J. (1989, November). *Transnational educational anthropology: The case of Mexican immigrant students.* Paper presented at the American Educational Research Association Conference, San Francisco.

Mantsios, G. (1995). Class in America: Myths and realities. In P. S. Rothenberg (Ed.), *Race, class, and gender in the United States: An integrated study* (3rd ed., pp. 131–143). New York: St. Martin's Press.

Masahiko, M. (1994). *Asian narrative* (Report No. FL-022-370). East Lansing, MI: National Center for Research on Teacher Learning. (ERIC Document Reproduction Service No. ED 372 652)

McCardle, P., & Walton, J. H. (1995, December). *A preliminary analysis of English phonological trends in Mississippi Choctaw children.* Paper presented at the American Speech and Hearing Association Conference, Orlando, FL.

McCollum, P. A., & Walker, C. L. (1990). The assessment of bilingual students: A sorting mechanism. In S. Goldberg (Ed.), *Readings on equal education: Vol. 10. Critical issues for a new administration and Congress* (pp. 293–314). New York: AMS Press.

McDonald, D. (1989, August 2). Stuck in the horizon: A special report on the education of Native Americans. *Education Week, 9,* 1–16.

Medicine, B. (1979). Bilingual education and public policy: The cases of the American Indian. In R. V. Padilla (Ed.), *Ethnoperspectives in bilingual education research: Bilingual education and public policy in the United States* (pp. 395–407). Ipsilanti: Eastern Michigan University.

Mercer, J. (1973). *Labeling the mentally retarded.* Los Angeles: University of California Press.

Michaels, S. (1981). "Sharing time": Children's narrative styles and differential access to literacy. *Language in Society, 10,* 423–442.

Miyanaga, K. (1991). *The creative edge: Emerging individualism in Japan.* New Brunswick, NJ: Transaction Publishers.

Moore, R. B. (1995). Racism in the English language. In P. S. Rothenberg (Ed.), *Race, class, and gender in the United States: An integrated study* (pp. 376–386). New York: St. Martin's Press.

National Coalition of Advocates for Students. (1985). *Barriers to excellence: Our children at risk.* Boston: Author.

Native American Languages Act of 1992, 106 Stat. 3434 (1993).

Nieto, S. (1992). *Affirming diversity: The sociopolitical context of multicultural education.* New York: Longman.

Oakes, J. (1985). *Keeping track: How schools structure inequality.* New Haven, CT: Yale University Press.

Office of Civil Rights. (1978). *1976 elementary and secondary schools civil rights survey.* Washington, DC: U.S. Department of Education.

Office of Civil Rights. (1980). *1978 elementary and secondary schools civil rights survey*. Washington, DC: U.S. Department of Education.

Office of Civil Rights. (1982). *1980 elementary and secondary schools civil rights survey*. Washington, DC: U.S. Department of Education.

Office of Civil Rights. (1984). *1982 elementary and secondary schools civil rights survey*. Washington, DC: U.S. Department of Education.

Office of Civil Rights. (1988). *1986 elementary and secondary schools civil rights survey*. Washington, DC: U.S. Department of Education.

Office of Civil Rights. (1990). *1988 elementary and secondary schools civil rights survey*. Washington, DC: U.S. Department of Education.

Office of Civil Rights. (1992). *1990 elementary and secondary schools civil rights survey*. Washington, DC: U.S. Department of Education.

Ovando, C. J., & Gourd, K. (1996). Knowledge construction, language maintenance, revitalization, and empowerment. In J. A. Banks (Ed.), *Multicultural education: Transformative knowledge and action*. New York: Teachers College Press.

Owens, R. E., Jr. (1992). *Language development*. New York: Merrill/Macmillan.

Paulston, C. B. (1980). *Bilingual education: Theories and issues*. Rowley, MA: Newbury House.

Perkins, D. (1995). *Outsmarting IQ: The emerging science of learnable intelligence*. New York: Free Press.

Persell, C. H. (1993). Social class and educational equality. In J. A. Banks & C. A. M. Banks (Eds.), *Multicultural education: Issues and perspectives* (2nd ed., pp. 297–322). Needham Heights, MA: Allyn & Bacon.

Philips, S. U. (1972). Participant structures and communicative competence: Warm Springs children in community and classroom. In C. B. Cazden, V. P. John, & D. Hymes (Eds.), *Functions of language in the classroom* (pp. 370–394). New York: Teachers College Press.

Philips, S. U. (1983). *The invisible culture: Communication in classroom and community on the Warm Springs Indian reservation*. White Plains, NY: Longman.

Philips, S. U., Steele, S., & Tanz, C. (Eds.). (1987). *Language, gender and sex in comparative perspective*. New York: Cambridge University Press.

Poplin, M. (1989, May). *Education and the revitalization of America*. Paper presented at the President's Forum, Claremont Graduate School, CA.

Poplin, M. (1992). Educating in diversity. In P. F. Drucker (Ed.), *Educating for results* (pp. 18–24). Baltimore: National School Boards Association.

Ramirez, M., & Castañeda, A. (1974). *Cultural democracy, bicognitive development and education*. New York: Academic Press.

Reyes, M. de la Luz. (1987). Comprehension of content area passages: A study of Spanish/English readers in third and fourth grade. In S. R. Goldman & H. T. Trueba (Eds.), *Becoming literate in English as a second language* (pp. 107–126). Norwood, NJ: Ablex.

Reyes, M. de la Luz. (1991). The "one size fits all" approach to literacy. *Invited Symposium on Literacy and Cultural Diversity: Voices, visibility, and empowerment*. Paper presented at the American Educational Research Association Conference, Chicago.

Reyes, M. de la Luz. (1992). Challenging venerable assumptions: Literacy instruction for linguistically different students. *Harvard Educational Review*, *62*(4), 427–446.

Reyhmer, J. (1992). Policies toward American Indian languages: A historical sketch. In J. Crawford (Ed.), *Language loyalties: A source book on the official English controversy* (pp. 41–47). Chicago: University of Chicago Press.

Rigg, P. (1989). Language experience approach: Reading naturally. In P. Rigg & V. G. Allen (Eds.), *When they don't all speak English: Integrating the ESL student into the regular classroom* (pp. 65–76). Urbana, IL: National Council of Teachers of English.

Roseberry-McKibbin, C. A., & Eicholtz, G. E. (1994). Serving children with Limited English Proficiency in the schools: A national survey. *Language, Speech, and Hearing Services in the Schools, 25*, 156–164.

Rosier, P., & Holm, W. (1980). *The Rock Point experience: A longitudinal study of a Navajo school program*. Washington, DC: Center for Applied Linguistics.

Ruiz, N. (1989). An optimal learning environment for Rosemary. *Exceptional Children, 56*(2), 130–144.

Sadker, M., & Sadker, D. (1994). *Failing at fairness: How America's schools cheat girls*. New York: Scribner.

Sadker, M., & Sadker, D. (1995). Sexism in the schoolroom of the eighties. *Psychology Today*, pp. 54–57.

Samuda, R. J., & Lewis, J. (1992). Evaluation practices for the multicultural classroom. In C. Diaz (Ed.), *Multicultural education for the 21st century* (pp. 97–111). Washington, DC: National Education Association.

Saravia-Shore, M., & Arvizu, S. F. (1992). *Cross-cultural literacy: Ethnographies of communication in multiethnic classrooms*. New York: Garland.

Schieffelin, B. B. (1979). Getting it together: An ethnographic approach to the study of the development of communicative competence. In E. Ochs & B. B. Schieffelin (Eds.), *Developmental pragmatics* (pp. 73–108). New York: Academic Press.

Sewell, W. H. (1971). Inequality of opportunity for higher education. *American Sociological Review, 36*(5), 793–809.

Siddle, E. V. (1986). *A critical assessment of the natural approach to teaching writing*. Unpublished qualifying paper, Harvard University, Cambridge, MA.

Skutnabb-Kangas, T. (1981). *Bilingualism or not: The education of minorities*. Clevedon, England: Multilingual Matters.

Slavin, R. E. (1983). *Cooperative learning*. New York: Longman.

Slobin, D. (1983). *The acculturation and development of language in Mexican American children* (National Institutes of Education Publication No. G-81-0103). Washington, DC: U.S. Department of Education.

Steffensen, M. S., Joag-dev, C., & Anderson, R. C. (1979). A cross-cultural perspective on reading comprehension. *Reading Research Quarterly, 15*(10), 10–29.

Stigler, J., & Perry, M. (1988). Mathematics learning in Japanese, Chinese, and American classrooms. In G. Saxe & M. Gearhart (Eds.), *Children's mathematics* (pp. 27–54) (Vol. 41 in *New directions for child development* series). San Francisco: Jossey-Bass.

Stockman, I. (1986). Language acquisition in culturally diverse populations: The black child as a case study. In O. L. Taylor (Ed.), *Nature of communication disorders in culturally and linguistically diverse populations* (pp. 114–155). San Diego: College Hill.

Swain, M. (1985). Communicative competence: Some roles of comprehensible input and comprehensible output in its development. In S. Gass & C. Madden (Eds.), *Input in second language acquisition* (pp. 235–253). Cambridge, MA: Newbury House.

Takada, N., & Hanahan, E. (1995, December). *Japanese-influenced English*. Paper presented at the American Speech and Hearing Association Conference, Orlando, FL.

Tannen, D. (1986). *That's not what I meant! How conversational style makes or breaks your relations with others*. New York: Morrow.

Tannen, D. (1990). *You just don't understand: Women and men in conversation*. New York: Ballantine.

Tannen, D. (1993). *Gender and conversational interaction*. New York: Oxford University Press.

Tannen, D. (1994). *Gender and discourse*. New York: Oxford University Press.

Tannen, D. (1997). Women and men talking: An interactional sociolinguistic approach. In M. R. Walsh (Ed.), *Women, men, and gender* (pp. 82–90). Rensselaer, NY: Hamilton.

Taylor, O. L., Payne, K. T., & Anderson, N. B. (1987). Distinguishing between communication disorders and communication differences. *Seminars in Speech and Language*, 8(4), 415–427.

Tharp, R. G. (1989). Psychocultural variables and constants: Effect on teaching and learning in schools. *American Psychologist, 44*(2), 349–359.

Tharp, R. G., Dalton, S., & Yamauchi, L. A. (1994). Principles for culturally compatible Native American education. *Journal of Navajo Education, 11*(3), 33–39.

Valdes, G. (1986). *Brothers and sisters: A closer look at the development of "cooperative" social orientation in Mexican-American children*. Paper presented at the 37th Annual Convention of the California Association of School Psychologists, Oakland.

Vasquez, O. A. (1993). A look at language as a resource: Lessons from La Clase Magica. In M. B. Arias & U. Casanova (Eds.), *Bilingual education: Politics, practice, and research* (pp. 1–14). Chicago: University of Chicago Press.

Willig, A., & Swedo, J. (1987). *Improving teaching strategies for exceptional Hispanic limited English proficient students: An exploratory study of task engagement and teaching strategies*. Paper presented at the annual meeting of the American Educational Research Association, Washington, DC.

Wong Fillmore, L. (1991). Second language learning in children: A model of language learning in social context. In E. Bialystok (Ed.), *Language processing in bilingual children* (pp. 49–69). Cambridge, England: Cambridge University Press.

Worth, S., & Adair, J. (1972). *Through Navajo eyes*. Bloomington: University of Indiana Press.

Ebonics and Hispanic, Asian, and Native American Dialects of English

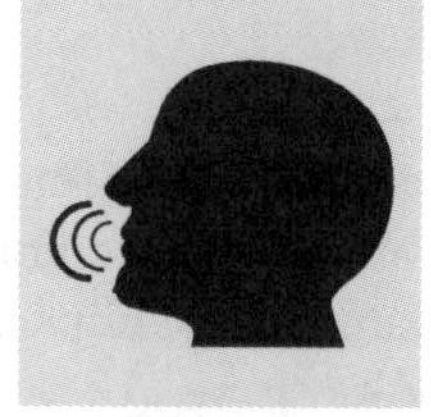

Chapter 6

D. Kim Reid

As noted in Chapter 5, the most efficacious approach to teaching students whose native language or dialect is not Standard American English (SAE) is to accept and respect the languages or dialects of their homes and build metacognitive bridges that promote understanding of the relationships that exist between the home dialect or language and SAE (Gee, 1990). Otherwise, we either denigrate the home culture or limit the students' opportunities to acquire the goods and services that, for better or worse, in our society are linked to the competent and appropriate use of the dominant language—SAE.

Consequently, general education teachers and specialists (i.e., bilingual, English as a Second Language [ESL], and special education teachers, and speech–language pathologists [SLPs]) must both learn about the material existence of the students they teach (Friere, 1998)—that is, gain some understanding of what their lives are like and the factors that support or impinge on their learning—and have some understanding of the ways that the students' native languages and cultures work. Proper assessment and instruction depend on the use of strategies that take the nature of the first language into account. For example, the prevalence of communication disorders among Native American students was estimated to be 5 to 15 times the rate of the general population, until researchers discovered that their phonological "errors" were predictable from the characteristics of their ancestral language (McCardle & Walton, 1995). Consequently, teachers and SLPs cannot make decisions about what is a predictable and rule-governed deviation from SAE and what constitutes a communication disorder without learning something about the characteristics of the child's home language.

Furthermore, because no teacher or SLP can learn about the full range of dialects or languages that students might bring to the classroom (in some school districts 100 or more languages are spoken), educationists are often dependent for help on other school personnel or older students, peers, parent volunteers, and so forth—anyone who knows a particular student's language and is available to help. This chapter is designed to introduce teachers (both of general and special education) and SLPs to some of the more salient characteristics of the communication patterns used by speakers of common "other-language" groups in the United States—African, Hispanic, Asian, and Native Americans.

Some General Comments

In his review of the literature on dual language acquisition, Garcia (1995a) noted that children who learn two languages simultaneously during their first 8 years of life typically have little difficulty acquiring both. Sometimes, early on, they mix the two languages together, but, by school age, grammatical forms develop independently. Although the languages are learned in parallel, one language may develop more rapidly than the other or be preferred over the other, or the two languages may develop at about an equal pace. There is no indication that learning one language interferes with learning another for those who are developing normally. There was some fear during the early 1970s that perhaps learning two languages would be associated with social or cognitive delays (Garcia, 1995a; Peters-Johnson, 1995), but that is not the case. Of course, those children with language disorders of one kind or another may experience difficulties.

Furthermore, although we tend to focus on the differences that dialects and languages make, those differences are more limited than was previously thought. All languages make use of the major language systems, such as phonology, morphology, and syntax or their equivalent (e.g., the motor productions of sign language). Additionally, some universals appear to exist among these systems. Semantic and pragmatic abilities, although their nature certainly varies across cultures, develop in a similar fashion regardless of the particular language or dialect that the child learns to speak. For example, Stockman and Vaughn-Cooke (1995) concluded that students tend to use the same semantic categories whether they speak SAE, Ebonics, Finnish, Italian, Serbo-Croatian, Samoan, or Turkish. The experience and maturation that accrue with age are more important to semantic development than the particular language spoken, and variations tend to occur within linguistic groups as a function of home environment. Similarly, Peters-Johnson (1995) concluded that students, regardless of the particular language or dialect they speak, develop the same types of pragmatic skills (e.g., those for initiating, maintaining, repairing, and terminating a conversation), although there may be some variation in the nature, rate, scope, or sequence of that development. Pragmatics development co-occurs with other social, cognitive, and linguistic developments. In short, any language/dialect is as good as any other in promoting social, cognitive, and linguistic growth. As noted in the discussion on Ebonics that comes later in this chapter, the perspective for making judgments about the value of any given language is actually ideological. As linguists are fond of saying, it is he who has the guns (i.e., the power) who determines what the standard language will be ("Linguists Find the Debate over 'Ebonics' Uninformed," 1997).

As noted in Chapter 5, when there is a clash between home and school languages or dialects, difficulties often arise. In this case, the native language or dialect may be treated as if it were somehow unacceptable, may be lost, or may influence the learning of a second language. Some students maintain or prefer the home language. Some, because there is no longer any instruction in the first language or because they have learned to be ashamed of it, come to prefer the second. Some never learn either language very well, or some, like the Puerto Ricans in the northeastern United States, may develop a dialect that combines two or more other languages or dialects.

In the United States today, because many new immigrant groups as well as other-language groups who have lived here for generations openly strive to maintain their identities, there is a strong movement among conservatives to pass English-only legislation, that is, to make English the official language (Baron, 1990). About one third of U.S. states have an English-only or an English-plus (English plus one other language) law. Many others have legislation pending. Still others, although they do not have "official language" statutes, do require English for official notices, legislation, and schooling. Proponents of English-only legislation are trying to (a) make certain that English remains the unifying language of the land and (b) simultaneously protect "American culture" as they understand it.

Influenced English

Languages are always in a state of flux. They are changed from the inside by native speakers and from the outside by contacts with speakers of other languages. Usually, the impact of native speakers is more restricted—that is, limited to more specific and more narrowly defined changes—but it is also most often permanent and passed on to subsequent generations. One common example is the current widespread acceptance of a grammatical construction previously considered to be incorrect: "Everybody must bring their lunch" (instead of the technically correct "Everybody must bring his or her lunch"). Changes imposed by other-language speakers tend to be more idiosyncratic—that is, related to their personal stage of English acquisition and the structures and mores of their native tongues.

Wolfram (1995a) illustrated the kinds of changes that affect each of the English language systems. Some grammatical changes, such as the omission of the 's' on third-person singular verbs (e.g., "she walk" instead of "she walks"), are equally apparent among native and other-language speakers. The reason is that they are simplifications that regularize usage and eliminate irregularities. Other changes related to grammar, such as those related to word order or the use of pronouns and auxiliary verbs, are more highly associated with speakers of English as a second language and are dependent on the rules of the original language. For example, speakers of Japanese or Vietnamese, whose languages do not include the articles *the* and *a,* may drop the article in English (e.g., "Old man saw bird in park"). Or, Navajos may change the word order from the traditional English subject–verb–object sequence (e.g., "The woman likes the class") to a more typically Navajo subject–object–verb format (e.g., "The woman the class likes").

Wolfram (1995a) noted that phonological differences also exist across languages and within a given language across time and distance. Different ways of producing particular sounds are what give us our "accents." We notice these differences as early as 3 to 5 years of age and they often complicate our spelling. For example, the *gh* in *through* or *bought* had its own pronunciation (something akin to an 'x' sound) in the English spoken centuries ago, but that sound has now been lost, although the form of the written word remains unchanged. Phonological differences in English are also apparent among native speakers of other languages. For example, Latinos do not differentiate between the sounds of *v* and *b,* Vietnamese between *sh* and *s,* and speakers of some Southern and Puerto Rican dialects retain the old English pronunciation of certain words (e.g., *ask* is pronounced as "aks"). Consonant clusters, such as *-st* in *west, sch* in *school,* are particularly vulnerable to change. Very few other languages in the world use these clusters, so they are typically dropped or modified by speakers of English as a second language. Vietnamese Americans, for example, might say "lap" for *lapse* and, like their Hispanic American neighbors, are likely to add an 'e' before an initial consonant cluster: *school* becomes "eschool." Understanding something about the speakers' first language is, therefore, essential in determining what is a "normal" deviation and what might be a clue to a language or articulation deficit or disability.

Finally, Wolfram (1995a) reminded us that language usage varies across languages and dialects, time, and place. There are differences, for example, in how direct we expect people to be. Southerners tend to regard the directness of Northeasterners as rudeness, for example, whereas Asians often fail to achieve their communicative purposes because they are so indirect that the message does not come through to native speakers of English (e.g., "I was happy to take the test" actually is intended to mean "May I please have the scores?"). Similarly, ritualized behaviors, such as greetings (e.g., "How are you?"), may be intended to open a conversation in one culture, but to ask for information in another. Permissible topics of conversation vary from culture to culture (e.g., an Asian may comment that a woman has gained weight) and the means of securing and yielding conversational turns vary as well. I can remember telephoning the family with whom I lived one summer in Guatemala and nervously talking and talking and talking, because I did not know how to terminate the phone conversation. When I subsequently visited, I asked my hostess and learned that "Bueno" is the signal you give to indicate that you are preparing to hang up.

Teachers and SLPs, then, must be willing (and learn how) to determine speakers' underlying intentions in conversation and to resist the temptation to respond to other-language speakers with the same sensibilities that they apply when interacting with native English speakers, especially those from the same region who speak the same dialect. It has been noted repeatedly in the literature, for example, that European American, middle class teachers who expect class members to be silent until called on and to raise their hands to obtain permission to speak are often disconcerted by more spontaneous African and Hispanic American students who tend to talk more, without invitation, and at different times. In the following sections I examine some of the characteristics of languages and dialects that teachers and SLPs are likely to encounter in U.S. schools.

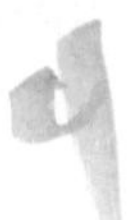

Ebonics

Ebonics, sometimes also called Black Vernacular English or Black English, is a highly controversial language spoken predominantly by working class African Americans (Labov, 1972), although it is also the language of some Puerto Ricans, European Americans, and Native Americans who live in certain urban and rural areas (Dillard, 1972; Wolfram, 1972, 1973). As noted previously in Chapter 1, for years, people have thought of Ebonics as "bad English" or "street English," but in fact most linguists now agree that it is a language (with many West African linguistic structures) in its own right—or at least a creole (Dillard, 1972; Stewart, 1970) and what distinguishes between a language and a creole is still open to debate ("Linguists," 1997). One of the reasons that Ebonics is so controversial is that the general public's attitudes toward this language are confounded by the emotionalism of widespread racism and classism. Furthermore, there is more overlap between English and Ebonics than, for example, English and Spanish or Japanese. Additionally, because of their constant exposure to and immersion in the SAE of the dominant society, some African Americans mix dialects. They even may shift between Ebonics and SAE within the same situation (Cole, 1995a). Nevertheless, Ebonics is a coherent language with its own regularities; its rules differ in at least 37 ways from SAE (Owens, 1999).

Although the use of Ebonics is typically associated with social class, one cannot simply assume that an inner-city, poor African American child, for example, uses Ebonics. Many, depending on aspirations, family history, and so forth, acquire SAE. Probably the best strategy is to visit with the student's primary caretaker to determine what language or dialect is being learned at home, and to remember that developmental phenomena apply. One cannot expect a young speaker of Ebonics to have mastered the full range of sounds and structures that are common to adult speakers. Furthermore, there is not one form of Ebonics. Ebonics, like other languages, has various dialects. The Gullah dialect of the coastal islands of South Carolina and Georgia, the Haitian and Jamaican dialects, and the dialects of Trinidad and the Virgin Islands are only a few examples. There are, in addition, subtle variations in other regional dialects within the United States. For example, Seymour and Seymour (1995) detected dialectal differences between the Ebonics of African Americans in Massachusetts and those in New York.

Cole (1995b; see also Labov, 1966, 1972; Owens, 1999) noted that the comparisons between Ebonics and SAE can be clustered into five categories: common features, non-obligatory features, regularized features, alternative features, and differences. Tables 6.1 through 6.5 present a sampling of those comparisons (please note that some of the structures differ in the Caribbean dialects). Common features (see Table 6.1) refer to those aspects of Ebonics and SAE that are the same (e.g., verb tenses, question types, word order). Because the greatest proportion of features of the two languages are the same, their speakers are mutually intelligible. Features required in SAE that are non-obligatory in Ebonics (see Table 6.2) include markers for pluralization, possession, past tense, and the verb *to be*. In some instances, Ebonics regularizes forms that are irregular in SAE, such as the consistent use of *a* whether or not the following word begins with a vowel (see Table 6.3). In the table on alternative features (Table 6.4), replacements, transformations, and semantic components that are roughly equivalent in the two languages are illustrated. Finally, in Table 6.5, examples of structures that have no equivalents in SAE are presented (e.g., ending a question that begins with *where* with the word *at*). Although these are only a few of the significant differences between Ebonics and SAE, the teacher and SLP can begin to develop some expectations for the language forms students might use in school and, therefore, be able to say to

Table 6.1
Some Important Features Shared by Ebonics and Standard American English

Vocabulary	Word order	Stress and intonation
Conjunctions	Gender	Clauses
Tense	Number	Modifiers
Prepositions	Person	Question types

Note. Adapted from *Black English in the United States and the Caribbean,* by L. Cole, 1995 (December), paper presented at the annual meeting of the American Speech-Language-Hearing Association, Orlando, FL.

Table 6.2
Features Required in Standard American English, but Non-obligatory in Ebonics

1. Count nouns need not be pluralized by adding *-s* or *-es.* Pluralization can be denoted by a number or other linguistic cue.

   Example: six desk

2. Possession need not be marked by *-'s* or *-s'.*

   Example: Tom aunt

3. There is no need to mark past tense when the verb ends with a consonant cluster, such as the *-st* in *west, -nd* in *find,* or *-ld* in *cold.*

   Example: He hand me the plate.

   When the verb ends with *-t* or *-d* and is followed by an infinitive phrase or a participle, the final consonant is dropped and the *-ed* reduced to simply *d.*

   Example: They started playing. (Remove final *-t* sound and omit *i* sound.)

   They stard playing.

4. *Is* and *are* are optional in content questions and interrogative reversals, but the question intonation is retained.

   Examples: It a big house?
   That your house?

Note. Adapted from *Black English in the United States and the Caribbean,* by L. Cole, 1995 (December), paper presented at the annual meeting of the American Speech-Language-Hearing Association, Orlando, FL.

Table 6.3
Irregular Standard American English Forms Regularized in Ebonics

1. In SAE, speakers add *-s* to the third-person singular, as in "He walks." That marker is redundant, because we know from *he* that the verb is in the third-person singular form. Ebonics regularizes the verb form, dropping the *-s*.

   Example: I talk, you talk, he talk, we talk, you talk, they talk
2. Similarly, use of the verb *to be* in the past tense shifts from *was* to *were* in all but the first- and third-person singular forms. Again the shift denotes a double, or redundant, marking, because of the presence of the pronoun. Ebonics regularizes the form.

   Example: I was, you was, he was, we was, you was, they was
3. In SAE, there are two forms of the indefinite article: *a* and before a vowel *an*. Ebonics regularizes the form.

   Example: a angle
4. In SAE, reflexive pronouns are formed by adding the syllable *self* to the possessive pronoun (e.g., *myself, yourself*), except for the third-person singular and plural forms in which the objective form of the pronoun is used (e.g., *himself, itself, themselves*). In Ebonics, those forms are regularized.

   Example: myself, yourself, herself, himself, itself, ourself, themself
5. In SAE, *those* is the demonstrative pronoun used in subjects and *them* is the form used as an object. In Ebonics, only the form *them* is used.

   Example: them apples
6. In SAE, all pronouns indicate number (e.g., *I, she, he, it, we, they*) except the second person in which *you* is used to indicate both singular and plural. In Ebonics, the form is regularized.

   Example: you (singular form), you all (plural form)

Note. Adapted from *Black English in the United States and the Caribbean,* by L. Cole, 1995 (December), paper presented at the annual meeting of the American Speech-Language-Hearing Association, Orlando, FL.

students, "In Ebonics, you say it this way. In English, it looks like this." Drawing such metacognitively explicit comparisons helps students learn to cross linguistic boundaries.

The controversy over the acceptance of Ebonics as a legitimate language continues to rage. During the fall of 1997, the Oakland, California, Board of Education received national media attention ("A Crisis in Any Language," 1997; "Ebonics," 1997; Fox, 1997; Gibbs, 1997; Golden, 1997; Hitchens, 1997; Leland & Joseph, 1997; Leo, 1997; Menand, 1997; "Oakland School Board,"

Table 6.4
Features Roughly Equivalent in Standard American English and Ebonics

1. In the first-person singular future, the forms *going to* or *gonna* replace the verb *will.* In Ebonics, *I'm gonna* often becomes contracted to *I'ma* or *I'mo.*
2. In SAE, to form the negative of the verb *to be* or auxiliary verbs, such as *have, not* is added in contracted or uncontracted forms: *am not, hasn't.* In Ebonics, *ain't* is often substituted.

   Examples: I ain't goin.

   He ain't told me nothin.
3. In SAE, double negatives are not permissible; in Ebonics the more negatives, the more negative the meaning.

   Example: I ain't gonna go no more no how!
4. In SAE, a clause that raises a question is embedded by changing it to its declarative form (e.g., The question "Is it raining?" becomes the statement, "It is raining") and then adding the word *if* or *whether* (e.g., "He wondered if it is raining"). In Ebonics, the question is simply added, without the transformation to a statement and without the use of a subordinator (i.e., *if* or *whether*).

   Example: He wanna know is it rainin.
5. In SAE, the verb *to be* can be replaced by the verb *to go* to indicate a change in location (e.g., "Here we go." "There goes the bus."). In Ebonics, *go* can be substituted without implying a change in location.

   Example: Here we go. (meaning "Here we are.")

   There go the store. (meaning "There is the store.")
6. In SAE, the superlative is formed by adding *-est* or by the formation of an adverbial phrase (e.g., *very fast*). In Ebonics, reduplication is used.

   Example: Sam run fast-fast-fast.

   Some days it cold-cold.

Note. Adapted from *Black English in the United States and the Caribbean,* by L. Cole, 1995 (December), paper presented at the annual meeting of the American Speech-Language-Hearing Association, Orlando, FL.

1997; Sowell, 1997, White, 1997) when it proposed educating teachers about the characteristics of Ebonics—not, as the media implied, to replace SAE with Ebonics, but as a way of educating teachers to the structure of the language so that they would understand how it works, be more accepting of it, learn that it was not deficient English, and be able, through that knowledge, to help students make the transition to SAE. The misrepresentation of the School Board's intent led to condemnations from African and European Americans alike. The

Table 6.5
Ebonics Forms for Which There Are No Standard American English Equivalents

1. In SAE, aspect—the distribution of an action or state across points in time—is denoted by the use of an adverb (e.g., *sometimes, frequently*) or an adverbial phrase (e.g., *most of the time*). In Ebonics, *be* is used to denote a state or action intermittently distributed over time.

   Example: He be talking on the phone.
   (meaning "He frequently talks on the phone.")

2. In SAE, speakers use *has* or *have* to show that an event or state that began in the past continues to have an effect in the present (e.g., "He has had that car for a very long time"). In Ebonics, the form *been* is used as an auxiliary verb.

   Example: He been had that car.

3. In SAE, the use of *at* at the end of a question that begins with *where* is considered redundant. In Ebonics, it is used at the end of a question that begins with *where* and at the end of an embedded question formed with *where.*

   Example: Where is my jacket at?
   I wonder where my jacket is at?

4. There are some forms in Ebonics that are considered overcorrections of SAE forms.

   Examples: childrens (which is plural without the -*s*)
   mine's (which is possessive without the -*'s*)

Note. Adapted from *Black English in the United States and the Caribbean,* by L. Cole, 1995 (December), paper presented at the annual meeting of the American Speech-Language-Hearing Association, Orlando, FL.

American Society of Linguists ("Linguists," 1997), however, putting ideological considerations aside, unanimously passed a resolution that called the Oakland proposal "linguistically and pedagogically sound" for the reasons that have been stated repeatedly in this book: Students learn best and most rapidly when educationists begin by accepting the language or dialect of the home and teach them SAE through immersion and metacognitive instruction.

Spanish-Influenced English and Dialects

The first area of what is now the United States was settled in 1508 by Ponce de León, only 15 years after the arrival of Columbus. Consequently, Spanish was in use in what is now Florida and the Southwest even before English became the language of the colonies. Although today most people consider the United States to be an English-speaking nation, it is also the fifth largest Spanish-speaking country in the world (Dato, 1995). Six major Spanish dialects are represented on the mainland—those associated with Mexico and the Southwestern United States, Central America, the Caribbean, the Highlands, Chile, and Southern South America (i.e., Paraguay, Uruguay, and Argentina). The most widely used dialects, however, are those of the Southwest and the Caribbean.

As might be expected, the most highly influenced English is that of native Spanish speakers who are learning English. What are often interpreted as "errors" made by given speakers are usually a reflection of both their specific dialect and their stage of development in learning English. Before they master the rules of English, Spanish speakers frequently transfer the rules for use of their mother tongue to their use of English. A sampling of specific characteristics associated with Spanish-influenced English are presented in Table 6.6 (see Owens, 1999, for a more complete listing). By the second generation, although there are distinctive dialects of English that characterize, for instance, Chicano from Puerto Rican English, those dialects adhere much more closely to the standard regional dialect or to the national dialect (the English of schooling and TV, i.e., SAE) and many of the Spanish influences apparent in the English of first-generation immigrants are lost. Thompson (1974) pointed out that the problem then becomes not one of Spanish interfering with or competing with English, but one of a *nonstandard dialect competing with SAE*.

Chicano English

Penalosa (1995) summarized the research on Chicano English. Chicano English is the first and only language of many hundreds of thousands of residents of California, Texas, and other areas of the Southwest. It is a dialect that is obviously related to Spanish, but is nevertheless independent from it. Although it resulted from the dialect that was created by attempts of Mexicans to learn English as a second language and showed marked influences from Spanish, Chicano English now serves as the only means of communication in many Hispanic American communities where Spanish is no longer spoken.

Not surprisingly, because of widespread prejudices, Chicano English suffers from low prestige and the fact that its speakers are often isolated from the mainstream linguistic community. With few exceptions, Chicanos use syntactic and morphological styles consistent with expectations for their socioeconomic class. Among the few syntactic deviations specific to their dialect are the occasional use of Spanish sentence structure ("Is hot today"); the pluralization of

Table 6.6
Hispanic American English

Phonological Differences

Hispanic American English	Standard American English
beeg	big
cet	cat
cot	cut
choe	shoe
butch	bush
soo	zoo
tum	thumb
dough	though
ban	van
rin	ring
sin	sing
gick	kick
lok	log

Syntactic Differences

1. The verb *to be* is eliminated.

   Example: He goin.

2. *Has* and *have* are substituted for *to be.*

   Example: He has 8 year.

3. The third-person singular present is regularized.

   Example: He talk.

4. Past-tense marker is omitted.

   Example: I work yesterday. (meaning "I worked yesterday.")

5. Adverbs of place are put close to the verb.

   Example: He put below the pot.

6. Use of adjectives rather than the comparative *(-er)* and superlative *(-est)* forms.

   Example: more big

7. Subject pronouns are frequently omitted, when the meaning is clear without it.

   Example: Bob got a car. I think will like it.

8. Articles are often omitted.

   Example: He is handsome kid.

9. *Do* is omitted in questions.

   Example: You want to go?

10. *No* is used as the form of the negative.

    Example: No leave the room.

Note. Adapted from *Language Disorders: A Functional Approach to Assessment and Intervention* (3rd ed.), by R. E. Owens, 1999, Needham Heights, MA: Allyn & Bacon. Copyright 1999 by Allyn & Bacon. Adapted with permission.

nominalized adjectives, such as "the bads"—a literal translation of the Spanish "los malos"; and the tendency to use Latin cognates (e.g., *wash* rather than *do* the dishes). Chicano English is much less formal than SAE. One of its most distinctive characteristics is its intonation, which Cheech and Chong used to great advantage to create satirical humor in their movies.

Several decades ago, Sawyer (1970) reported that Chicanos in Texas were so concerned about "corrupting" their English that they would not even use the terms from Spanish that have been assimilated into English (e.g., *patio, bronco, burro, plaza*). Today, however, many Chicano youth, especially college students and other intellectuals, use Spanish pronunciations of place names and other Spanish words, even when speaking unaccented SAE.

Puerto Rican English

Wolfram (1995b) studied the English of second-generation Puerto Rican youth growing up in New York City. He reported that Puerto Rican English shares many of the characteristics of the Ebonics spoken by the surrounding community—dropping of final consonants, reduction of consonant clusters, elimination of the verb *to be* in sentences such as "You ugly," the sole use of *a* as the indefinite article, inclusion of multiple negatives, regularizing of irregular verbs, and so forth.

Some dialectal characteristics are, however, distinctly Puerto Rican. For example, words ending in *-s* plus *p, t,* or *k* add *-es* (rather than *-s*) to form the plural. As a result, *desk, ghost,* and *wasp* become in their plural forms *desses, ghosses,* and *wasses*. Like Chicano English, Puerto Rican English is characterized by its intonation and also its rhythms. Spanish intonation spans a smaller range of highs and lows than English, so Puerto Rican English tends to sound monotonal to English speakers. Furthermore, Wolfram explained that in Spanish the pronunciation of each syllable is given an equal amount of time (called *syllable-timing*), whereas in English speakers tend to lengthen the duration of a stressed word (called *phrase-timing*). For example, if one were to say "The boy pet the DOG," the words preceding dog would be uttered more quickly than the word *dog*. Similarly, if one were to say "The boy PET the dog," the word *pet* would receive the longest duration. When compared to the rhythmical phrase-timing of English, the syllable-timing of the Puerto Rican dialect gives the impression of a short and choppy cadence. Finally, the word *no* is used in place of all forms of English negation among Spanish-influenced English speakers. Even among second-generation speakers there are still some vestiges of this exclusive use of *no*, especially when *don't* would be the standard English form. Thus, a Puerto Rican would be likely to say, "They no like it."

Teachers and SLPs must keep this process of linguistic evolution in mind—from Spanish (or other language), to Spanish-influenced English, to nonstandard dialect—when assessing the language skills of Hispanic American (and other) children. *Even though parents report that English is the language of the home, the linguistic environment to which the children are exposed is often not SAE.* Consequently, procedures for assessing language competency and performance of second-generation students entering school must approximate those of students whose home language is not any form of English. Assessment is facilitated when the SLP or psychologist is also a member of the Chicano, Puerto Rican, or other speech community. However, when that is not the case, Eblen (1995) recommends that the tester invite a parent or other family member to the testing session, so that a model of the adult phonological and communication patterns is available. That way, the educational team (i.e., teacher, SLP, psychologist, and, if warranted, perhaps a bilingual, ESL, or special education teacher) can sort out what are nonstandard patterns established in the child's speech community and what is idiosyncratic and, hence, more likely problematic. Failure to recognize the linguistic needs of such students has led many of them to "fall between the cracks"—exhibiting low achievement without qualifying for bilingual, ESL, or special education services, and therefore not getting the language instruction they need on how to cross the boundaries between Chicano, Puerto Rican, or other dialects and SAE. On the other hand, many of these students are diagnosed with special learning needs, when they are simply language different. Both outcomes are costly to the children, their families, and the nation.

In addition, Garcia (1995b) advocates that teachers and SLPs who work with Hispanic American children be reasonable in their expectations. For example, nearly all Hispanic Americans pronounce *para* (meaning *for* or *to*) as "pa" and conjugated forms of the verb *estar* (meaning *to be*) without the first syllable, for example "ta" (*esta* = *is*) or "taba" (*estaba* = *was*). Similarly, English speakers commonly say, "I'm gonna" ("I'm going to") or "Not par-ti-cu-ly" (rather than "not par-ti-cu-lar-ly"). Those who are teaching students must accept such "incorrect," but commonly used pronunciations and not hold students to higher standards of usage and pronunciation than are used in the linguistic community.

Finally, Hispanic American dialects, like Ebonics and SAE, are rule-governed and highly organized systems of communication, rather than poor approximations of SAE. Therefore, teaching must begin with a positive, respectful, and nonpaternalistic attitude toward the student's first language—whatever it may be. Wolfram (1995b) suggests that it is attitudes toward these dialects and not the dialects themselves that are the biggest problem Latino students face.

Asian-Influenced English

As with Latinos, we also tend to categorize Asians as a single cultural–linguistic group, when in fact they represent many, highly varied cultures. Their ancestral groups and histories, as well as their histories in this country, differ markedly. Many Chinese, for example, were imported as laborers during the middle of the 19th century, mostly to complete the transcontinental railroad. Takada and Hanahan (1995) noted that there are six different groups of Japanese currently in the United States with very different language profiles—some speak Japanese-influenced English, some use Hawaiian English, some are fluent in both Japanese and English, and others speak SAE as their first language. The Vietnamese, as a group, tend to be relatively recent immigrants and their numbers are small.

Linguistically, patterns similar to those of Hispanic Americans adhere: First-generation immigrants tend to develop a dialect of English that is heavily influenced by their native tongues. The second generation, however, typically acquires a nonstandard English dialect or SAE. In fact, rates of assimilation among linguistic groups have not changed much throughout the history of our nation (Baron, 1990). Asian languages tend to be quite different from English in phonology and syntax. Many are tonal; that is, a modulation in pitch can change the meaning of a word that is written and pronounced the same way. In the following sections I delineate some of the most salient characteristics of Chinese, Japanese, and Vietnamese that affect the ways in which their native speakers use English.

Chinese-Influenced English

There are 35 different dialects in the Chinese language, each with its own set of subdialectal variations. Unlike most of the dialects that have developed in the United States, Chinese dialects are *not mutually intelligible*; that is, speakers of one dialect cannot communicate with speakers of another. Nevertheless, these dialects *share a single system of writing*. Consequently, any given graphic character is associated with a host of oral realizations. Furthermore, word meaning is encoded by tones as well as phonemes.

Some of the other differences from English are summarized in Table 6.7 (Cheng, 1995). Chinese word forms remain stable, because inflections are not used. Instead, separate words are used to mark time, plurality, and questions. Whereas in English the basic sentence structure is subject–verb–object, Chinese uses two structures: subject–verb–object and subject–object–verb. Of course, as with any language there are differences in the use of idiomatic ex-

Table 6.7
Characteristics of Chinese that Influence English Usage

1. The plural in Chinese is marked by using a number word, rather than by adding a bound morpheme. Consequently, Chinese are likely to omit the final *-s, -es.*

   Example: two book

2. Tense is marked by a separate word. The past tense in the Mandarin, for example, is marked by adding *le* after the verb at the end of the sentence.

   Example: ta lai le (He come already.)

   Another way to express tense is to use an adverb of time, such as *yesterday* or *tomorrow.* Note that the form of the verb does not change.

   Example: wo min tien chu (I tomorrow go)
   wo zuo tien chu (I yesterday go)

3. Sentences are not transformed in order to form interrogatives. A questions marker *(ma)* is added.

   Example: ta gau ma (Is he tall?)

   Another way to form an interrogative is by coupling positive and negative forms.

   Example: ta gau bu gau? (He tall, not tall. = Is he tall?)

4. Chinese does not mark gender, such as *he, she,* and the neuter form, *it.*

   Example: He and his husband eat.

5. Chinese does not use the verb *to be.*

   Example: hwa hen mel (Flower very beautiful)

6. Chinese does not use the indefinite article.

   Example: I take lesson today.

Note. Adapted from *Chinese-Influenced English,* by L.-R. Cheng, 1995 (December), paper presented at the annual meeting of the American Speech-Language-Hearing Association, Orlando, FL. Adapted with permission.

pressions and conversational rules. In Chinese, for example, it is considered impolite for students to interrupt a teacher to ask questions or for a child to speak at the dinner table. Chinese are not encouraged to be emotionally demonstrative, and a giggle is more likely a sign of shyness than amusement.

Japanese-Influenced English

Takada and Hanahan (1995) articulated the major differences between English and Japanese. Probably the most significant is the importance of marking social stratification in Japanese. Speakers must select the proper level of politeness by taking into account the listener's age, gender, and social position; the occasion for the conversation; and the degree of familiarity between the conversants. Because they are often uncertain both about such relations in U.S. culture and about expressing such relations in English, Japanese speakers often prefer silence to small talk. A second striking difference is that the major purpose for communication among Japanese people is to create harmony and reach consensus. Accordingly, the negative marker does not appear in a sentence until just before the verb, which is always in the final position—a convenience that enables a speaker monitoring listeners' reactions to change his or her mind about using the negative. Takada and Hanahan also mention that, because of the focus on consensus in Japanese culture, Japanese tends to be much less precise than English, except in expressions that describe nature and natural phenomena. There are, for example, 10 words for rice.

English word order tends to be difficult for Japanese students to master. Their language is highly inflected, with subject, direct object, and indirect object markers attached to individual words. Attaching these endings enables them intelligibly to put particular words just about anywhere in the sentence, as long as the verb is last. Like Chinese, a sentence is made interrogative by adding a word (*ka*) at the end of a sentence. Some other differences, which we have also seen as characteristic of other languages, include using a number word to mark a plural, no plural form of demonstrative pronouns, differences in preposition usage, and the simplification of the third-person singular verb. In addition, speakers of Japanese often omit the verb altogether. See Table 6.8 for other differences that tend to affect the structure of English spoken specifically by the Japanese.

Japanese has 5 vowels and 35 consonants. The vowels approximate vowels in English, but there are several consonants in English that do not appear in Japanese (e.g., *f, v, l, r*) and *p, t,* and *b* are not aspirated to the same extent. Many consonant clusters in English are formed with *r* and *l*, but since these sounds are not distinguished in Japanese, all of those clusters present pronunciation problems for Japanese speakers learning English. Furthermore, every sound in Japanese is accompanied by a vowel (i.e., they use a consonant–vowel syllable structure as in *ka-ta-ka-na,* the name for one of the Japanese writing systems). As in most Spanish-influenced dialects, Japanese speakers also give equal stress to each syllable, creating a staccato-like impression.

Most English vocabulary is unknown to the Japanese (i.e., there are fewer cognates than there are with Spanish or French), but they have borrowed a few English words. These words are assimilated into the language in a variety of ways. For example, some are used as they are in English with Japanese pronunciations (*mo-no-re-e-ru = monorail*) and some are shortened by combining two

Table 6.8
Characteristics of Japanese that Influence English Usage

1. Word order is flexible, because inflected endings mark the grammatical function of various words: *wa* is the subject marker, *o* the direct object marker, and *ni* the indirect object marker.

   Example: Yesterday Sue-wa Bill-ni candy-o gave.
   Sue-wa Bill-ni candy-o yesterday gave.

2. Articles are absent in Japanese and are, therefore, likely to be left out in English.

   Example: Every day he take walk.

3. *Do* is not used as an auxiliary verb, so it is likely to be omitted in English.

   Example: What he carry to school?

4. When answering negative questions, speakers of Japanese respond to the correctness of the *person* asking the question, whereas English speakers respond to the correctness of the question itself.

   Example: Question: You're not coming?
   Answer: Yes, I am not coming. (English answer: No, I'm not.)

5. The impersonal *it* is not used in Japanese, so it is likely to be eliminated in English.

   Example: To bake take one hour.
   (English equivalent: It takes one hour to bake.)

6. The Japanese use gerunds and infinitives interchangeably, so they may not be distinguished in English sentences.

   Example: I am helping painting.
   (English equivalent: I am helping to paint.)

Note. Adapted from *Japanese-Influenced English,* by N. Takada and E. Hanahan, 1995 (December), paper presented at the annual meeting of the American Speech-Language-Hearing Association, Orlando, FL.

English words into one Japanese word (*waa-pu-ro* = *word processor* shortened from *waa-do pu-ro-se-saa*) (Takada & Hanahan, 1995).

For writing, the Japanese use three different systems. *Kanju* is their name for the system of Chinese ideographs or characters, and *hir-ra-ga-na* is a phonetic system used in combination with *kanju*. It takes knowledge of about 5,000 characters to be considered fully literate. The third system, *ka-ta-ka-na*, is also phonetic and is used to represent natural sounds and to indicate foreign words. The examples of their words for *monorail* and *word processor*, then, would be written in *ka-ta-ka-na*. Japanese is written from the top to the bottom of the page and from the right side to the left; however, because mathematics texts are written horizontally from left to right, Japanese children are usually familiar with the directionality of the English writing system, which typically presents no problem for them. When English is taught in Japan, as a transition step, Takada and Hanahan (1995) report that the students write Japanese sentences phonetically with the English alphabet.

Finally, the Japanese are socialized to be quite reserved, seldom revealing their emotions. Eye contact is not expected when answering teachers' questions. Asking a question is interpreted as questioning the teacher's authority or as showing off. However, Japanese students are also taught that learning requires diligence and hard work, which will eventually be rewarded.

Vietnamese-Influenced English

Hoi and Bich (1995) have written about Vietnamese-influenced English. One of the points they stress is that there are enormous differences in phonology between English and Vietnamese, which may have contributed to the fact that, although large numbers of U.S. troops were in Vietnam from 1959 to 1975 and interacted daily with the Vietnamese population, a Vietnamese–English pidgin never developed. To illustrate how extensive this difference is, the Center for Applied Linguistics (1981) reported that there are phonemes in English that do not exist in Vietnamese (e.g., *th* as in *thin*, usually pronounced by Vietnamese as *tin; j* as in *jump;* the *z* sound in *pleasure*) and phonemes that are distinguished in Vietnamese but not in English (e.g., the aspirated vs. nonaspirated *t,* (as in the contrast between *tip* and *Tom*). Furthermore, the Vietnamese do not use initial consonant clusters, so they are likely to insert a short vowel between the consonants (e.g., *stop* becomes "si-top") or, like Latinos, add a short vowel before the cluster (e.g., "es-pecial"). Neither do they use final consonant clusters or pronounce the final consonant of words. This difference between the two languages causes serious problems, because many final clusters in English are grammatical markers (e.g., *girls*). To complicate matters even more, Vietnamese is a tonal language like Chinese and, although they have 11 vowels, the 5 English vowels do not exist among them. Some of the more important morphological and syntactic differences are summarized in Table 6.9.

Summary

Asian languages contrast more sharply with English in phonology and structure than do Ebonics or Spanish: There are fewer overlaps between the respective sound systems and fewer cognates. Some Asian languages convey meaning

Table 6.9
Characteristics of Vietnamese that Influence English Usage

1. Vietnamese is essentially monosyllabic. Many words do consist of more than one syllable, but they are written as separate syllables, sometimes with and sometimes without hyphens. There are bound (e.g., *un-*) and free (e.g., *tie*) morphemes. Nevertheless, the language is noninflectional. Context and specific markers are used to denote tense, plurals, possessives, and so on.

   Example: Yesterday I go to school.

2. Although Vietnamese uses subject–verb–object word order, speakers put the adjective after the noun.

   Example: desk high

3. Vietnamese speakers eliminate the verb *to be.*

   Examples: He teacher.
   They happy yesterday.

4. Speakers of Vietnamese use the verb *done* to indicate past action.

   Example: I done visit my uncle.

5. There is no *to* in the infinitive form.

   Example: He learn sing?

6. Vietnamese forms the interrogative by placing *no* at the end of the sentence.

   Example: You want play, no? (meaning "Do you want to play?")

Note. Adapted from *Vietnamese-Influenced English,* by D. T. Hoi and N. N. Bich, 1995 (December), paper presented at the annual meeting of the American Speech-Language-Hearing Association, Orlando, FL.

through changes in tone, and many use markers to indicate grammatical structures rather than word inflections. Similarly, cultural differences have the potential to complicate communication between Asians and Westerners quite significantly. The two cultural groups are grounded in diametrically opposed values—the rugged individualism of the West versus the harmonious interpersonal focus of the East.

The English of Native Americans

There is not one dialect of English spoken by Native Americans. There are many, each with its own history, its own grammatical and lexical rules, and its own standards of usage within specific speaking situations. As Leap (1995) wrote,

> American Indian English is not a deficient form of English nor does it represent a faulty adaptation or imperfect imitation of standard language constraints. Each variety of American Indian English contains a fully developed, well ordered set of grammatical and phonological rules; speaker use of these rules shows no evidence of limitation in expressiveness or explicitness. Speaker use does, however, show ample evidence of the "Indianness" of the speaker's background. (p. 1)

Leap (1995) noted further that features of the speaker's ancestral language are typically evident in the English of Native Americans even if they are not fluent in, or even familiar with, their ancestral tongue, just as SAE has been influenced by the word choices, images, metaphors, and strategies for oratory of its past speakers. Native American dialects, however, have been derived from the more than 500 different languages and dialects that were in use prior to contact with the Europeans, and this diversity accounts for their richness and variety today. Some of the more interesting linguistic, ancestral practices that Leap delineated include (a) distinctions in vocabulary use, pronunciation, and inflectional endings between male and female speech patterns within some Indian speech communities; (b) age-related patterns that had elders using language forms totally different from those of their grandchildren; and (c) specific speaking styles for tribal activities, such as ceremonials, political decision making, and dispute settlement.

Most interesting of all is that "variants of . . . maritime pidgin, and not the English vernaculars spoken by the colonists themselves, formed the core of the English first learned by some of the tribes along the Eastern seaboard" (Leap, 1995, p. 4). These pidgins were used only in certain circumstances, such as trading and communicating with English speakers and were, therefore, used only by the very few members of the ancestral group who interacted with outsiders. Although, as mentioned in the previous chapter, the United States established government schools early with the purpose of eradicating Indian languages by teaching English, tribal language was the first language and English the second language of most Native Americans until the 1930s. Even today among a number of Native American groups, the ancestral tongue continues to be the first language, with students acquiring SAE or Indian English dialects beginning with school entrance (i.e., Head Start, kindergarten, or first grade). Many learn several nonstandard dialects and use them with other Native Americans and non-Indians alike. Some of the distinguishing characteristics of Native American dialects are summarized in Table 6.10.

Table 6.10
Characteristics of Native American English Dialects

1. It is common across many, but not all, Native American dialects for speakers to drop final consonants and to reduce final consonant clusters, but the *rules* for doing so vary in complex ways across ancestral groups. The rules also vary from those of other language communities (e.g., African and Hispanic Americans) and are influenced by the particular characteristics of the ancestral tongue.
2. Use of the negation parallels structures used in SAE and in other nonstandard dialects. There is evidence to suggest, however, that the placement of the negative may reflect different rules. Among Isletans, for example, the placement is used to convey a highly precise meaning and is not governed by rules related to language form.

   Examples: The Isleta man does not do anything like that. (meaning that Isleta women may)

   The Isleta man does not do nothing like that. (meaning that the Isleta man will do something else)
3. Many of the deviations from Standard American English pronunciations are predictable from the phonological characteristics of Native American languages. Consequently, these features do not constitute error patterns.

Note. Adapted from *American Indian English,* by W. L. Leap, 1995 (December), and from *A Preliminary Analysis of English Phonological Trends in Mississippi Choctaw Children,* by P. McCardle and J. H. Walton, 1995 (December), papers presented at the annual meeting of the American Speech-Language-Hearing Association, Orlando, FL.

Conclusion

School personnel must keep in mind that one language or dialect is not in any inherent way better than any other. All are rule governed; sufficient to promote intellectual, social, and spiritual and emotional growth; and able to express the full range of concepts and ideas. We get the impression that one dialect is superior to others, because it is the dialect used by the powerful and associated with education and affluence. In the United States today, that language or dialect is SAE. The issue of dominance in language, therefore, is a political and ideological matter, rather than a linguistic one.

It is precisely because language is politically and ideologically privileged that we must teach all of our children SAE: It is their passport to the American dream. Darder (1991), Friere (1985, 1998), Giroux (1988), Macedo (1994), and other critical theorists have argued that we cannot ignore the role that public education plays in maintaining the status quo, privileging the children of the powerful and marginalizing those of the underclasses. Language is the major vehicle for keeping people "in their place." The way schools are currently configured, those who arrive there speaking the dominant language typically enjoy success; those who do not often struggle, and some eventually drop out. But, if language is the vehicle for oppression, it can also be the key to a more equitable future.

Collier (1995) reported that characteristics of successful programs for language-minority students include (a) integrated schooling with students who use SAE, (b) high expectations, (c) equal status being accorded to the two languages or dialects, (d) home–school cooperation, and (e) continuous support for staff development. Furthermore, she noted that traditional ESL pullout in the early grades is the "least successful program model for students' long-term academic success" (p. 9). Instead, language should be taught through cognitively complex content using problem solving and discovery learning in highly interactive classrooms. When first-language support cannot be offered, she recommends that SAE be taught through meaningful academic content with a conscious focus on teaching thinking and problem-solving strategies.

Similar recommendations have been made by Echevarria (1995) for special education teachers who are monolingual but teach students with special needs who also demonstrate limited English proficiency. Her approach includes a variety of techniques that are designed to make the curriculum content accessible to language-diverse students (including those with special needs), while simultaneously facilitating their acquisition of SAE. Some of these techniques include the use of a slower rate of speech and controlled vocabulary, contextualizing instruction through the use of visual supports and hands-on activities, and making curriculum adaptations.

Finally, immersion in SAE through contact with native speakers is essential but not sufficient for instruction of English as a second language or dialect. The development of students' metacognitive knowledge is crucial (Gee, 1990). Over time, they must come to understand and be able to compare and contrast important aspects of the first language or dialect with usage in SAE—the production of phonemes, variations in morphological and syntactic structures, rules governing stress and intonation, and differences in pragmatic expectations that are dictated by the two cultures. It is only when students can cross linguistic boundaries at will, acquiring SAE without sacrificing their mother tongues, that we will have achieved educational equity.

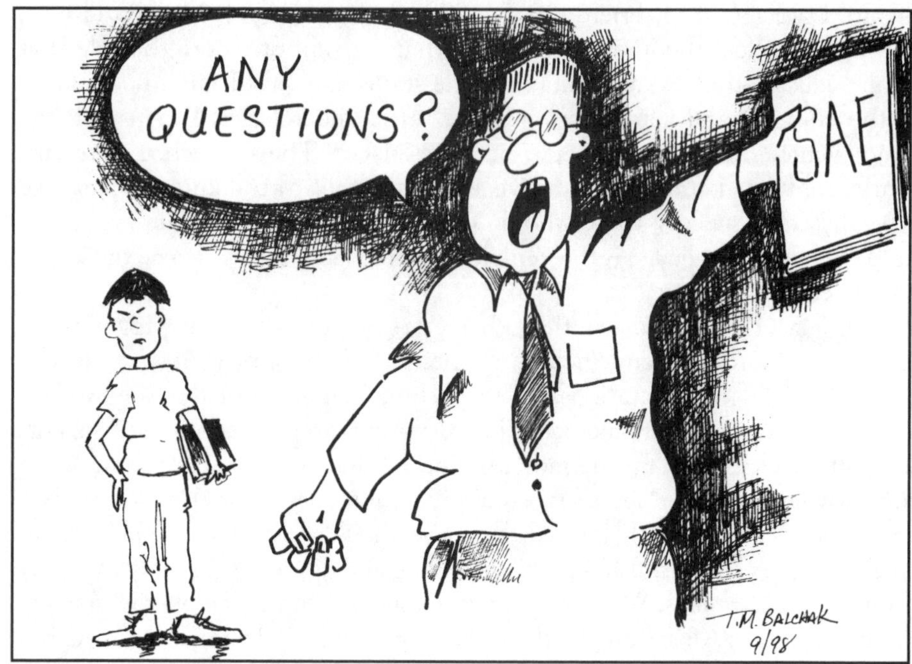

As linguists are fond of saying, it is he who has the guns (i.e., the power) who determines what the standard language will be.

References

Baron, D. E. (1990). *The English only question: An official language for Americans?* Binghamton, NY: Vail-Ballou Press.

Center for Applied Linguistics. (1981). *English pronunciation exercises for speakers of Vietnamese* (Refugee Education Guide #7). Washington, DC: Author.

Cheng, L.-R. (1995, December). *Chinese influenced English*. Paper presented at the annual meeting of the American Speech-Language-Hearing Association, Orlando, FL.

Cole, L. (1995a, December). *Black English in children: A developmental analysis of grammatical forms*. Paper presented at the annual meeting of the American Speech-Language-Hearing Association, Orlando, FL.

Cole, L. (1995b, December). *Black English in the United States and the Caribbean*. Paper presented at the annual meeting of the American Speech-Language-Hearing Association, Orlando, FL.

Collier, V. P. (1995). Acquiring a second language for school. *Directions in Language and Education, 1*(4). Washington, DC: The National Clearinghouse for Bilingual Education.

A crisis in any language: Oakland, Calif. plan to use Ebonics to teach standard English. (1997, January 13). *U.S. News & World Report*, p. 13.

Darder, A. (1991). *Culture and power in the classroom: A critical foundation for bicultural education*. Westport, CT: Bergin & Garvey.

Dato, D. P. (1995, December). *Spanish speakers in the United States*. Paper presented at the annual meeting of the American Speech-Language-Hearing Association, Orlando, FL.

Dillard, J. L. (1973). *Black English*. New York: Random House.

Eblen, R. E. (1995, December). *Some observations on the phonological acquisition of Hispanic-American children*. Paper presented at the annual meeting of the American Speech-Language-Hearing Association, Orlando, FL.

Ebonics: Rush to judgment? (1997). *The Education Digest*, *62*, 24–28.

Echevarria, J. (1995). Sheltered instruction for students with learning disabilities who have limited English proficiency. *Intervention in School and Clinic*, *30*, 302–305.

Fox, S. (1997). The controversy over Ebonics. *Phi Delta Kappan*, *79*, 237–240.

Friere, P. (1985). *The politics of education: Culture, power, and liberation*. Westport, CT: Bergin & Garvey.

Friere, P. (1998). *Teachers as cultural workers: Letters to those who dare teach*. Boulder, CO: Westview Press.

Garcia, E. E. (1995a, December). *Dual language acquisition*. Paper presented at the annual meeting of the American Speech-Language-Hearing Association, Orlando, FL.

Garcia, E. E. (1995b, December). *The development of Spanish morphology and syntax among Hispanic children in the United States*. Paper presented at the annual meeting of the American Speech-Language-Hearing Association, Orlando, FL.

Gee, J. P. (1990). *Social linguistics and literacies: Ideology in discourse*. Bristol, PA: Falmer Press.

Gibbs, W. W. (1997). A matter of language. *Scientific American*, *276*, 25–27.

Giroux, H. A. (1988). *Teachers as intellectuals: Toward a critical pedagogy of learning*. New York: Bergin & Garvey.

Golden, T. (1997, January 14). Oakland scratches plan to teach black English. *New York Times*, p. A10.

Hitchens, C. (1997, March). Hooked on Ebonics. *Vanity Fair*, p. 88.

Hoi, D. T., & Bich, N. N. (1995, December). *Vietnamese-influenced English*. Paper presented at the annual meeting of the American Speech-Language-Hearing Association, Orlando, FL.

Labov, W. (1966). *The social stratification of English in New York City*. Washington, DC: Center for Applied Linguistics.

Labov, W. (1972). *Sociolinguistic patterns*. Philadelphia: University of Pennsylvania Press.

Leap, W. L. (1995, December). *American Indian English*. Paper presented at the annual meeting of the American Speech-Language-Hearing Association, Orlando, FL.

Leland, J., & Joseph, N. (1997, January 13). Hooked on Ebonics: Oakland, Calif. plan to teach Black English. *Newsweek*, pp. 78–79.

Leo, J. (1997, January 20). Ebonics? No thonics! *U.S. News & World Report*, p. 20.

Linguists find the debate over "Ebonics" uninformed. (1997, January 17). *Chronicle of Higher Education*, pp. A16–A17.

Macedo, D. (1994). *Literacies of power: What Americans are not allowed to know*. Boulder, CO: Westview Press.

McCardle, P., & Walton, J. H. (1995, December). *A preliminary analysis of English phonological trends in Mississippi Choctaw children*. Paper presented at the annual meeting of the American Speech-Language-Hearing Association, Orlando, FL.

Menand, L. (1997, January 13). Johnny be good: Ebonics controversy in Oakland, California. *The New Yorker*, pp. 4–5.

Oakland school board approves black English program and sparks nationwide debate. (1991). *Jet, 91*, 12.

Owens, R. E. (1999). *Language disorders: A functional approach to assessment and intervention* (3rd ed.). Needham Heights, MA: Allyn & Bacon.

Penalosa, F. (1995, December). *Chicano English.* Paper presented at the annual meeting of the American Speech-Language-Hearing Association, Orlando, FL.

Peters-Johnson, C. (1995, December). *Pragmatic development: Cross-cultural or universal?* Paper presented at the annual meeting of the American Speech-Language-Hearing Association, Orlando, FL.

Sawyer, J. B. (1970). Spanish–English bilingualism in San Antonio, Texas. In G. Gilbert (Ed.), *Texas studies in bilingualism* (pp. 171–191). Berlin: Walter de Gruyter.

Seymour, H. N., & Seymour, C. M. (1995, December). *Black English and standard American English contrasts in consonantal development of four- and five-year-old children.* Paper presented at the annual meeting of the American Speech-Language-Hearing Association, Orlando, FL.

Sowell, T. (1997). Ebonics: Follow the money. *Forbes, 159*, 48.

Stewart, W. (1970). Sociolinguistic factors in the history of American Negro dialects. In F. Williams (Ed.), *Language and poverty: Perspectives on a theme* (pp. 353–362). Chicago: Markham.

Stockman, I. J., & Vaughn-Cooke, F. B. (1995, December). *Semantic development: Cross-cultural or universal?* Paper presented at the annual meeting of the American Speech-Language-Hearing Association, Orlando, FL.

Takada, N., & Hanahan, E. (1995, December). *Japanese-influenced English.* Paper presented at the annual meeting of the American Speech-Language-Hearing Association, Orlando, FL.

Thompson, R. M. (1974). Mexican American language loyalty and the validity of the 1970 Census. *International Journal of the Sociology of Language, 2*, 7–18.

White, J. E. (1997, January 13). Ebonics according to Buckwheat. *Time*, p. 62.

Wolfram, W. (1972). Linguistic assimilation in the children of immigrants. *The Linguistic Reporter, 14*, 1–3.

Wolfram, W. (1973). *Linguistic assimilation: A study of Puerto Rican English in New York City.* Arlington, VA: Center for Applied Linguistics.

Wolfram, W. (1995a, December). *Grammatical, phonological and language use differences across cultures.* Paper presented at the annual meeting of the American Speech-Language-Hearing Association, Orlando, FL.

Wolfram, W. (1995b, December). *Puerto Rican English.* Paper presented at the annual meeting of the American Speech-Language-Hearing Association, Orlando, FL.

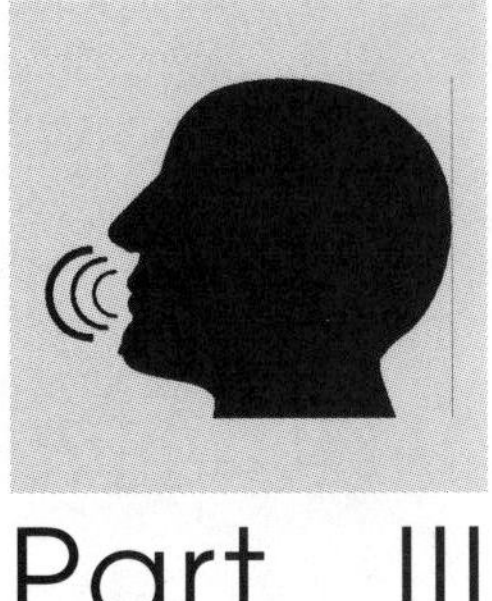

Part III

Language Disorders

Language Acquisition Problems Exhibited in Classrooms

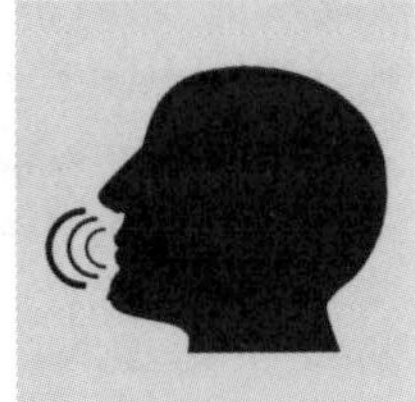

Chapter 7

Kathleen R. Fahey

Most children learn their native language during their first 5 years as opportunities and experiences to use language occur during everyday interactions with family and community members. They develop the oral language system (i.e., articulation and phonology, suprasegmental aspects, morphology and syntax, semantics, pragmatics, metalinguistics) and learn to use it in a variety of discourses (i.e., conversations, stories, explanations) and modes (i.e, oral and written) throughout their school years. Language acquisition is influenced by race, social class, and gender, and by the linguistic characteristics of the particular language or dialect used within the speaking community. Thus, the children with whom teachers and speech–language pathologists (SLPs) work in schools represent a broad range of language characteristics.

Unfortunately, about 10% of children do not develop language according to the typical trends (American Speech-Language-Hearing Association Committee on Language, Speech, and Hearing Services in Schools, 1982) described in the previous chapters. Some experience language *delay* (i.e., slower development) or language *disorders* (i.e., atypical or uneven emergence of language systems). Both cause them difficulty communicating and learning in classrooms. Teachers recognize students with language problems in their own classrooms, but may not understand fully how the problems interfere with academic learning and social development. Further, although they are interested in finding effective ways of fostering language growth and academic success, teachers must rely on special educators and SLPs to help in the assessment and intervention processes.

This chapter first discusses the causes and general characteristics of language acquisition disabilities, then considers eight specific language problems including definitions, characteristics, and implications for learning. They are (1) language learning disabilities, (2) central auditory processing disorders, (3) attention-deficit/hyperactivity disorder, (4) mental retardation, (5) traumatic brain injury, (6) pervasive developmental disorder and autism, (7) fetal exposure to substance abuse, and (8) maltreatment. The chapter is useful as a resource for general and special educators as well as SLPs as they explore together each student's language and learning strengths and weaknesses, and educational needs.

Problems with Language Acquisition and Usage

Language acquisition and usage problems are often recognized by parents, other caregivers, and preschool teachers during the preschool years. Even though some adults are reluctant to compare children in the home, neighborhood, or school, it is natural to see differences in youngsters' development, especially as they interact with each other. Despite knowing that problems exist, however, it is difficult to ascribe them to specific causes. Problems in language and learning can result from several factors. According to Nelson (1993), no clear and predictable causal patterns have emerged through research efforts, and causal factors are heterogeneous, changeable, layered, multifaceted, and interactive. They include biological conditions (e.g., syndromes, injury, neurological problems), linguistic system development, situational conditions, cognitive abilities, and social interaction factors. Thus, each child requires careful observation and study to reveal the specific factors contributing to his or her individual language and learning problems.

It is also important to note that causal factors can co-occur, making diagnosis more difficult. Mixed conditions, such as language delay and emotional problems, present myriad confounded characteristics that impact on students' linguistic, social, and academic performance. To complicate matters even more, physical, environmental, social, and linguistic factors change over time. For example, a child with an early history of ear infection and fluctuating conductive hearing loss may have language delay during the toddler and preschool years. Although correction of the physical problem through rigorous medical management and maturation can restore normal hearing, early hearing loss impacts both early and later stages of language development (Gravel & Wallace, 1995; Roberts & Medley, 1995).

As changes occur over time, a student's needs may also change. Consider a child with a severe expressive language disorder who in the early grades successfully uses manipulatives, gestures, and direct support from peers and teachers to interact within the classroom. Such a child will likely find that by third grade these supports are not as readily available and will experience greater demands to listen, speak, read, and write. If this student is not able to adjust her expressive language to increasingly complex linguistic and curricular demands, she may experience increasing academic failure. Often, students who have been labeled as having language disability are reclassified as having language learning problems.

Despite our inability to determine causes in every case, we still *attempt* to categorize causal factors and characteristics associated with language problems. One benefit in doing so is our ability to encourage prevention, such as advocating helmet use during participation in sports in the case of a child who experienced trauma, seeking genetic testing when a syndrome is present in a family, and eliminating neglect and abuse in families. Categories also help general and special educators and SLPs to describe characteristics of students with language problems, thus increasing understanding and fostering communication both among themselves and with the students and their parents. For example, a child with Down syndrome is likely to have below average cognition and language abilities, whereas a child with a label of specific language impairment has average (or nearly average) cognition, but below average language abilities. Such categorical distinctions facilitate the selection of in-depth diagnostic procedures and possibly even intervention approaches. The use of categories also enables research on specific causes and their relation to other factors and permits interested persons to form advocacy groups. While these benefits seem to support the use of categories, we should also keep in mind the artificial nature of categories and know the dangers in using stereotyped labels to discuss the challenges that specific children bring to school. Educators must remember that the particular speech, language, and learning characteristics of individuals, *and not their classification labels*, are the most important considerations in designing and delivering effective educational programs (Nelson, 1993; Paul, 1995). In other words, educators must develop interventions that treat the symptoms of language problems, not their causes.

In summary, language disabilities result from many causes, which are often difficult to determine. Although labels help educators define some general characteristics of problems in students, facilitate efforts in prevention and research, and foster discussion among professionals, the labels are not especially helpful in assessing language problems or in helping professionals design interventions to suit the needs of individual students.

The Characteristics of Language Acquisition Problems

Language acquisition problems are difficult to define, perhaps due to our own changing understandings of their nature. Various terms have been used to speak of such problems across decades of research, clinical practice, legislation, and service delivery in schools. Subcategories have been based on theories of underlying causes (e.g., mental retardation, traumatic brain injury), varied perspectives of professional disciplines (e.g., linguistics and sociolinguistics, psychology, speech–language pathology, special education, neurology), the evolution of symptoms within a child over time (e.g., language delay, learning disability), the co-occurrence of disorders occurring within a syndrome or separately (e.g., autism, attention-deficit disorder), and varied use of terminology across states and professional associations (Nelson, 1993). Thus, it is common to see and hear many different terms regarding language and learning problems in the professional literature, at Individualized Education Plan (IEP) meetings, and in the media. Some of these terms include *specific language impairment*, *developmental language disorder*, *language learning disability*, and even *dyslexia*.

Several categories of *language and learning problems* based on major characteristics associated with language, cognition, attention, memory, and social competence are discussed in this chapter. These include language learning disabilities of unknown origin, central auditory processing disorders, attention-deficit/hyperactivity disorder, mental retardation, traumatic brain injury, and pervasive developmental disorder and autism. Two other tragic, yet preventable environmentally based problems (i.e., fetal exposure to substance abuse, and child abuse and neglect) are discussed separately because of their unique characteristics. Other disorders associated with *speech problems* (that also impact language and social development) are discussed in the next chapter. These include hearing impairment and deafness, visual impairment and blindness, motor speech disorders (i.e., dysarthria and developmental verbal apraxia), cleft lip and palate, phonological and articulation disorders, stuttering and prosodic disturbances, and voice disorders.

Language Learning Disabilities of Unknown Origin

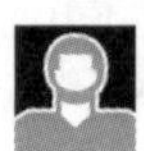

Paula

Paula is 8 years, 4 months old and in the second grade at a suburban school. She began kindergarten at age 6 because she seemed immature in her relationships with others and in her conceptual development. For example, she lagged behind her preschool peers in learning concepts, remembering sequences (as in counting and saying the alphabet), and putting her ideas into sentences. Paula loves to draw and paint, sitting for hours with art supplies, but she becomes upset and impatient when she tries to read or write. It seems as if she cannot remember what sounds go with what letters.

Definition and Characteristics

When a child such as Paula is confirmed to have difficulty acquiring and using language, one of the first questions parents and others ask is what caused the problem. As we have noted, however, even when a great deal is known about prenatal, birth, medical, environmental, and educational histories, much of the time professionals do not have an answer to this question. Language acquisition problems are often diagnosed when other conditions, such as cognitive deficits, social and emotional disorders, sensory problems (i.e., hearing, visual), and physical limitations have been ruled out. They include difficulties with the language structure (i.e., articulation and phonology, morphology and syntax), development of vocabulary and figurative language (i.e., semantics), functional use of language (i.e., pragmatics), and ability to manipulate language (i.e., metalinguistics), which significantly affect literacy. Further, problems in one or more of these areas can have broad-reaching effects that influence academic progress and social and emotional development. Refer to Table 7.1 (Ratner & Harris, 1994) for a detailed list of the linguistic, social, emotional, and academic problems related to language deficit.

The term learning disability is often used categorically in academic settings to describe language problems in school-age children and youth. Students labeled as having language learning disabilities (LLDs) typically exhibit problems in reading, writing, and/or mathematics learning. Debate has been lively on the exact nature and definition of learning disabilities (Simon, 1991). The definition of LLD approved by the National Joint Council on Learning Disabilities (1991), a group of professional organizations whose members work with and study LLD, emphasizes its intrinsic physiological cause, its existence across the life span, and its possible co-occurrence with other conditions and across cultural and socioeconomic environments:

> Learning disabilities is a generic term that refers to a heterogeneous group of disorders manifested by significant difficulties in the acquisition and use of listening, speaking, reading, writing, reasoning, or mathematical abilities. These disorders are intrinsic to the individual and presumed to be due to central nervous system dysfunction. Even though a learning disability may occur concomitantly with other handicapping conditions (e.g., sensory impairment, mental retardation, social and emotional disturbance) or environmental influences (e.g., cultural differences, insufficient/inappropriate instruction, psychogenic factors), it is not the direct result of those conditions or influences. (p. 19)

Students with language learning disabilities vary considerably in the linguistic problems they demonstrate. The problems can be mild, moderate,

(*text continues on page 255*)

Table 7.1
Problems Related to Language Deficits

Linguistic Problems: Difficulty with Understanding and/or Expression

Language Structure:

- Omissions and distortions of speech sounds
- Omissions of parts of words
- Sounds or syllables of words out of sequence
- Omissions of morphological endings of words
- Immature syntax
- Limited ability with complex sentences
- Undeveloped age-appropriate grammar
- Unintelligibility: can't be understood

Language Meaning:

- Difficulty with directions
- Confusion with concepts and ideas
- Difficulty with questions
- Paucity of vocabulary
- Literal interpretation of words and concepts
- Difficulty with figurative language, humor, slang, and double meanings of words
- Poor word classification and association skill

Language Use:

- Difficulty initiating, maintaining, and terminating conversational exchanges
- Immature turn-taking strategies
- Inadequate code-switching—change of language to suit specific person or situation
- Pauses, word fillers, word repetitions, and circumlocutions
- Difficulty assuming listener's point of view

Metalinguistics:

- Difficulty expressing ideas about language
- Poor syllabification skills
- Poor phonics skills
- Poor rhyming skills

(*continues*)

Table 7.1 *Continued.*

Social Problems: Difficulty Interacting Appropriately

Conversational Deficits:

- Poor eye contact
- Inappropriate comments and responses to questions
- Excessive pauses before responding
- Inappropriate voice quality: intonation
- Poor social language (e.g., please, thank you)
- Insufficient information for listener
- Redundancy

Social-Interaction Issues:

- Poor sense of fair play (e.g., sharing, win/lose rules)
- Inadequate setting of limits or boundaries
- Inconsistent responses and actions in social encounters
- Difficulty with new situations
- Inappropriate clinging, touching, and kissing
- Excessive demands for attention
- Inappropriate laughing and crying
- Difficulty expressing wants, needs, and ideas
- Inappropriate clowning

Emotional Problems: Difficulty Monitoring Behavior

Personal Issues:

- Egocentric
- Poor self-concept
- Limited repertoire of emotions
- Rigidity of routine
- Low frustration level
- Need for immediate gratification
- Impulsive
- Perseverative and repetitious
- Poor differentiation of fantasy and reality

(*continues*)

Table 7.1 *Continued.*

Emotional Problems: Difficulty Monitoring Behavior *Continued.*

Emotional-Interaction Issues:

- Inability to accept responsibility
- Dependency (i.e., on parent, teacher)
- Gullible; easily led
- Sensitive to criticism
- Withdrawn or acting out
- Poor coping strategies
- Unpredictable

Classroom Issues:

- Poor retention of material; need for constant repetition
- Problems in organization and planning
- Difficulty problem solving
- Left/right confusion
- Symbol reversals: numbers and letters
- Difficulty expressing known information
- Poor generalization of information to novel situations
- Difficulty with inferences and deductions
- Poor judgment and understanding of cause and effect
- Inability to self-monitor and self-correct
- Poor integration of information
- Poor short- and/or long-term memory

Metacognition:

- Inability to verbalize about academic tasks
- Inability to self-regulate behaviors

Academic Problems: Difficulty Learning and/or Retaining Information

Sensory Deficits:

- Hyper- or hypo-sensitivity to smell, touch, or taste
- Immature body image
- Underdeveloped sense of one's position in space
- Distractions by visual and auditory stimuli
- Over- or under-reactions to sight and sound

(*continues*)

Table 7.1 *Continued.*

Academic Problems: Difficulty Learning and/or Retaining Information *Continued.*

Sensory Deficits:

- Attentional deficits
- Auditory and visual perception, discrimination, and memory deficits, including figure–ground and sequence problems

Associated Physiological Issues:

- Awkward gait
- Excessive eye blinking
- Hyper- or hypo-activity
- Poor motor coordination: fine and gross
- Allergies and asthma
- Poor posture
- Restlessness
- Slow processing and response time

Note. From *Understanding Language Disorders: The Impact on Learning* (pp. 171–174), by V. L. Ratner and L. R. Harris, 1994, Eau Claire, WI: Thinking Publications. Copyright 1994 by Thinking Publications. Reprinted with permission.

or severe, and can affect one or more language systems. Language deficits commonly observed among students with learning disabilities include problems in (a) phonology, (b) syntax or morphology, (c) semantics, (d) discourse processing, (e) metalinguistics, and (f) pragmatics (Gerber, 1993). Further, students may find one mode (e.g., oral language) more functional than another (e.g., reading or writing) and have difficulty with listening comprehension, comprehension monitoring, nonverbal communication, and social behaviors (Ratner & Harris, 1994). Subtle learning style preferences, as well as cultural differences, can make learning appear different from other students and can cause teachers to question the presence of learning disability in particular children. Considering all of these possible problems, it is impossible to predict what language strengths and weaknesses particular children will demonstrate.

The linguistic problems such students exhibit include how information is perceived and stored, especially during reading and writing. Research has shown that reading and writing problems are not to be the result of visual perception difficulties, but rather stem from poor verbal memory and deficient verbal knowledge (Gerber, 1993). Students with language learning problems have shown slower response times to verbal information and a more global, diffused, and less differentiated language perception style (Merzenich et al., 1996; Tallal, 1988; Tallal et al., 1996). They may have difficulty with verbal learning and recall (Shear, Tallal, & Delis, 1992), speech sound discrimination problems, and deficits in phonological awareness that are related to reading disability (Gerber, 1993).

Attentional disorders can occur separately, yet often co-occur with language and learning problems. Signs of distractibility, impulsivity, hyperactivity, poor organization, inadequate planning, and slower processing have been noted in children labeled as having learning disabilities (Gerber, 1993). Some attribute attentional problems in students with learning disabilities to poor modulation of the attention system (Rudel, 1988), inefficient or ineffective allocation of attentional resources to tasks (Barkley, 1990a; Hamlett, Pellegrini, & Conners, 1987), more effortful and less automatized processing and retrieval of information (Barkley, 1995), or slower processing by the central processing system (Richards, Samuels, Turnure, & Ysseldyke, 1990). Attention-deficit/hyperactivity disorder as a unique problem is discussed later in this chapter.

Students with language learning problems can have difficulty storing and retrieving information. Debate exists about whether memory problems suggest limited capacity for storage of input. Many researchers have investigated the nature of memory problems in children with learning problems to determine whether such problems are the result of limited strategies for organizing and storing information (e.g., Swanson & Cooney, 1991). Short-term and long-term memory problems have been attributed to limited memory span for sequential verbal materials (e.g., letters, words) (Torgeson, 1988), restricted use of verbal codes to store and retrieve information (Swanson, 1993; Vellutino & Scanlon, 1985), inefficient use of working memory during high-effort verbal tasks (Swanson, Ashbaker, & Lee, 1995), and differences in semantic knowledge, semantic coding, and mnemonic performance (Gerber, 1993). Problems in short- and long-term memory are closely tied to linguistic knowledge and the use of such knowledge for academic learning. The higher the linguistic complexity of information, the more apparent are difficulties in storage and retrieval processes (Gerber, 1993).

Psychosocial problems can co-exist in students with language and learning disabilities. For some they can arise from the "failure cycle" that occurs as they attempt to survive academically and socially in classrooms (Gerber, 1993). The cumulative impact of linguistic, cognitive, and metacognitive deficits; the resultant academic failure and low self-esteem; and the consequent drop in motivation can provide a self-perpetuating spiral of continued failure in classrooms. However, it is interesting to note that this cycle typically occurs exclusively within academic settings; in other social arenas the students' psychosocial health and behavior are similar to their peers' (Cooley & Ayers, 1988). Recall that the definition of learning disabilities excludes emotional problems as either a cause or a significant attribute of the overall characteristics. Secondary emotional problems (e.g., poor self-esteem, anxiety, depression) may exist, but are not necessarily caused by the language learning problems. Rather, they are by-products of how the disability limits full and successful participation in academic settings.

Implications for the Classroom

Considering the range of problems that can exist in students with language learning disabilities, general and special education teachers and SLPs must carefully observe their students to determine the presence and extent of linguistic strengths and weaknesses. If diagnostic information in these areas is lacking, general education teachers should refer students for assessment by the speech–language pathologist (SLP), school psychologist, or special education teacher. The IEP meeting provides a forum for collaborative discussion and consensus-reaching about the student's needs by teachers, parents, and the special educators or SLPs who provide service to the child. Whenever possible, students also should take part in the IEP meetings. During classroom instruction, each student's needs should be considered and instructional strategies offered that support and advance student achievement. Specific ideas for children with language and learning disabilities are presented and discussed in Chapter 10 on intervention strategies.

Summary

Students who have language learning problems face challenges as they develop language, especially upon entry into school. Such students often have impoverished language systems, which limit their abilities to participate fully in classroom activities as well as in social settings within and outside the classroom. Students often struggle to acquire reading and writing abilities, which results in further academic difficulties. In addition to an impoverished linguistic system, students who have LLD can also have attentional or memory difficulties that further complicate successful learning. Secondary psychosocial or emotional problems can result from repeated failure in academic and social situations. Thus, teachers, SLPs, and other professionals and parents must work together to clearly define the nature and extent of each student's problems through assessment, and develop appropriate interventions within the classroom.

Central Auditory Processing Disorders

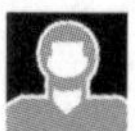

Matthew

Matthew is 10 years old and in the fifth grade. Although his hearing is normal now, he had many ear infections during his first 4 years that caused intermittent hearing loss and language delay. Matthew liked his first 2 years in school, although he lagged behind his peers. His attitude toward school changed during the second grade and is now quite negative. Matthew does his best academic work in quiet environments when he can watch others. He has the most difficulty during listening activities, often understanding or remembering only part of what is said. He misunderstands quite often and these misunderstandings cause him embarrassment and even anger. For example, he came to school prepared for a field trip which was not to occur until the following week. Matthew is very interested in animals and wants to be a veterinarian, yet he is beginning to question whether he is smart enough for this profession.

Definition and Characteristics

For children such as Matthew, peripheral hearing is normal, yet they have difficulty processing the meanings of information as it proceeds along the auditory neural pathways in the brain stem to the auditory reception areas in the cortex. This complicated transmission of information can be compromised at several different levels, leading to some behavioral signs common to central auditory processing disorders (CAPD). Table 7.2 contains a definition of CAPD from the Task Force on Central Auditory Processing Consensus Development (1996). It is beyond the scope of this chapter to provide a detailed description of the behavioral phenomena included in the definition.

Not all audiologists, SLPs, and psychologists agree on the existence of CAPD. It is controversial because of its focus on a single modality (i.e., auditory) as the cause of language comprehension problems. Arguments against CAPD as a category of language disability favor the idea that prior knowledge and experience, in combination with automatic and conscious processing, determine how people process incoming verbal information (M. Lahey, 1988). Proponents of CAPD as a separate category of language disability support the idea that specific deficits in auditory perception lead to linguistic difficulties (Bellis, 1996; Chermak & Musiek, 1997). Despite the controversy about whether CAPD exists and whether it leads to language disabilities, teachers do note that some students have particular problems with verbal information, especially during noisy situations. Table 7.3 lists behaviors that teachers and SLPs can readily observe in the classroom while children are listening, speaking,

Table 7.2
Definition of Central Auditory Processing and Central Auditory Processing Disorder

---

Central Auditory Processes

Several mechanisms and processes are responsible for auditory behavioral phenomena that allow individuals to respond to nonverbal as well as verbal signals. As such, they affect many areas of function, including speech and language. These processes include:

- Sound localization and lateralization
- Auditory discrimination
- Temporal aspects of audition (e.g., resolution, masking, integration, ordering)
- Auditory performance decrements with competing acoustic signals
- Auditory performance decrements with degraded acoustic signals

Central Auditory Processing Disorder

CAPD is an observed deficiency in one or more of the behavioral phenomena. It can occur from problems within the auditory system, or it can be associated with attention-deficit/hyperactivity disorder. Speech-language development and academic performance problems occur as students attempt to learn in classrooms.

Note. Adapted from "Central Auditory Processing: Current Status of Research and Implications for Clinical Practice," by Task Force on Central Auditory Processing Consensus Development, 1996, *American Journal of Audiology, 5*(2), pp. 41–54.

learning, and paying attention. Note that when students are observed during classroom activities that require listening, they seem to miss important information, especially in noisy situations. This reduced access to verbal information has a cumulative effect over time because it results in reduced knowledge (through faulty receptive language) and incomplete understandings (semantic knowledge). Teachers and SLPs can observe students having difficulty in speaking situations, especially when information is being exchanged between one or more parties. Dialogues require the ability to listen, derive meaning, and quickly formulate a response that makes sense in context. Yet, even when students understand what is being said, their impoverished expressive language systems and delays caused by slow processing deny them sophisticated interactions.

Students who have CAPD also show signs of attentional problems in classrooms. In fact, distractibility and poor attention lead SLPs, teachers, and parents to

Table 7.3
Classroom Behaviors Typical of Children with Central Auditory Processing Disorders

Listening

- Says "huh" or "what" frequently
- Often misunderstands what is said
- Constantly requests that information be repeated
- Has difficulty following oral directions
- Has difficulty listening in the presence of background noise
- Has poor receptive language
- Confuses words that sound alike
- Learns poorly through the auditory channel

Speaking

- Gives inconsistent responses to auditory stimuli
- Has poor expressive language across some or all of the language systems
- Gives slow or delayed responses to verbal stimuli

Learning and Attention

- Has poor auditory attention
- Is easily distracted
- Has difficulty with phonics and speech sound discrimination
- Has poor auditory memory span and sequence
- Has reading, spelling, or other academic problems
- Exhibits behavior problems

Note. Adapted from *SCAN: A Screening Test for Auditory Processing Disorders,* by R. Keith, 1986, San Antonio, TX: The Psychological Corporation. Adapted with permission.

question whether particular students have attention-deficit/hyperactivity disorder. Some students do have coexisting auditory processing and attention conditions, but for others, the presumed attention difficulties are symptomatic of the difficulty they have listening to and understanding information. In addition, poor attention to verbal information during reading and writing instruction can make awareness of the segments of the language (e.g., letter–sound correspondence, breaking words into syllables) obscure. Not all children with CAPD have reading and writing difficulties, but SLPs, teachers, and parents should be alert to potential problems in literacy development.

As was true of language and learning disabilities, students with CAPD do not comprise a homogeneous group. Four subtypes have been identified and described according to common language and learning characteristics (see Table 7.4): (1) auditory decoding deficit, (2) integration deficit, (3) associative deficit, and (4) output-organizational deficit (Bellis, 1996; Katz & Smith, 1991). Even these discrete categories have overlapping symptoms, but are named based on how children respond during intensive audiological and language testing. Subcategories can be useful for audiologists, SLPs, and general and special educators when determining teaching and learning strategies in classrooms.

Implications for the Classroom

Upon referral by the teacher or parent, checklists such as *The Classroom Communication Skills Inventory* (1993), *Fisher's Auditory Problems Checklist* (Fisher, 1985), and the *Children's Auditory Processing Performance Scale* (CHAPPS) (Smoski, 1990) are completed by parents; the student, if appropriate; general and special education teachers; and any other educational or health care providers familiar with the student's language and learning characteristics. If more detailed assessment is needed, a multidisciplinary team approach is considered the best practice for determining the presence and nature of CAPD (Colorado Task Force on Central Auditory Processing Disorders, 1997).

The goal of the assessment is to identify strengths and weaknesses in auditory processing, speech and language, and achievement areas. Audiological evaluation should include assessment of peripheral hearing (e.g., acuity, speech recognition), middle ear function (tympanogram), and specific behavioral auditory measures of the phenomena listed in Table 7.2. The speech–language evaluation should include standardized and nonstandardized measures of expressive and receptive language functions, with specific attention given to comprehension of verbal and nonverbal information both in the classroom and under more favorable listening conditions, such as in a testing room or with a personal listening system. The school psychological evaluation should include formal and informal measures of cognitive development and academic achievement.

A profile of strengths and weaknesses based on the outcome of the observations and tests can be used to design appropriate interventions for each student's individual needs. There are four general avenues that practitioners can access for the development of an intervention plan: (1) classroom accommodations and modifications, (2) environmental modifications in the home and classroom, (3) instructional practices, and (4) speech–language therapy (Bellis, 1996; Chermak & Musiek, 1997; Colorado Task Force on CAPD, 1997). These interventions are discussed in Chapter 10.

Table 7.4
Common Language and Learning Characteristics of Central Auditory Processing Disorders by Subtypes

Auditory Decoding Deficit

- Poor auditory closure when parts of the signal are distorted or absent
- Poor phonemic representation resulting in articulation errors
- Poor sound recognition, blending, discrimination, and retention
- Problems with the development of reading, writing, and spelling
- Difficulty understanding speech in noisy environments and possible distraction from background noise
- May ask for repetition of verbal information
- Good comprehension when information is decoded

Integration Deficit

- Difficulty with tasks involving verbal or nonverbal information when more than one modality (auditory, visual, tactile, kinesthetic) is involved
- Delays in responding to information
- Poor phonemic representation of information
- Difficulty recognizing and using gestalt patterns for sight word recognition and spelling
- Impairment in the suprasegmental aspects of speech
- Difficulty with tasks requiring hemispheric cooperation (e.g., dancing to music, drawing from verbal description)
- Poor music ability

Associative Deficit

- Good ability to repeat verbal instruction
- Difficulty applying the rules of language to incoming information, particularly when messages are complex (e.g., passive voice, compound and complex sentence structure)
- Difficulty attaching meaning to phonemic units of speech leading to poor word recognition
- Receptive language deficits in vocabulary, semantics, and syntax
- Possibly poor pragmatic and social skills
- Appropriate early academic achievement, but general academic difficulties as language complexity increases

(*continues*)

Table 7.4 *Continued.*

Output-Organizational Deficit

- Difficulty in sequencing, planning, and organizing responses due to problems acting on incoming information
- Poor discrimination of speech in noisy environments
- Poor ability to follow directions
- Poor organizational skills
- Sequencing errors and sound blending errors in speech
- Poor spelling and writing due to complexity of these tasks along with good reading comprehension
- Poor fine and gross motor planning

Summary

CAPD is a language disorder presumably caused by inefficient perception of information received through the auditory mechanism. It results in difficulties in listening and comprehending language, especially when the listening environment is noisy, but it can also result in expressive language problems because of inadequate input. Because CAPD is a difficult disorder to assess, a multidisciplinary team of professionals (e.g., audiologist, SLP, psychologist, teachers) must work collaboratively. Appropriate interventions must assist the student to effectively participate within the classroom and to improve language comprehension and expressive abilities.

Attention-Deficit/Hyperactivity Disorder

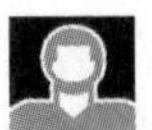

Tommy

Tammy, a 14-year-old eighth grader, has always been very restless and highly active. She is often disciplined at home for rough play with her younger sister. She likes to play outside where she rides her bike, climbs trees, and runs races with neighborhood children. School has been difficult for Tammy. She has trouble remaining seated for even short periods of time and is constantly handling objects such as paper, pencils, and other students' supplies. She calls out answers in class, even after repeated instruction to raise her hand and wait to be acknowledged. The other children become irritated with her and avoid her whenever possible. Tammy is interested in many topics, but has difficulty paying attention to the teacher. She is falling behind in her schoolwork, because she does not get her work done on time (or sometimes not at all). Her schoolwork is highly disorganized and she often forgets to take assignments home.

Definitions and Characteristics

Attention-deficit/hyperactivity disorder (ADHD) is included in this chapter because for some children it coexists with language disorders. For other children, it can interfere with the self-regulation of language and metacognitive abilities.

ADHD is characterized by a persistent pattern of inattention, hyperactivity-impulsivity, or both. It is a syndrome thought to be of neurobehavioral origin that describes a heterogeneous group of children and adults. Incidence figures in school-age children vary considerably in the literature due to the high rate of coexisting problems, including deficits in language, learning, and emotional disturbance. Estimates of ADHD in the school population are as low as 3% to 5% (American Psychiatric Association, 1994; Shelton & Barkley, 1994) and as high as 10% to 20% (Shaywitz & Shaywitz, 1988), and ADHD is far more common in boys (3 to 9 times greater) than in girls (Conti, 1991).

The American Psychiatric Association's (1994) *Diagnostic and Statistical Manual of Mental Disorders, Fourth Edition* (DSM–IV) includes three categories of attentional disorders reflecting distinctions among individuals who are inattentive, those who are hyperactive and impulsive, and those demonstrating all three characteristics. The categories are called ADD, Predominantly Inattentive Type; ADHD, Predominantly Hyperactive–Impulsive Type; and ADHD, Combined Type. Table 7.5 includes the DSM–IV criteria for these categories. The inattention category has been associated with metacognitive difficulties, whereas the hyperactivity–impulsivity category has been associated with behavioral difficulties (Shaywitz, Fletcher, & Shaywitz, 1994). For a diagnosis to be made, at least 6 of the total 18 behaviors must be present prior to age 7 in at least two settings (e.g., home and school) and must interfere with developmentally appropriate social, academic, or occupational functioning (Westby & Cutler, 1994).

Inattention is a problem that teachers and SLPs can observe in classrooms. Attention problems can occur when a student is (a) selectively focusing on tasks or verbal messages; (b) sustaining attention and mental effort once focus is achieved in order to engage in and complete tasks; (c) organizing materials, tasks, or activities; and (d) storing and remembering information. Thus, inattention can result in difficulty during academic and social interactions. Contrary to the popular belief that students with ADD are always distracting, some children with inattention appear passive and demonstrate little movement.

Table 7.5
Diagnostic Criteria for Attention-Deficit/Hyperactivity Disorder

A. Either (1) or (2):

(1) six (or more) of the following symptoms of **inattention** have persisted for at least 6 months to a degree that is maladaptive and inconsistent with developmental level:

Inattention

(a) often fails to give close attention to details or makes careless mistakes in schoolwork, work, or other activities

(b) often has difficulty sustaining attention in tasks or play activities

(c) often does not seem to listen when spoken to directly

(d) often does not follow through on instructions and fails to finish schoolwork, chores, or duties in the workplace (not due to oppositional behavior or failure to understand instructions)

(e) often has difficulty organizing tasks and activities

(f) often avoids, dislikes, or is reluctant to engage in tasks that require sustained mental effort (such as schoolwork or homework)

(g) often loses things necessary for tasks or activities (e.g., toys, school assignments, pencils, books, or tools)

(h) is often easily distracted by extraneous stimuli

(i) is often forgetful in daily activities

(2) six (or more) of the following symptoms of **hyperactivity-impulsivity** have persisted for at least 6 months to a degree that is maladaptive and inconsistent with developmental level:

Hyperactivity

(a) often fidgets with hands or feet or squirms in seat

(b) often leaves seat in classroom or in other situations in which remaining seated is expected

(c) often runs about or climbs excessively in situations in which it is inappropriate (in adolescents or adults, may be limited to subjective feelings of restlessness)

(d) often has difficulty playing or engaging in leisure activities quietly

(e) is often "on the go" or often acts as if "driven by a motor"

(f) often talks excessively

(*continues*)

Table 7.5 *Continued.*

Impulsivity

(g) often blurts out answers before questions have been completed

(h) often has difficulty awaiting turn

(i) often interrupts or intrudes on others (e.g., butts into conversations or games)

B. Some hyperactive–impulsive or inattentive symptoms that caused impairment were present before age 7 years.

C. Some impairment from the symptoms is present in two or more settings (e.g., at school (or work) and at home).

D. There must be clear evidence of clinically significant impairment in social, academic, or occupational functioning.

E. The symptoms do not occur exclusively during the course of a Pervasive Developmental Disorder, Schizophrenia, or other Psychotic Disorder and are not better accounted for by another mental disorder (e.g., Mood Disorder, Anxiety Disorder, Dissociative Disorder, or a Personality Disorder).

Code based on type

314.01 Attention-Deficit/Hyperactive Disorder, Combined Type: if both Criteria A1 and A2 are met for the past 6 months

314.00 Attention-Deficit/Hyperactivity Disorder, Predominantly Inattentive Type: if Criterion A1 is met but Criterion A2 is not met for the past 6 months

314.01 Attention-Deficit/Hyperactivity Disorder, Predominantly Hyperactive-Impulsive Type: if Criterion A2 is met but Criterion A1 is not met for the past 6 months

Coding note: For individuals (especially adolescents and adults) who currently have symptoms that no longer meet full criteria, "In Partial Remission" should be specified.

Note. From *Diagnostic and Statistical Manual of Mental Disorders* (4th ed., pp. 83–85), by American Psychiatric Association, 1994, Washington, DC: Author.

They can be daydreaming (which leads to missed information in the classroom) and may be socially withdrawn from others. Because they are quiet and nondisruptive, they may be an underidentified group (Ratner & Harris, 1994; Shaywitz & Shaywitz, 1988).

The symptoms common to *hyperactivity–impulsivity* include (a) excessive movements while sitting or standing; (b) the need to be on the go regardless of environmental demands; (c) feelings of restlessness; (d) excessive talking; and (e) difficulty controlling verbal responses and conversational turns. Shelton and Barkley (1994) defined hyperactivity as a deficiency in response inhibition. Toddlers with ADHD are described as being overly active in gross motor physical movements, such as running and jumping on furniture, and have difficulty listening to stories or engaging in other nonphysical activities. School-age children have similar difficulties, but the problems are typically less frequent and intense. They move their limbs and fidget with objects, talk excessively, and get up frequently. Older students demonstrate continued difficulties with attention and following instructions, and they display oppositional behaviors such as arguing and irritability. Adolescent students with hyperactivity also have higher uses of tobacco and alcohol. Their academic outcomes are considerably poorer than their normal peers, with at least three times as many hyperactive students failing a grade (Barkley, 1990a; Barkley, Fischer, Edelbrock, & Smallish, 1990; Fischer, Barkley, Edelbrock, & Smallish, 1990).

Impulsivity is a deficiency in sustained attention and in inhibiting behaviors in response to situational demands. Characteristics such as impatience, difficulty awaiting one's turn, blurting out thoughts or answers to questions when others are speaking, and intruding on others cause difficulty in school, home, and in other settings. Infants and preschool children exhibit restlessness and irritability. In school-age children, their nonreflective cognitive style and behavioral impulsivity lead them to make quick and sometimes poor decisions (Cantwell & Baker, 1985, 1991). The term *distractibility* is often used to describe children with ADHD, and other factors such as poor self-regulation, decreased persistence of effort, and difficulty inhibiting responses are also considered hallmarks (Barkley, 1990b; Shaywitz & Shaywitz, 1994).

ADHD can co-occur with psychiatric conditions such as oppositional defiant disorder (ODD) and conduct disorder (CD). Estimates of 40% (child) to 65% (adolescents) for co-occurrence of ODD and 21% (child) to 50% (adolescents) for co-occurrence of CD are reported in the literature (Barkley, 1990a). Although these problems coexist in many children and adults, their causes are considered to be from different influences. ADHD is likely to be a disorder of cognitive or neuromaturational development, whereas ODD and CD are likely to reflect problems in temperament and negative family and social influences (Barkley, 1990b).

Psychiatrists, pediatricians, and physicians in family practice become involved in the diagnosis and treatment of ADHD because of the link between the disorder and metabolic and neurotransmission difficulties. Thus, when diagnosis occurs, some children receive psycho-stimulant drugs which act to stimulate neurotransmitters, making concentration longer. Ritalin (methylphenidate), Cylert (pemoline), and Dexedrine (dextroamphetamine) are common names of such stimulants (Gadow, 1986). The dosages of such medications vary with the needs of the child and the behavioral outcomes of trial therapy. Cylert is used more frequently with adolescents, perhaps because it has a longer duration, thereby decreasing the need for a dosage during school hours. Typically, children take the medication only during school hours when concentration demands are the highest; however some children, who have negative effects from taking medication periodically or difficulty sleeping, take it during the evenings and on weekends or even during vacations as well (Gadow, 1986).

Psycho-stimulant drugs do have side-effects that parents and teachers should be alert to so that dosages can be adjusted. The two most common adverse reactions are insomnia and loss of appetite. These problems can be managed through the timing of dosages or the use of other medications. Other side-effects include headache, stomachache, nausea, moodiness (e.g., weepiness) or the suppression of adaptive behavior, irritability or euphoria, talkativeness, and marked decrease in activity (Gadow, 1986). Cognitive side-effects that occur for some children regardless of dosage or for others when the dosage is too high include poorer performance on thinking and problem-solving tasks, yet this outcome is unusual (Gadow, 1985, 1986). Other unusual and infrequent side-effects include facial grimaces, spasms or twitching of facial muscles, jerking or writhing movements of limbs, and twisting of the head and neck (Gadow, 1986). Caregivers should be in contact with the physician if side-effects occur so that dosages can be adjusted or medications can be changed (Gadow, 1986).

Several decades of research have shown that stimulants improve many aspects of behavior, including activity level in classrooms, motor steadiness and balance, handwriting, visual and auditory vigilance, reaction times, impulsivity, and short-term memory and paired-associate learning. However, despite such behavioral improvements, there is little evidence that stimulant therapy improves academic achievement (B. Lahey, Carlson, & Frick, 1992). Rather, the benefits appear to be related more to controlled social behavior, improved interpersonal relationships, and perhaps suppression of conduct problems. As children gain better control over their activity levels and behaviors, family members, peers, and teachers provide less controlling and less intense behavioral responses (Barkley, 1990a).

Some children have ADHD without coexisting language problems, whereas others have language and learning difficulties (Batshaw & Mercugliano, 1992; Conti, 1991; Shaywitz & Shaywitz, 1988; Silver, 1990). The link between ADHD and these other problems remains unclear. However, researchers attribute coexisting attention, linguistic, and reading problems to subtle differences in neurological brain substrates (Hynd et al., 1995; Hynd et al., 1993; Hynd, Semrud-Clikeman, Lorys, Novey, & Eliopulos, 1990).

Westby and Cutler (1994) regard inattention, hyperactivity, and impulsivity as primarily pragmatic and metacognitive deficits, which are language-based, rule-governed behaviors. Difficulties may occur in metacognitive processes that involve organizing and monitoring behavior, response inhibition, and self-regulation. Developmental impairments in these executive functions are thought to relate to problems in using verbal mediation for planning and engaging in goal-directed behavior (Shelton & Barkley, 1994). These complex interactions between attention, thinking, and self-regulation impact language, learning, and social-emotional success in school. The social-emotional aspects of pragmatic and metacognitive deficits associated with ADHD are listed in Table 7.6.

Weaver (1993) suggested that ADHD be viewed as a systemic problem affecting many areas of functioning. She proposed that biologically caused inattention–disorganization and impulsivity–hyperactivity characteristics ulti-

Table 7.6
Metacognitive and Pragmatic Problems Associated with Attention-Deficit/Hyperactivity Disorder

Metacognition

- Displays less knowledge and is immature in social skills
- Displays inappropriate behavior with others
- Makes decisions outside of social expectations
- Demonstrates aggression, disruption, intrusion, or domination in social relationships
- Views events that happen as outside of personal control
- Interprets others to have negative or hostile intentions

Pragmatics

- Lacks use of self-talk to control and organize interpersonal behavior
- Misreads or ignores verbal, nonverbal, and situational cues
- Displays awkwardness or inattention during verbal conversation
- Displays frequent talking but diminished response to questions or interaction
- Demonstrates verbal dysfluencies when organization is required
- Lacks variability in communication strategies according to task and setting
- Becomes easily frustrated and cries when language demands increase

Note. Adapted from "Language and ADHD: Understanding the Basis and Treatment of Self-Regulatory Deficits," by C. E. Westby and S. K. Cutler, 1994, *Topics in Language Disorders, 14*(4), pp. 58–76.

mately interfere with social appropriateness and acceptability. Thus, the disorder should be managed from a medical and sociological perspective that enables children to improve concentration while expectations and demands in educational settings are adjusted to each student's needs. Weaver also stated that behavioral approaches are not effective because they constrain and control student learning. Such approaches should be replaced with a combination of medication, when needed, and "a curriculum that keeps language and learning whole and meaningful, that offers students choice and ownership of learning, and that supports learners in taking more responsibility for their own learning and behavior" (p. 84).

Implications for the Classroom

When parents, teachers, SLPs and others suspect that ADHD is present in a student, careful observation within several settings must occur. Checklists such as the *Conners' Rating Scales–Revised* (Conners, 1997) are useful in the identification of symptoms and help physicians and the educational team members note the scope, variability, and consistency of the behaviors exhibited. For students whose problems also include language, a comprehensive assessment can involve several professionals including a physician, the school psychologist, the student's teachers, and an SLP (American Speech-Language-Hearing Association, 1997). Input from the classroom and special education teacher(s) is very important, since the classroom environment is often the most difficult for students with ADHD. Once the diagnosis is made, checklists are useful in documenting positive or negative outcomes of medication and behavioral and educational techniques implemented in the home and classroom. Careful and persistent documentation based on observation can greatly assist the educational team in modifying the academic plan and preventing hit-and-miss interventions.

Language intervention for children who also have ADHD must include strategies that facilitate self-monitoring, self-talk, and think-aloud techniques (Paul, 1995). Intervention should focus on activities that direct students' attention to the language and thinking abilities they use as they perform language-based tasks (Wallach & Miller, 1988). Such activities bring the student's awareness of language to a higher level and helps them stay focused.

Summary

Students who exhibit attention problems often have associated passivity, hyperactivity, or impulsivity. When left untreated, older students may develop related psychiatric conditions, such as oppositional defiant disorder or conduct disorder. Treatment for attention problems may consist of the use of psychostimulant medications or behavioral and cognitive therapy. Attention problems can coexist with language disorders and reading delays, presumably because of faulty development of some neural areas in the brain. Attention problems affect students' social use of language, as well as their ability to use metacognitive strategies during learning situations. Thus, students with ADHD require a collaborative approach to assessment and intervention. Teachers, SLPs, school psychologists, and parents must determine the appropriate educational strategies that result in better attention, self-regulation, and self-monitoring abilities during learning opportunities.

Mental Retardation

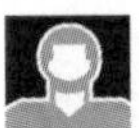

Jason

Jason is 7½ years old. He was full term and had a normal birth, yet he required oxygen. Jason was very slow in accomplishing developmental milestones. He sat unsupported at 9 months, crawled at 12 months, and walked without support around 17 months. He is currently not bladder or bowel trained. His motor skills appear delayed and he is awkward when eating, using crayons and pencils, and running. Jason is an affectionate child, seeking hugs and kisses from family members and others. He plays with toys that make noise or action and is beginning to attend to picture books. He likes to listen to stories before sleeping. Jason is putting words together into four- and five-word combinations. His use of pointing and gestures to make his wants and needs known is decreasing as he learns new vocabulary.

Definitions and Characteristics

Persons like Jason exhibit (a) intellectual functioning that is in the subaverage range (intellectual quotient of 70 or below); (b) limitations in adaptive behavior such as academic learning, personal independence, and social responsibility with respect to chronological age and cultural expectations; and (c) manifestations of the problem during the first 18 years of life (American Psychiatric Association, 1994). Mental retardation occurs in about 1% of the total population (Nelson, 1993).

Cognitive impairments in persons with mental retardation can range from mild to profound. Intelligence quotient ranges are used to determine the following categories: mild (55 to 70), moderate (40 to 55), severe (25 to 40), and profound (below 25). Most persons with mental retardation (89%) are mildly affected, whereas 10% fall in the moderate range and 2% to 5% fall in the severe and

Table 7.7
Performance Descriptions of Persons with Mental Retardation by Severity Categories

Mild Retardation

- Delays in social and communication abilities
- Minimal delays in sensorimotor abilities
- Acquisition of academics to approximately the sixth-grade level during teenage years
- Special education particularly in secondary school
- Social and vocational independence
- Supervision required for some social or economic situations
- Acquisition of reading and writing

Moderate Retardation

- Delays in communication abilities and poor social awareness
- Fair motor development in preschoolers
- Acquisition of academics to approximately the fourth-grade level during teen years
- Special education in all grades
- Unskilled or semiskilled occupational employment
- Supervision required for social and economic situations
- Acquisition of some reading and writing

Severe Retardation

- Minimal speech development and limited communication abilities
- Poor motor development and acquisition of self-help abilities
- May learn to communicate through alternative or augmentative systems
- Nonacademic educational opportunities in self-help and self-protection
- Supervision required for social situations

Profound Retardation

- Minimal functioning communication and sensorimotor areas
- Some motor development may occur, but total care is required from others
- Minimal benefits from training self-help skills
- Continous supervision required

profound range (American Psychiatric Association, 1994). Table 7.7 lists some general performance descriptions of persons with mental retardation (Chinn, Drew, & Logan, 1975; Nelson, 1993). Levels of language, motor, social, self-help, and academic abilities are highly associated with the severity of the mental retardation.

Several factors are associated with the occurrence and severity of mental retardation: biological factors, such as chromosomal or infectious processes; nutritional and metabolic factors; gestational factors; pregnancy and birth complications; and gross disorders of the central nervous system. Additionally, contributing factors such as information processing problems and social interaction correlate with the severity of mental retardation (Nelson, 1993).

The incidence of hearing loss is high in children with mental retardation. For example, children with Down syndrome have structural malformations of the face, head, middle ear, and eustachian tube, which can result in recurrent middle ear infections (otitis media) and chronic conductive hearing loss (Ratner & Harris, 1994). The biological factors that cause mental retardation are also causes of hearing loss, such as oxygen deprivation during birth or the presence of a genetic syndrome. Because hearing loss further complicates language development in children who have cognitive deficits, such children require a hearing evaluation early in life, regular medical checkups, medical management of ear infections, and annual hearing evaluations.

Language development in children with mental retardation is related to cognitive development. *Mental age* is a term often used to describe the cognitive abilities of individual children. Educationists sometimes adjust a person's chronological age to his or her mental age based on estimated intellectual functioning, so that educational planning occurs according to the needs of the child. For example, a 5-year-old child with an intelligence score of 70 may have a mental age of 4 years. Mental ages are often compared with language abilities demonstrated by the children (see Nelson, 1993, pp. 216–217, for a discussion of problems with such comparisons). However, it is sometimes difficult to estimate cognitive functioning in children, particularly when language delay is substantial. The interpretation of intelligence and achievement test scores is confounded by the verbal nature of many of these tests. Thus, careful observation of each child's language, nonlinguistic abilities, social and self-help development, and problem-solving abilities in toy manipulation and drawing can provide important information that can be used in educational planning.

Children with mental retardation demonstrate a wide range of language abilities. Compared to others with language problems, they have (a) higher incidence of articulation disorders; (b) greater difficulty comprehending and producing prefixes and suffixes; (c) difficulty using simple sentence structures with less flexibility to vary the structure; and (d) concrete, literal, and restricted word meanings. They have also been observed to be less verbally assertive than children without mental retardation (Nelson, 1993; Owens, 1989).

Implications for the Classroom

Educational options for children with mental retardation have expanded significantly during the past decade. These children are now being included in public education within general classrooms and in resource rooms. Careful observation, assessment, and intervention planning in accord with each child's changing needs require that general education teachers, special educators, SLPs, and parents work closely together with the child whenever possible.

Summary

Students who are mentally retarded exhibit cognitive impairments from the mild to the profound range and have delays in language abilities, motor coordination, social relationships, self-help abilities, and academic learning. Because of the high incidence of hearing loss in children with mental retardation, especially those who have Down syndrome, it is essential that regularly scheduled hearing evaluations and treatment for otitis media occur. The extent of language delay in persons with mental retardation relates to their degree of cognitive ability. Because assessment tools are highly verbal in nature, it is often difficult to accurately determine cognitive level; thus, educationists must use a combination of standardized and observational tools to estimate the levels of cognitive and linguistic functioning. Language development continues into adulthood for persons who are mentally retarded, just as it does for persons who are not mentally retarded. Consequently, language intervention must be an ongoing process as individuals learn to listen, speak, read, and write.

Traumatic Brain Injury

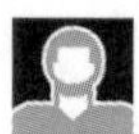

Sean

Sean is 16 years, 3 months old. He was hit by a car while riding his bicycle when he was 6½ years old. Sean sustained a closed head injury to the left frontal and temporal lobes. During his 3-month hospitalization, he received intensive speech–language therapy, physical therapy, occupational therapy, and psychological services. All these special services continue to be maintained on a less intensive basis. Sean is now able to walk, yet he is awkward in both gross and fine motor coordination. He communicates his ideas in simple, concrete sentences. His articulation is mildly impaired because of oral motor incoordination, and he has difficulty making connections between ideas and relating known information with new concepts. Sean understands what others say when sentences are short and concrete and when gestures or pictures are used with verbal language. He can follow one- and two-step directions that involve repetitive daily living tasks. Sean is successfully included in his eighth-grade classroom.

Definitions and Characteristics

Brain injury is the leading cause of death in pediatric populations, and traumatic brain injury (TBI) is the most common cause of brain injury in children and adolescents, as with Sean. A TBI is defined as "a nonpenetrating injury to the brain usually associated with motor-vehicle, motor-pedestrian, motor-bicycle, or sports-related injuries, or falls" (Chapman, 1997). The highest risk group for TBI is the young adult population (19 to 25 years); however, 30% of all severe head injuries are sustained by children and adolescents ages 19 and younger (Gross, Wolf, Kunitz, & Jane, 1985; Ylvisaker, Kolpan, & Rosenthal, 1994).

TBI is sudden and unexpected. Consequently, the entire family system is suddenly involved in acute treatment, followed by involvement in the rehabilitation process, and finally the person's reintegration into the community. The family's ability to respond positively and effectively to these challenges depends on a variety of factors: (a) roles and responsibilities assumed by family members; (b) the communication styles of family participants; (c) ethnic and cultural background, which may affect family beliefs about disability; (d) the stages within the life cycle of family participants; (e) the family's willingness and ability to access community resources; (f) the availability of resources; and (g) the age of the family member with TBI (DePompei & Williams, 1994). DePompei and Williams (1994) proposed a family-centered model of interdisciplinary collaboration. In this model, family members can participate in the assessment and intervention processes as information providers, advocates, expert communication partners, and those who develop their vision for their future.

As with other language acquisition disabilities, children with TBI represent a heterogeneous group. The variability in language characteristics after TBI is associated with the severity of the injury, the site(s) and extent of the injury, as well as the language, cognitive, emotional, personality, and environmental characteristics of the child *prior* to the TBI (Chapman, Levin, & Culhane, 1995).

A summary of the common language problems characteristic of children with TBI is provided in Table 7.8. Notice that language structure (i.e., phonology, morphology, and syntax) and the ability to comprehend language are typically not disturbed, especially when lesions are in the frontal lobe (the most common site). However, damage to the frontal lobe often results in language and cognitive deficits (Chapman, 1997; Chapman et al., 1992; Levin, Goldstein, Williams, & Eisenberg, 1991; Levin et al., 1993) that interfere with learning, thinking, and integrating information. Children with TBI find it difficult to (a) keep pace with the rate and amount of information; (b) integrate

Table 7.8
Language Problems Common in Children with Traumatic Brain Injury

- Language comprehension is typically not impaired
- Sentences are well formed and of average complexity
- Word finding and naming deficits may be present
- Injury to the left hemisphere results in specific language impairments
- Language problems occur on tasks requiring timed responses or cognitive manipulation for problem solving
- Impairment in narrative discourse when manipulation of extended units of language is required, such as for retaining information from stories and constructing or retelling stories
- Marked difficulty in paraphrasing discourse information into summaries or main ideas

Note. Adapted from "Cognitive-Communication Abilities in Children with Closed Head Injury," by S. B. Chapman, 1997, *American Journal of Speech-Language Pathology, 6*(2), pp. 50–58.

information being studied; (c) use previously acquired knowledge; (d) use memory and attention processes effectively; (e) acquire new information; and (f) construct, retell, or paraphrase ideas (Chapman, 1997).

Brain injury can occur from causes other than TBI. Focal acquired lesions caused by strokes (cerebral vascular accidents), convulsive disorder (Landau-Kleffner syndrome), and infection or irradiation of tumors can result in language problems. The term *aphasia* is sometimes used to label the profile of receptive and expressive language problems resulting from these conditions (Nelson, 1993). The incidence of their occurrence is too low to warrant more attention in this chapter, as most teachers and school-based SLPs will not encounter students with aphasia.

Implications for the Classroom

TBI can result in profound consequences in language, learning, social-emotional skills, and physical growth and development. It can impact a child's current and future development. Formal tests for language disability and other areas do not always show the nature or extent of the difficulties associated with TBI (Ylvisaker et al., 1994). Therefore, Szekeres and Meserve (1994) recommended that educators, SLPs, and other specialists adopt a conceptual framework in which TBI is seen as "an often enduring educational disability requiring ongoing identification, assessment, and intervention within the school setting. Such a framework must allow for flexible assessment, management, and delivery of curriculum and instruction in a variety of school settings and include a strong family service component." (p. 23). This framework requires collaboration among members of the educational team (classroom teacher, SLP, special education teachers, school psychologist, etc.) and family members, and careful deliberation about the needs of the student with TBI. The cognitive and linguistic demands of activities within the classroom should be analyzed so that appropriate accommodations and modifications maximize the student's success and provide the best use of educational resources.

Summary

Traumatic brain injury occurs most often in young people prior to their high school graduation. This sudden and life-changing event has far-reaching consequences for the members within the family and the student with TBI who must reintegrate into school and other community settings. Language problems associated with TBI tend to occur when the student attempts to learn, think, and integrate information. Because TBI is an enduring educational disability, flexible and ongoing assessment and intervention are necessary for students to effectively participate in classrooms.

Pervasive Developmental Disorder and Autism

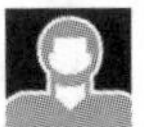

Andrew

Andrew is a 5-year-old, strong, stocky child. He seeks food often and smells everything before eating. His parents lock cupboards and the refrigerator at home, because Andrew gets sick when he eats too much. Andrew is aggressive with other children when they get too close to his food, personal property, or activities. He does seek attention, affection, and physical comfort by giving and receiving brief hugs or high-fives. When Andrew is angry or frustrated, he hits himself in the head or bites the backs of his hands. Andrew began to use a few single words at about 13 months, including "Hi," the family dog's name "Buttons," and "Okay." He stopped using these around his second birthday and currently does not speak. Andrew's attention is captured by noise from airplanes and trucks, but he responds by covering his ears when the phone rings or the dog barks. Andrew is very neat; he organizes his shoes and toys in his closet daily. During school, he sorts objects and arranges pictures. He recognizes about 10 printed words and can print his name.

Definition and Characteristics

Pervasive developmental disorder (PDD) is a broad and general classification for a group of severe and pervasive impairments affecting social interaction and communication, often accompanied by stereotyped behaviors, interests, and activities (American Psychiatric Association, 1994). Disorders within the PDD category include autism (Andrew's problem), Rett's disorder, childhood integration disorder, Asperger's disorder, and PDD not otherwise specified. Autism is the focus in this chapter, because it is the most common of the PDD disorders.

Autism occurs in 2 to 5 per 10,000 individuals. Although its incidence is low, it is more common than the other types of PDD and more is understood about its characteristics. The diagnostic criteria for autistic disorder (see Table 7.9) include four main areas: (1) qualitative impairment in social interaction with others; (2) qualitative impairment in verbal and nonverbal communication; (3) markedly restricted repertoire of activities and interests; and (4) onset during infancy or childhood. Persons with autism can have cognitive abilities within the average or low average ranges; however, up to 60% have measured IQs below 50, which is in the severe and profound range. Table 7.10, summarizing contemporary research, shows the many contributing factors such as cognitive, biological, linguistic, environmental, and information-processing variables that are associated with autism (Nelson, 1993).

The behavioral signs of autism are numerous and well known. Children may engage in repetitive movements, such as rocking, hand flapping, head banging, hand biting, spinning, and abnormal postures and gait. Movement and motor planning problems are hypothesized to be responsible for these repetitive movements (Maurer & Damasio, 1982). Behaviors associated with hypersensitivity include blocking the ears during loud or high-pitched sounds, shielding the eyes in bright light, and taking off tight-fitting or new clothing (Bauman, 1993; Courchesne, 1989). In addition, lack of eye contact, aloofness, passivity, lack of self-awareness, need for structure and routine, ritualistic and compulsive behavior, and social isolation are descriptions often made about children with autism (Ratner & Harris, 1994).

Many of the communication and social-interaction characteristics of autism are quite different from those that accompany children with other language or cognitive impairments. Some children produce some words early on, but between 18 and 30 months these words are lost and not replaced by new ones. It is estimated that 50% do not develop functional language production. Of those who speak, many differences have been observed in (a) the use of *echolalia* (i.e., immediate or delayed repetition of part or all of someone else's language); (b) improper use of pronouns to refer to self (e.g., "you," "she,"

Table 7.9
Diagnostic Criteria for Autistic Disorder

A. A total of six (or more) items from (1), (2), and (3), with at least two from (1), and one each from (2) and (3):
   (1) qualitative impairment in social interaction, as manifested by at least two of the following:
      (a) marked impairment in the use of multiple nonverbal behaviors such as eye-to-eye gaze, facial expression, body postures, and gestures to regulate social interaction
      (b) failure to develop peer relationships appropriate to developmental level
      (c) a lack of spontaneous seeking to share enjoyment, interests, or achievements with other people (e.g., by a lack of showing, bringing, or pointing out objects of interest)
      (d) lack of social or emotional reciprocity
   (2) qualitative impairments in communication as manifested by at least one of the following:
      (a) delay in, or total lack of, the development of spoken language (not accompanied by an attempt to compensate through alternative modes of communication such as gesture or mime)
      (b) in individuals with adequate speech, marked impairment in the ability to initiate or sustain a conversation with others
      (c) stereotyped and repetitive use of language or idiosyncratic language
      (d) lack of varied, spontaneous make-believe play or social imitative play appropriate to developmental level
   (3) restricted repetitive and stereotyped patterns of behavior, interests, and activities, as manifested by at least one of the following:
      (a) encompassing preoccupation with one or more stereotyped and restricted patterns of interest that is abnormal either in intensity or focus
      (b) apparently inflexible adherence to specific, nonfunctional routines or rituals
      (c) stereotyped and repetitive motor mannerisms (e.g., hand or finger flapping or twisting, or complex whole-body movements)
      (d) persistent preoccupation with parts of objects

B. Delays or abnormal functioning in at least one of the following areas, with onset prior to age 3 years: (1) social interaction, (2) language as used in social communication, or (3) symbolic or imaginative play.

C. The disturbance is not better accounted for by Rett's Disorder or Childhood Disintegrative Disorder.

Note. From *Diagnostic and Statistical Manual of Mental Disorders* (4th ed., pp. 70–71), by American Psychiatric Association, 1994, Washington, DC: Author.

Table 7.10
Associated Factors Within Autism

Biological

- High levels of the neurotransmitter serotonin
- High amounts of peptides, making children less prone to seek physical affection and comfort
- Soft neurological signs including low muscle tone, poor coordination, and toe-walking
- Abnormal patterns of brain activity
- Structural abnormalities in the brain, including small size and cellular irregularities in the cerebellum

Linguistic and Social Interaction

- Delayed and qualitatively different communication, which results in social interaction problems
- Often impaired cognitive development, which can lead to linguistic development problems
- Autism is a neurological disorder, not a psychogenic disorder
- Disturbances in social interaction

Cognitive and Information Processing

- Cognitive impairments, ranging from IQ below 50 to IQ above 70
- Wide scatter within cognitive abilities within individuals
- Cerebellar abnormalities that may cause hyper- or hyposensitivity to auditory, visual, tactile, and kinesthetic processes
- Various information processing mechanisms may function independently rather than in concert, resulting in problems with integration of multisensory information, and less ability to use meaning and sentence structure for recall and formulation of language

Note. Adapted from *Childhood Language Disorders in Context: Infancy Through Adolescence,* by N. W. Nelson, 1993, New York: Merrill.

"he"); (c) repetitive speech without apparent functional value; (d) monotonous inflection, rhythm, pitch, rate, and articulation; (e) confusion in grammar and meanings; and (f) impaired understanding of nonverbal gestures, facial expressions, and physical distance from others.

Students who are autistic often demonstrate characteristics similar to those of students with language and learning disorders. For instance, comprehension problems occur with abstract concepts such as time, space, quantity, or direction. Figurative language (e.g., metaphors, idioms, jokes) is interpreted literally, frequently causing misunderstandings and hurt feelings. Reading may develop in some individuals, but comprehension problems interfere with progress, and difficulties with writing occur in the integration of the meaning (Nelson, 1993).

Implications for the Classroom

The unique characteristics of students with autism make assessment and educational planning challenging for educators, SLPs and other specialists, and parents. Many factors must be taken into consideration (e.g., cognitive, linguistic, behavioral, and the social-emotional status of each individual) to determine the least restrictive and most appropriate settings, instructional methodologies, and interactions needed for maximum learning opportunities. Early intervention, student and family involvement in all aspects of the educational plan, and consistent support from peers are essential ingredients to providing each student opportunities to develop social and communicative competence. Students with autism who do not speak may benefit from alternative or augmentative communication strategies, such as sign language or (low- or high-technology) communication devices.

Summary

Autism is a complex disorder that affects several aspects of development, including language, cognition, social relationships, and academic learning. Students who are autistic may be verbal or nonverbal. Those who have verbal language have difficulty developing each of the language systems and using language for social interactions with others. Additionally, low cognitive abilities often result in poor comprehension of abstract concepts and figurative language forms. Some children may develop written language, yet poor comprehension and low pragmatic understanding can interfere with progress. A collaborative team of professionals, parent participation, and consistent educational support enhances the student's success in grade-level classrooms.

Fetal Exposure to Substance Abuse

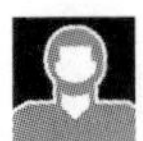

Cindi

Cindi is 12 years old and has been in foster care since birth. She was born prematurely, weighing 4 pounds, and had a cocaine addiction at birth. She has petit mal seizures, which are controlled by Tegretol, and her vision is poor. Cindi began physical and speech–language therapies around her first birthday. Her motor development was slow, with walking occurring at 3 years. She has difficulty running and lacks coordination when dancing. Cindi's language development was also slow, with first words occurring at 2½ years. She currently speaks in sentences; however, grammatical structure is often immature and vocabulary is weak. She has difficulty understanding complex directions and loses concentration when others are speaking. Cindi is often irritable and appears sleepy and disinterested in her surroundings.

Definition and Characteristics

Legal and illegal chemical substances taken singly or in combination during pregnancy include alcohol, tobacco, cocaine, marijuana, heroin, and amphetamines. Substance abuse by women and men crosses all socioeconomic levels; however, poverty and participation in the drug culture lead many women (and their developing fetuses) to further complications from undernourishment, risk of infectious diseases, and lack of prenatal care during pregnancy (Kronstadt, 1991; Sparks, 1993).

Physical irregularities are linked to exposure to chemicals in utero. Table 7.11 compares the effects of abuse of alcohol, crack/cocaine, tobacco and environmental smoke, and marijuana on birth, early physical development, and physical problems. Possible results include pregnancy complications; prematurity; low birth weight; malnutrition; growth deficiencies; underdevelopment of the brain; neurological problems; malformations of the face or limbs; cardiac problems; motor, sensory, and attentional problems; and even death (Ratner & Harris, 1994). In other cases, the babies are born normal and develop normally.

The effects of substance abuse on the developing child are numerous. The amount, timing of ingestion during fetal development, and type of substance have differential effects on fetal development. The potential problems with hearing and vision, cognition, attention and memory, language, social skills and behavior, and academic performance can have lasting effects on a student during school and throughout his or her lifetime.

Implications for the Classroom

For children exposed in utero to toxic substances, early intervention and a positive, drug-free environment are essential for improving physical and developmental levels. Health and social service professionals must educate parents

(*text continues on page 286*)

Table 7.11
The Effects of Fetal Exposure to Substance Abuse on Child Development

Effect	Fetal Alcohol Syndrome and Fetal Alcohol Effects	Crack/Cocaine	Tobacco and Environmental Smoke	Marijuana
Birth and early physical development	Prematurity Low birth weight Postnatal growth retardation	Prematurity Growth retardation in utero Low birth weight and malnutrition Sexually transmitted disease Small head circumference	Prematurity Low birth weight Pregnancy complication (bleeding, rupture of membranes) Decreased head circumference and birth length	Infant tremors
Malformations and other physical problems	Malformations in heart, limbs, palate, or brain Unusual facial formation Delayed motor development	Increased blood pressure, small strokes, heart attacks, and seizures Poor health Poor feeding patterns Limb reduction, urinary tract defects	Higher fetal and infant death rates Poor fine and gross motor skills Acute and chronic respiratory disease Impaired postnatal lung development Middle ear infections	
Sensory problems	Hearing problems Vision problems	Visual tracking sensitivity and responsiveness difficulties Auditory pathways impairments	Decreased visual alertness Difficulty orienting to voice	Sensory difficulties Unresponsive to visual stimuli

(*continues*)

Table 7.11 *Continued.*

Effect	Fetal Alcohol Syndrome and Fetal Alcohol Effects	Crack/Cocaine	Tobacco and Environmental Smoke	Marijuana
Cognitive development	Delayed intellectual development Conceptual confusion Difficulty predicting consequences Normal to severe intellectual deficits	Difficulty with abstract concepts Disorganized and less representational in play	Poor performance on cognitive tasks	
Attention and memory and others	Short attention, distractibility, and hyperactivity	Sleeping difficulties Reduced memory Excitability, depression, irritability, hypersensitivity Difficulty organizing and maintaining alertness Problems with self-regulation		Sleep disturbances Reduced performance on memory tasks Attention deficits in school-age children
Language development	Delayed language Sparse early vocabularies Shallow word meanings Reduced sentence length	Difficulty comprehending and expressing language Deficiencies in gazing and turn-taking Poor pragmatics	Poor language performance	Reduced performance on verbal tasks

(*continues*)

Social development and behavioral difficulties	Immature play routines Lack of skills for friendships Inappropriate use of language Avoidance of conversation in social situations	Unresponsive to interactions from caregivers Difficulty forming secure attachments Immature play routines Abrupt, inappropriate changes in behavior Reduced recognition of emotional states in self, others Higher incidence of autism	
Academic performance	Difficulties in comprehension, abstract thinking, visual/spatial memory, problem solving, conceptualization	Academic performance may decline with age Learning disabilities	Less advanced verbal, reading, and math scores

Note. Adapted from *Understanding Language Disorders: The Impact on Learning,* by V. L. Ratner and L. R. Harris, 1994, Eau Claire, WI: Thinking Publications.

(biological or adoptive) about the effects of the drug(s) and the physical and developmental problems associated with substance abuse. The daily physical care and the complex developmental and behavioral problems these children demonstrate make early education and intervention with parents very important.

Teachers and specialists can also make a positive difference in decreasing the incidence of substance abuse through education of youngsters (and their parents) about the dangers of drugs and their effects on persons and the community (e.g., legality, side-effects, addiction, economic and cultural effects). Drug Abuse Resistance Education (DARE) police officers are available in some states to provide education, prevention, and decisive action regarding drug use. Teachers must alert authorities and social service providers when there is suspicion of drug exposure in the home, and enforce strict and consistent policies of nontolerance for any drugs (legal or illegal) at school-sponsored activities.

Problems with senses (both hearing and vision) and across all aspects of development require detailed assessment, including observation in several settings (e.g., home, playground, classroom); formal hearing and vision testing; and formal and informal measures of cognition, language, social skills, and academics. A collaborative approach to assessment and intervention brings together the expertise of general and special educators, health care professionals, SLPs and other specialists, and parents so that a comprehensive understanding of each student's needs can be considered in the educational plan.

Summary

Some pregnant women expose their unborn fetuses to legal and illegal chemical substances that cause addiction or developmental problems. For some newborns, these toxic substances affect numerous aspects of development, including physical health, the senses, cognitive ability, and language development. As children grow, the effects involve attention, written language development, and academic performance. Early intervention for such children is vital to improve the physical and developmental consequences of substance abuse. In addition, educationists and other professionals in the community must educate students and their parents about the adverse effects of drugs on children's development. Teachers must carefully observe students who were victims of substance abuse and design appropriate interventions that target the specific needs of each child.

Maltreatment of Children: Abuse and Neglect

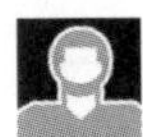

Bradley

Bradley is 5 years old and attends kindergarten. He is of slight build, appears malnourished, and has low energy. Bradley wears worn-out tennis shoes without socks, dirty jeans, and one of three short-sleeved shirts daily. He is quiet among peers and very polite with adults, but appears reticent to interact with others. He has little knowledge of concepts (e.g., numbers, letters, colors), story structure, or phonological awareness. Recent bruising on his arms and face provoked a report to social services about possible abuse and neglect in the home.

Definitions and Characteristics

Maltreatment occurs in children who suffer abuse (physical, sexual, emotional) or neglect (physical, emotional) within or outside of their families. It is thought to result from complex and multiple influences involving attributes of parents and families, the children themselves, and the setting (Knutson & Sullivan, 1993). Although maltreatment can and does occur in all social classes of society, the incidence is higher in lower socioeconomic strata, perhaps because of inadequate economic resources, housing, and nutrition, and lower levels of educational achievement and employment (Coster & Cicchetti, 1993). The type of maltreatment, age of the student during maltreatment, family influences, and nature of the physical and social environment are factors that influence the nature and extent of the problems exhibited by children who suffer abuse or neglect.

Children with disabilities, the largest minority in the United States, comprise a high-risk group for maltreatment, both abuse and neglect. Medical problems, physical mobility limitations, and developmental difficulties in cognition, behavior, and communication have been linked to additional stress within family systems, which may lead to maltreatment. Knutson and Sullivan (1993) cautioned, however, that research regarding cause–effect relationships is difficult to conduct. They wrote, "it is often impossible to determine whether the handicapping condition contributes to the occurrence of abuse or is a consequence of abuse" (p. 2). For example, physical abuse can result in head trauma, which can lead to cognitive, behavioral, and communication problems. These developmental problems can further increase stress, which may contribute to further abuse, thus making children with disabilities susceptible as victims.

Table 7.12
Communication Problems of Children Who Are Maltreated

Infants and Toddlers

- Elevated rates of insecure attachments, including insecure/avoidant or disorganized/disoriented patterns
- Signs of apprehension in the presence of the caregiver
- Reduced participation in interactions with others
- Reduced ability to make cause–effect connections between social cues and environmental responsiveness
- Reduced mean length of utterance
- Limited expressive vocabulary during interactions with the mother or caregiver
- Less communication directed at exchanging information about feelings or about their own activities
- Less reference to persons or events outside the immediate context
- Shorter instances of continuous contingent discourse
- Less use of language as a medium for social or affective exchanges
- Restricted use of language to communicate needs and feelings, to convey abstractions, and to sustain dialogue and construct narratives

Preschool and School-Age Children

- Low normal performance on linguistic tasks
- Inadequate ability to convey thoughts and feelings
- Decreased verbal language performance and reading achievement
- Depressed cognitive levels
- Lack of experience in verbal problem-solving methods
- Limited experience attending to complex communications
- Difficulty extracting key ideas from lengthy narratives
- Decreased motivation and frustration tolerance
- Overcompliance or passivity
- Increased prevalence of behavior problems including aggression, noncompliance, depression, and lack of motivation

Note. Adapted from "Research on the Communicative Development of Maltreated Children: Clinical Implications," by W. Coster and D. Cicchetti, 1993, *Topics in Language Disorders, 13*(4), pp. 25–38.

Because the acquisition of language is intertwined with cognitive and social-emotional development, it is not surprising that maltreated children have developmental delays and difficulties in interactive communication (Coster & Cicchetti, 1993). Table 7.12 shows the communication problems that have been observed in children who are maltreated. For infants and toddlers, the interaction patterns suggest problems with security, trust, and predictability. For school-age children, the problems reflect impoverished linguistic experiences and difficulties in using language for problem solving and academic learning. Thus, language difficulties have the potential to impact a wide range of abilities in school, from establishing satisfactory peer relationships to acquiring literacy. In fact, nonoptimal home environments can influence all areas of achievement.

Language difficulties in children who are maltreated have consequences for how children respond in communicative situations with other children and adults. One troublesome situation is reporting and testifying in court about their maltreatment. In particular, the courtroom discourse requires that children produce narrative accounts and recounts, answer repeated questions about details, and understand the nature of questions being asked. These high language expectations can be difficult for children who have developmental problems resulting from maltreatment (Snyder, Nathanson, & Shaywitz, 1993).

Implications for the Classroom

Professionals who work with children have a legal and ethical responsibility to watch for and report suspicion of maltreatment. State laws define child abuse, mandate who is required to report, describe standards and procedures for reporting, and establish consequences for failure to report (Berliner, 1993). Thus, teachers must exercise their responsibilities whenever maltreatment is suspected. In addition, teachers can confer (while maintaining confidentiality) with other teachers, the principal, and other professionals within the community to seek advice and gain insight about a problem (Berliner, 1993).

Several steps can be taken to preserve or even build a working relationship between professionals and families when a report of abuse or neglect is to be made. Berliner (1993) suggested that a consent-for-care document be signed by all parents and kept in the school file for each student stating that a report of child abuse or neglect is possible. Open-ended interviews of parents and students, and informing the parents and the student when a report is being made (if it is appropriate to do so) can improve understanding and allow the family to become a part of the dialogue.

Teachers, SLPs, health care providers, and community agencies should be actively engaged in education efforts to prevent violence and neglect. Strict policies prohibiting violence in schools can heighten awareness about the nature of violence and teach students that negative social consequences are tied to violent acts.

Finally, signs of communication delay and interaction problems should be documented so that further investigation of contributing factors can occur. If emotional problems appear to be present, referral for psychological assessment and intervention is appropriate. Speech–language and achievement assessment, based on teacher observation of students in the classroom and interactions with peers, may be recommended.

Summary

The final category of students who have difficulty with language that I discuss in this chapter are those who suffer from maltreatment or neglect. The nature of the language problems demonstrated by these students depends on the many factors associated with the maltreatment or neglect. However, such children have been observed to have difficulties in interactive communication, the development of the linguistic system, and use of language in problem-solving situations and in academic learning. Children with disabilities are at particular risk for maltreatment and neglect. While some researchers attribute this problem to increased stress within families, others point out that maltreatment and neglect contribute to both developmental and physical disabilities. All professionals within schools are legally and ethically responsible by law for reporting suspicion of maltreatment and neglect. They also share, with other community professionals, the responsibility for educating students and their parents about the adverse effects of maltreatment and neglect and for enforcing strict policies prohibiting violence in schools. When a student has language and other developmental problems associated with maltreatment and neglect, the educational team must work to fully understand the scope of problems and develop interventions that focus on growth in language, learning, and social-emotional health.

Summary and Conclusion

This chapter has highlighted eight types of problems that have concomitant linguistic implications. Several factors within the child (e.g., biological, genetic, neurological) and the environment (e.g., toxins, educational opportunity, maltreatment) contribute to the types of language problems children with disabilities manifest. These problems impact the development of cognition, language, academic achievement, and social relationships as children mature. The language acquisition and usage problems in school-age children result in reduced success in classroom participation, weak knowledge of content-area information, and underdevelopment of reading and writing abilities.

Educationists, health care professionals, and social service providers have a role in the prevention of disabilities related to language acquisition and usage. It is vitally important that those professionals who work with students and their families create and use opportunities to inform them about the negative effects of poor prenatal care, drug and alcohol abuse, violence, poor safety practices, and environments lacking in rich social interaction. Through education about risk factors and strict public policies regarding physical safety, drug abuse, and violence, the incidence of some of these disorders could decrease.

In addition to preventive measures, professionals who work with children have the responsibility to observe when language acquisition and usage disabilities are present and make appropriate referrals for assessment. Once the nature and extent of the problems are defined, general and special educators and SLPs should work collaboratively to design interventions that help students become successful in classrooms. All team members should understand federal and state laws and local policies so that the educational plan is constructed in an informed and complete manner with the best interests of children and families in mind. Once the educational plan is determined, its effectiveness should be monitored and changes made regularly to maximize learning in all areas of academic and social growth. Ways to engage in collaboration will be explained in Chapter 9. Chapter 8 continues the discussion of disabilities by focusing on language problems related to speech production.

TODAY'S WORK
• READING 56-64
TEXT
QUESTIONS 1-5
DISCUSSION
• MATH
CHAPT. 3
PROBLEMS
WHAT'S A TEXT?
WHERE'S MY PENCIL?
T.M. BALCHAK
9/98

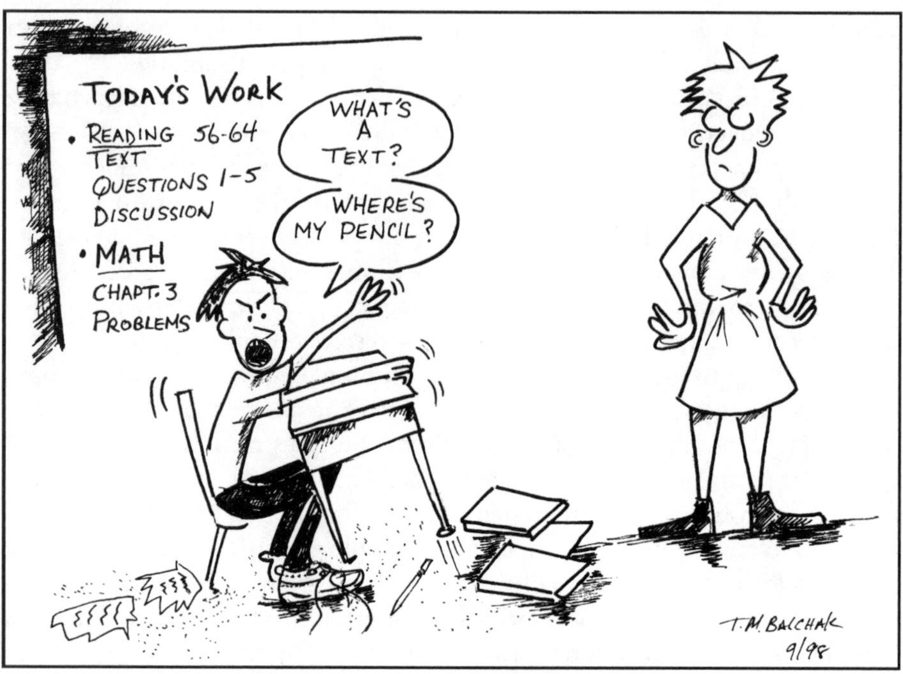

Complex interactions between attention, thinking, and self-regulation impact language, learning, and social-emotional success in school.

References

American Psychiatric Association. (1994). *Diagnostic and statistical manual of mental disorders* (4th ed.), Washington, DC: Author.

American Speech-Language-Hearing Association. (1997, Spring). Position statement: Roles of audiologists and speech–language pathologists working with persons with attention deficit hyperactivity disorder. *Asha, 39* (Suppl. 17), 14.

American Speech-Language-Hearing Association Committee on Language, Speech, and Hearing Services in Schools. (1982). Definitions: Communication disorders and variations. *Asha, 24*, 949–950.

Barkley, R. A. (1990a). *Attention deficit hyperactivity disorder: A handbook for diagnosis and treatment*. New York: Guilford.

Barkley, R. A. (1990b). A critique of current diagnostic criteria for attention deficit hyperactivity disorder: Clinical and research implication. *Journal of Developmental and Behavioral Pediatrics, 11*, 343–352.

Barkley, R. A. (1995). Delayed responding and attention deficit hyperactivity disorder: A unified theory. In D. K. Routh (Ed.), *Disruptive behavior disorders in children: Essays in honor of Herbert Quay*. New York: Plenum.

Barkley, R. A., Fischer, M., Edelbrock, C. S., & Smallish, L. (1990). The adolescent outcome of hyperactive children diagnosed by research criteria: I. An 8 year prospective follow-up study. *Journal of the American Academy of Child and Adolescent Psychiatry, 29*, 546–557.

Batshaw, M., & Mercugliano, M. (1992). Attention deficit hyperactivity disorder. In M. Batshaw & Y. Perret (Eds.), *Children with disabilities: A medical primer* (pp. 387–406). Baltimore: Brookes.

Bauman, M. (1993). An interview with Dr. Margaret Bauman. *Advocate: Autism Society of America, 24*(4), 1–14.

Bellis, T. J. (1996). *Assessment and management of central auditory processing disorders in the educational setting*. San Diego: Singular.

Berliner, L. (1993). Identifying and reporting suspected child abuse and neglect. *Topics in Language Disorders, 13*(4), 15–24.

Cantwell, D. P., & Baker, L. (1985). Psychiatric and learning disorders in children with speech and language disorders: A descriptive analysis. In K. D. Gadow (Ed.), *Advances in learning and behavioral disabilities* (Vol. 4). Greenwich, CT: JAI.

Cantwell, D. P., & Baker, L. (1991). Association between attention deficit–hyperactivity disorder and learning disorders. *Journal of Learning Disabilities, 24*, 88–95.

Chapman, S. B. (1997). Cognitive–communication abilities in children with closed head injury. *American Journal of Speech–Language Pathology*, 6(2), 50–58.

Chapman, S. B., Culhane, K. A., Levin, H. S., Harward, H., Mendelsohn, D., Ewing-Cobbs, L., Fletcher, J. M., & Bruce, D. (1992). Narrative discourse after closed head injury in children and adolescents. *Brain and Language, 43*, 42–65.

Chapman, S., Levin, H., & Culhane, K. (1995). Language impairment in closed head injury. In H. Kirschner (Ed.), *Handbook of neurological speech and language disorders* (pp. 387–414). New York: Marcel-Dekker.

Chermak, G. D., & Musiek, F. E. (1997). *Central auditory processing disorders: New perspectives*. San Diego: Singular.

Chinn, P., Drew, E., & Logan, D. (1975). *Mental retardation: A life cycle approach*. St. Louis: Mosby.

The Classroom Communication Skills Inventory: A listening and speaking checklist. (1993). San Antonio: Psychological Corp.

Colorado Task Force on Central Auditory Processing Disorders. (1997). *Central auditory processing disorders: A team approach to screening, assessment, and intervention practices*. Denver: Colorado Department of Education.

Conners, C. K. (1997). *The Conners' Rating Scales–Revised*. Austin, TX: PRO-ED.

Conti, R. (1991). Attention disorders. In B. Wong (Ed.), *Learning about learning disabilities*. New York: Academic Press.

Cooley, E. J., & Ayers, R. R. (1988). Self-concept and success–failure attributes of nonhandicapped students and students with learning disabilities. *Journal of Learning Disabilities, 21*, 174–178.

Coster, W., & Cicchetti, D. (1993). Research on the communicative development of maltreated children: Clinical implications. *Topics in Language Disorders, 13*(4), 25–38.

Courchesne, E. (1989). Neuroanatomical systems involved in infantile autism: The implications of cerebellar abnormalities. In G. Dawson (Ed.), *Autism: Nature, diagnosis, and treatment* (pp. 119–143). New York: Guilford Press.

DePompei, R., & Williams, J. (1994). Working with families after TBI: A family-centered approach. *Topics in Language Disorders, 15*(1), 68–81.

Fischer, M., Barkley, R. A., Edelbrock, C. S., & Smallish, L. (1990). The adolescent outcome of hyperactive children diagnosed by research criteria: II. Academic, attentional, and neuropsychological status. *Journal of Consulting and Clinical Psychology, 58,* 580–588.

Fisher, L. I. (1985). Fisher's Auditory Problem Checklist. In R. J. Van Hattum (Ed.), *Administration of speech–language services in the schools* (pp. 231–292). San Diego: College-Hill.

Gadow, K. D. (1985). Relative efficacy of pharmacological, behavioral, and combination treatments for enhancing academic performance. *Clinical Psychology Review, 5,* 513–533.

Gadow, K. D. (1986). *Children on medication: Volume 1. Hyperactivity, learning disabilities, and mental retardation.* Boston: College-Hill.

Gerber, A. (1993). *Language-related learning disabilities: Their nature and treatment.* Baltimore: Brookes.

Gravel, J. S., & Wallace, I. F. (1995). Early otitis media, auditory abilities, and educational risk. *American Journal of Speech–Language Pathology, 4*(3), 89–94.

Gross, C. R., Wolf, C., Kunitz, S. C., & Jane, J. A. (1985). Pilot "traumatic coma data bank: A profile of head injuries in children." In R. G. Dacey, R. Winn, & R. Rimel (Eds.), *Trauma of the central nervous system.* New York: Raven Press.

Hamlett, K. W., Pellegrini, D. S., & Conners, C. K. (1987). An investigation of executive processes in the problem-solving of attention deficit disorder–hyperactive children. *Journal of Pediatric Psychology, 12,* 227–240.

Hynd, G. W., Hall, J., Novey, E. S., Eliopulos, D., Black, K., Gonzales, J. J., Edmonds, J. E., Riccio, C., & Cohen, M. (1995). Dyslexia and corpus callosum morphology. *Archives of Neurology, 52,* 32–38.

Hynd, G. W., Hern, K. L., Novey, E. S., Eliopulos, D., Marshall, R., Gonzales, J. J., & Voeller, K. (1993). Attention deficit–hyperactivity disorder and asymmetry of the caudate nucleus. *Journal of Child Neurology, 8,* 339–347.

Hynd, G. W., Semrud-Clikeman, M., Lorys, A., Novey, E. S., & Eliopulos, D. (1990). Brain morphology in developmental dyslexia and attention deficit/hyperactivity. *Archives of Neurology, 47,* 919–926.

Katz, J., & Smith, P. (1991). The Staggered Spondaic Word Test: A ten minute look at the CNS through the ears. In R. Zapulla, F. F. LeFever, J. Jaeger, & R. Bilder (Eds.), *Windows on the brain: Neuropsychology's technical frontiers* (pp. 1–19). *Annals of the New York Academy of Sciences, 620,* 233–251.

Keith, R. (1986). *SCAN: A screening test for auditory processing disorders.* San Antonio: Psychological Corporation.

Knutson, J. F., & Sullivan, P. M. (1993). Communicative disorders as a risk factor in abuse. *Topics in Language Disorders, 13*(4), 1–14.

Kronstadt, D. (1991). Complex developmental issues of prenatal drug exposure. *The Future of Children, 1*(1), 36–49.

Lahey, B., Carlson, C., & Frick, P. (1992). Attention deficit disorders without hyperactivity: A review of research relevant to DSM–IV. In T. A. Widiger, A. J. Frances, H. A. Pincus, W. Davis, & M. First (Eds.), *DSM–IV Sourcebook* (Vol. 1). Washington, DC: American Psychiatric Association.

Lahey, M. (1988). *Language disorders and language development.* New York: Macmillan.

Levin, H. S., Culhane, K. A., Mendelsohn, D., Lilly, M. A., Bruce, D., Fletcher, J. M., Chapman, S. B., Harward, H., & Eisenburg, H. M. (1993). Cognition in relation to magnetic resonance imaging in head-injured children and adolescents. *Archives of Neurology, 50,* 897–905.

Levin, H. S., Goldstein, F. C., Williams, D. H., & Eisenberg, H. M. (1991). The contribution of frontal lobe lesions to the neurobehavioral outcome of closed head injury. In H. S. Levin,

H. M. Eisenberg, & A. L. Benton (Eds.), *Frontal lobe function and disfunction*. New York: Oxford University Press.

Maurer, R., & Damasio, A. (1982). Childhood autism from the point of view of behavioral neurology. *Journal of Autism and Developmental Disorders, 12*(2), 195–205.

Merzenich, M., Jenkins, W., Johnston, P., Schreiner, C., Miller, S., & Tallal, P. (1996). Temporal processing deficits of language-learning impaired children ameliorated by training. *Science, 271*, 77–81.

National Joint Council on Learning Disabilities. (1991). Learning disabilities: Issues on definition (A position paper of the National Joint Committee on Learning Disabilities). *Asha, 33*(Suppl. 5), 18–20.

Nelson, N. W. (1993). *Childhood language disorders in context: Infancy through adolescence*. New York: Merrill.

Owens, R. E., Jr. (1989). Mental retardation: Difference of delay? In D. K. Bernsterin & E. Tiegerman (Eds.), *Language and communication disorders in children* (2nd ed., pp. 229–297). Columbus, OH: Merrill/Macmillan.

Paul, R. (1995). *Language disorders from infancy through adolescence: Assessment and intervention*. Boston: Mosby.

Ratner, V. L., & Harris, L. R. (1994). *Understanding language disorders: The impact on learning*. Eau Claire, WI: Thinking Publications.

Richards, G. P., Samuels, S. J., Turnure, J. E., & Ysseldyke, J. E. (1990). Sustained and selective attention in children with learning disabilities. *Journal of Learning Disabilities, 23*, 129–136.

Roberts, J. E., & Medley, L. (1995). Otitis media and speech–language sequelae in young children: Current issues in management. *American Journal of Speech–Language Pathology, 4*(1), 15–24.

Rudel, R. G. (1988). Disorders of attention. In R. G. Rudel, J. M. Holmes, & J. R. Pardel (Eds.), *Assessment of developmental learning disorders* (pp. 51–74). New York: Basic Books.

Shaywitz, S. E., Fletcher, J. M., & Shaywitz, B. A. (1994). Issues in the definition and classification of attention deficit disorder. *Topics in Language Disorders, 14*(4), 1–25.

Shaywitz, S., & Shaywitz, B. (1988). Attention deficit disorder: Current perspectives. In J. Kavanagh & T. Truss, Jr. (Eds.), *Learning disabilities: Proceedings of the national conference* (pp. 369–523). Parkton, MD: York Press.

Shaywitz, S. E., & Shaywitz, B. A. (1994). Learning disabilities and attention disorders. In K. Swaiman (Ed.), *Pediatric neurology* (pp. 1119–1151). Baltimore: Mosby.

Shear, P. K., Tallal, P., & Delis, D. C. (1992). Verbal learning and memory in language impaired children. *Neuropsychologia, 30*, 451–458.

Shelton, T. L., & Barkley, R. A. (1994). Critical issues in the assessment of attention deficit disorders in children. *Topics in Language Disorders, 14*(4), 26–41.

Silver, L. (1990). Attention deficit hyperactivity disorder: Is it a learning disability or a related disorder? *Journal of Learning Disabilities, 23*(7), 394–397.

Simon, C. (Ed.). (1991). *Communication skills and classroom success: Assessment and therapy methodologies for language and learning disabled students*. Eau Claire, WI: Thinking Publications.

Smoski, W. (1990). Use of CHAPPS in a children's audiology clinic. *Ear and Hearing, 11*(5 Suppl.), 535–565.

Snyder, L. S., Nathanson, R., & Shaywitz, K. J. (1993). Children in court: The role of discourse processing and production. *Topics in Language Disorders, 13*(4), 39–58.

Sparks, S. (1993). *Children of prenatal substance abuse*. San Diego: Singular.

Swanson, H. L. (1993). Executive processing in learning-disabled readers. *Intelligence, 17*, 117–149.

Swanson, H. L., Ashbaker, M., & Lee, C. (1995). The effects of processing demands on working memory of learning disabled readers. *Journal of Experimental Child Psychology, 59*(2), 211–233.

Swanson, H., & Cooney, J. B. (1991). Learning disabilities and memory. In B. Y. L. Wong (Ed.), *Learning about learning disabilities* (pp. 103–127). San Diego: Academic Press.

Szekeres, S. F., & Meserve, N. F. (1994). Collaborative intervention in schools after traumatic brain injury. *Topics in Language Disorders, 15*(1), 21–36.

Tallal, P. (1988). Developmental language disorders. In J. F. Kavanagh & T. J. Truss, Jr. (Eds.), *Learning disabilities: Proceedings of the national conference* (pp. 181–272). Parkton, MD: York Press.

Tallal, P., Miller, S., Bedi, G., Byma, G., Wang, X., Nagarajan, S., Schreiner, C., Jenkins, W., & Merzenich, M. (1996). Language comprehension in language-learning impaired children improved with acoustically modified speech. *Science, 271*, 81–84.

Task Force on Central Auditory Processing Consensus Development. (1996). Central auditory processing: Current status of research and implications for clinical practice. *American Journal of Audiology, 5*(2), 41–52.

Torgeson, J. K. (1988). Studies of learning disabled children who perform poorly on memory span tasks. *Journal of Learning Disabilities, 21*, 605–612.

Vellutino, F. R., & Scanlon, D. M. (1985). Verbal memory in poor and normal readers: Developmental differences in the use of linguistic codes. In D. B. Gray & J. F. Kavanaugh (Eds.), *Biobehavioral measures of dyslexia* (pp. 177–214). Parkton, MD: York Press.

Wallach, G., & Miller, L. (1988). *Language intervention and academic success*. Boston: College-Hill.

Weaver, C. (1993). Understanding and educating students with attention deficit hyperactivity disorder: Toward a system theory and whole language perspective. *American Journal of Speech–Language Pathology, 2*(2), 79–89.

Westby, C. E., & Cutler, S. K. (1994). Language and ADHD: Understanding the basis and treatment of self-regulatory deficits. *Topics in Language Disorders, 14*(4), 58–76.

Ylvisaker, M., Kolpan, K. I., & Rosenthal, M. (1994). Collaboration in preparing for personal injury suits after TBI. *Topics in Language Disorders, 15*(1), 1–20.

Speech Problems in Classrooms

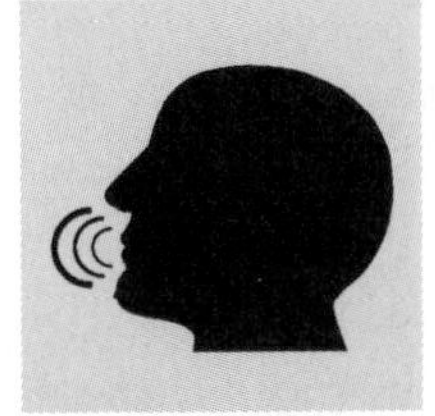

Chapter 8

Kathleen R. Fahey

In the previous chapter, the causes and characteristics of disabilities related to language acquisition and usage were presented and eight specific problems were defined and described. In this chapter, seven problems associated with speech production (and often also language) are discussed: (1) hearing impairment and deafness; (2) visual impairment and blindness; (3) motor speech disorders: dysarthria and developmental verbal apraxia; (4) cleft lip and palate; (5) phonological and articulation disorders; (6) fluency and prosody disorders; and (7) voice disorders. These problems are discussed according to definitions and characteristics, as well as the role of educators and speech–language pathologists (SLPs) in classroom prevention, identification, and planning.

Causes of Speech Problems

Speech is a verbal means of communicating resulting from specific motor behaviors of the oral mechanism in interaction with the hearing, vision, respiration, phonation, resonation, and neurological systems. Speech sounds are combined to form words and morphemes and, along with suprasegmental aspects (e.g., intonation, pauses, rate), convey meaning within the speaking community. When disorders in speech occur, individuals can experience decreased quality and quantity of interactions with others, producing impoverished acquisition of language and world knowledge, social and emotional difficulties, and academic problems.

Speech problems can result when any of the systems mentioned above are not structurally or functionally adequate. For example, hearing acuity problems greatly influence the development of speech sounds, as do structural malformations of the hard and soft palate in children born with cleft lip and palate. It is sometimes possible to determine the cause of a speech problem, especially when physical signs are present; however, for many children, the cause of speech difficulties remains unclear. This is because many different factors contribute to speech difficulties. As listed in the previous chapter, such factors include biological conditions, linguistic system development, situational conditions, cognitive abilities, and social interaction factors. In fact, speech disorders often coexist with language acquisition and usage problems; they are a part of the same linguistic system (Nelson, 1993).

As with language acquisition and usage problems, causal factors can co-occur. For example, motor control problems often lead to imprecise articulation, and hearing loss results in difficulty with resonance and loudness. Mixed conditions can make both diagnosis and intervention challenging. In addition, changing needs in communication expectations as children mature must lead to thoughtful modifications in the school and home so that students are able to participate as fully as possible in normal life events. For example, a communication picture board may provide a preschool student with severe motor limitations the opportunity to participate in limited interactions with peers and to express basic wants and needs in the classroom, but as the student advances to elementary school this device should be replaced with a computerized communication system, allowing for increased social interaction, continued linguistic development, and participation in learning activities in the classroom.

Both the type of speech problem (e.g., articulation, fluency, voice) and the causes of that problem (e.g., hearing loss, cleft lip and palate, cerebral palsy) are referred to by speech–language pathologists (SLPs) when individual children are described in assessment and progress reports; however, labels do not reveal severity, characteristics, or the needs of particular children. Careful assessment and intervention require collaborative efforts from members of the educational teams, the students, and their families.

Characteristics of Speech Problems

Speech problems can vary in severity from mild alterations to moderate, severe, or even profound disabilities. Generally, the severity of the problem relates to its cause and the extent to which the interrelated systems are affected. For instance, a child with moderate delays in the linguistic system, without accompanying problems from other systems, will likely have moderate phonological and developmental articulation difficulties. However, a child with severe motor speech problems caused from traumatic brain injury will likely have problems across the neurological, oral motor, respiratory, phonatory, and resonance systems, making speech very labored, distorted, and infrequent. The severity of speech problems should be considered during educational planning because severity impacts both language competence and performance, which in turn affect classroom participation and learning.

Speech problems can be described according to several characteristics: articulation, resonance, fluency or prosody, and voice. *Articulation* is the production—with accuracy (correct sound) and precision (clarity)—of speech sounds within words. Children and adults with speech disorders omit, substitute, distort, and add sounds to words, causing them to be mispronounced. Articulation problems can either be developmental or occur from sensory or oral-motor irregularities (Bernthal & Bankson, 1998).

Resonance is the quality of the voice as it travels from the vocal cords through the pharynx and oral and nasal cavities. Resonance problems occur when too much nasal resonance (hypernasality) or too little nasal resonance (hyponasality) is present during speech production. Resonance problems can result from hearing impairment or deafness, cleft lip and palate, damage to cranial nerves, and obstructions in the resonating cavities (Shprintzen & Bardach, 1995).

Normal *fluency* of speech and *prosody* (suprasegmentals) allow speech to flow smoothly with appropriate rate, sequence, intonation, and modulation of stress. Disruptions in fluency or prosody cause speech to be halting, disjunctive, too fast or slow, monotonous, or uncontrolled. Dysfluent speech can cause the speaker and listener difficulty in interactions and lead to feelings of anxiousness in speaking situations. A single cause of these problems has not been discovered; however, fluency and prosody problems can accompany language disabilities and articulation disorders (Bernstein Ratner, 1995; Hargrove, 1997).

Finally, *voice* disorders occur when the vocal cords in the larynx are damaged, put under excessive abuse or misuse, or changed structurally and functionally from growths. The voice can be described as hoarse, breathy, weak, strained, or tremulous depending on the nature of the problem and on its perception from listeners. Voice problems are often preventable. However, conditions such as hearing impairment, neurological disease or damage, and viral conditions produce secondary voice problems (Colton & Casper, 1996).

Hearing Impairment and Deafness

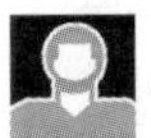

Alison

Alison, age 14½, attends the sixth grade. She has worn bilateral hearing aids since her moderate sensorineural hearing loss was diagnosed in kindergarten. Alison had numerous ear infections during infancy and through her preschool years. Some of the infections were treated with antibiotics, yet the family did not have health insurance or adequate access to health care. Alison's father and cousin also have hearing losses. Alison receives speech-language therapy to improve articulation, resonance, and grammar. She attended a total communication elementary school program where she learned sign language and is currently in an oral classroom.

Definitions and Characteristics

The degree of hearing loss in persons can be slight to profound, depending on the amount of remaining hearing sensitivity (acuity) measured by decibels (dB): normal 0 to 15 dB; slight 16 to 25 dB; mild 26 to 40 dB; moderate 41 to 65 dB; severe 66 to 95 dB; and profound 96+ dB (Northern & Downs, 1984). Three types of hearing impairment—conductive, sensorineural, and mixed—have specific causes and result in various degrees of hearing loss. The nature of the hearing loss, age of onset, and its severity are important variables in the speech characteristics that result.

A *conductive hearing loss* results when the transmission of sound is impeded as it travels from the outer and middle ear to the inner ear. Transmission problems can result from impacted wax in the ear canal, fluid in the middle ear, or mechanical difficulties affecting the efficiency of the small middle ear bones to transmit sound waves to the inner ear. *Otitis media*, a prevalent illness in early childhood, is a condition where inflammation and fluid in the middle ear leads to fluctuating hearing loss. When the fluid is not infected it is called otitis media with effusion (OME), and when it is infected it is called acute otitis media (AOM). A child may complain of pain, have a fever, and be irritable, but these symptoms are not always present. Further, the condition can fluctuate in the same child and can occur occasionally or chronically (Roberts & Clarke-Klein, 1994). Although otitis media is treatable through antibiotics or the insertion of pressure equalization tubes, a hearing loss continues as long as fluid is present, so diagnosing and treating the problems can prove difficult. This temporary loss can be mild (25 dB) to moderate (50 dB) depending on the quantity of fluid present.

Note that intermittent OME in and of itself may not constitute increased risk for language disorders, but such a problem may increase children's vulnerability to language problems when coupled with other risk factors (Klein & Rapin, 1992). However, persistent or recurrent otitis media influences development of speech and language and can have serious consequences on educational outcomes. Table 8.1 summarizes research findings regarding these relationships. Although conflicting reports appear in the literature, recent investigations provide more definitive results

Table 8.1
Relationship of Otitis Media to Speech, Language, and Educational Performance

- Low scores on tests of speech production, speech processing, receptive language, and expressive language
- Low scores on tests of intelligence and academic achievement
- Attentional and behavioral problems in school
- Grade-level retention
- May require support services

Note. Adapted from "Otitis Media and Speech–Language Sequelae in Young Children: Current Issues in Management," by J. E. Roberts and L. Medley, 1995, *American Journal of Speech–Language Pathology, 4*(1), pp. 15–24.

about the nature of these relationships (Roberts & Medley, 1995). One report suggests that otitis media and mild conductive hearing loss during the first year of life is associated with poorer academic abilities at school age than otitis media occurring after the first year. Gravel and Wallace (1995) proposed that the first year is critical for the development of auditory processing and auditory-based learning skills. Otitis media can delay auditory development and create significant problems in the use of these underdeveloped skills.

Mild to moderate hearing loss can also result in incomplete and inconsistent reception of speech and language segments. For example, phonemes produced with low energy or with high frequency (e.g., vowels, /s, z, ʃ, tʃ, dʒ, ʒ/) (see Chapter 3, Appendix 3.A for the phonetic alphabet), morphemes with light stress (e.g., plurals, past tense markers), and vocal inflections used in questions can be distorted or not heard. Additionally, children may develop problems attending to verbal communication, learning to tune out messages and decreasing interactions with others (Bernthal & Bankson, 1994).

Sensorineural hearing loss is the result of problems in the functioning of the inner ear (cochlea) or the eighth cranial nerve as sound travels through the auditory pathways. Causes include viral infection (e.g., meningitis, mumps), severe and prolonged otitis media, genetic syndromes, fetal development complications, birth trauma, and the influence of teratogenic factors such as drug abuse. Sensorineural hearing loss is permanent and the degree of loss does not fluctuate unless accompanied by periods of otitis media. This combination of sensorineural hearing loss and otitis media is known as a *mixed hearing loss*.

The acquisition of speech and language can be significantly delayed when sensorineural hearing loss is present yet unidentified in infancy and early childhood. Unfortunately, although technology is available to assess infant hearing, children typically are not identified as having hearing loss until between 12 months and 2 years of age (Bernthal & Bankson, 1994). Fortunately, this situation is changing as states pass legislation mandating universal infant hearing testing. Early identification of sensorineural hearing loss leads to parent education about hearing impairment, decisions about amplification through hearing aid technology, and choices regarding communication development (oral, sign, total communication).

The impact of sensorineural hearing loss on speech, language, and educational achievement depends on the severity of the loss, and whether or not amplification and speech and language intervention is provided to the child. Table 8.2 shows the relationships between severity of hearing loss, the amount of speech heard without amplification, the degrees of handicap without early intervention, and the probable needs of children who are identified (Northern & Downs, 1984).

Infants with hearing impairments vocalize shortly after birth and continue to vocalize as do hearing children. However, delays of 6 to 12 months have been found in the onset of babbling. Another difference in early speech development concerns the size, composition, and nature of the consonant inventories of children with hearing impairments as compared to children with normal hearing. The inventories are often smaller, have a reduced variety of sounds, and develop at slower rates (Stoel-Gammon & Kehoe, 1994). Young children with hearing impairments have difficulty engaging in vocal and verbal interactions, relying more on visual than auditory input.

Speech characteristics of children with severe hearing loss include (a) vowel and consonant distortions, substitutions, and omissions; (b) problems distinguishing between voiced (e.g., /b, v, g, z/) and unvoiced (e.g., /p, f, k, s/) consonants; (c) inappropriate nasalization of nonnasal consonants; and (d) deletion of final consonants in words. Other problems include inadequate breath control, excessive and inappropriate pausing, inappropriate vocal pitch, tenseness or harshness of the voice, inappropriate rate of speech, and nontypical duration of stressed and unstressed syllables (Paterson, 1994).

Children with profound to total loss of hearing are considered *deaf*. They face the challenge of learning language and engaging in interactions with others through manual communication or manual communication in combination with oral language. The decision about which modes are learned depends on student and parental attitudes (including their knowledge of such modes) and the hearing and speech professionals who are providing information and services. Children born to deaf parents are often taught *American Sign Language* (ASL) through natural interactions with their parents. This rule-governed language has different grammar and syntactic structure from spoken and written English. Therefore, oral speech does not accompany it. In ASL, all

Table 8.2
Hearing Handicap as a Function of Average Hearing Threshold Level of the Better Ear

Average Threshold Level at 500–2000 Hz (ANSI)	Description	Common Causes	What Can Be Heard Without Amplification	Degrees of Handicap (If not treated in 1st year of life)	Probable Needs
0–15 dB	Normal range		All speech sounds	None	None
16–25 dB	Slight hearing loss	Serous otitis, perforation, monomeric membrane, sensorineural loss, tympanosclerosis	Vowel sounds heard clearly, may miss unvoiced consonant sounds	Possible mild or transitory auditory dysfunction Difficulty in perceiving some speech sounds	Consideration of need for hearing aid Lip reading Auditory training Speech therapy Preferential seating Appropriate surgery
26–40 dB	Mild	Serous otitis, perforation, tympanosclerosis, monomeric membrane, sensorineural loss	Hears only some speech sounds; the louder voiced sounds	Auditory learning dysfunction Mild language retardation Mild speech problems Inattention	Hearing aid Lip reading Auditory training Speech therapy Appropriate surgery
41–65 dB	Moderate hearing loss	Chronic otitis, middle ear anomaly, sensorineural loss	Misses most speech sounds at normal conversational level	Speech problems Language retardation Learning dysfunction Inattention	All of the above, plus consideration of special classroom situation
66–95 dB	Severe hearing loss	Sensorineural loss or mixed loss due to sensorineural loss plus middle ear disease	Hears no speech or sound of normal conversations	Severe speech problems Language retardation Learning dysfunction Inattention	All of the above; plus assignment to special classes
96+ dB	Profound hearing loss	Sensorineural loss or mixed loss	Hears no speech or other sounds	Severe spech problems Language retardation Learning dysfunction Inattention	All of the above; probable assignment to special classes

ANSI = American National Standards Institute.
Note. From *Hearing in Children* (3rd ed., p. 89), by J. L. Northern and M. P. Downs, 1984, Baltimore: Williams & Wilkins. Copyright 1984 by Williams & Wilkins. Reprinted by permission.

concepts are expressed by altering and modulating movements of the hands, arms, facial expressions, and face and head (Ratner & Harris, 1994). Development of vocabulary through ASL occurs slightly more rapidly during the first year in deaf children than does oral language in hearing children. Similar acquisitions occur, however, in syntax and pragmatics (Orlansky & Bonvillian, 1988; Ratner & Harris, 1994; Spencer, 1993). Yet, gaps in language knowledge occur among deaf students, especially when they encounter oral speakers and begin to learn to read and write.

Manual Coded English is a sign system that uses the vocabulary and grammar of oral language. Its purpose is to make spoken language visible to children with severe hearing impairments. It is popular in the United States because parents and teachers find it easy to learn and use, especially when others in the home and school use spoken language. Simultaneous use of signed and spoken language promotes delayed but normal language development (Acredolo & Goodwyn, 1985; Holmes & Holmes, 1980). A less formal version of Manual Coded English, known as *Pidgin Sign English,* omits inflections such as tense and plural forms. This informal language is not considered conducive to language development because it is inconsistent and incomplete (Ratner & Harris, 1994).

Implications for Classrooms

Classroom teachers, special educators, and SLPs can help prevent ear problems and hearing loss in children. They can decrease the incidence of otitis media by minimizing the spread of germs within the classroom and they can reduce the prolonged nature of otitis media by being alert to symptoms and notifying parents when symptoms occur. Parents should be informed about the language development needs of children with hearing impairments and provided information on ways to provide extra language stimulation (Lahey, 1988). Educationists can also suggest names of health and hearing professionals when assessment and intervention for ear and hearing problems are required. They can educate children to the dangers of loud noise exposure and discuss ways to protect hearing when in noisy environments. See Chapter 10 for discussion of classroom implications and intervention practices for children with hearing impairments.

When a child is identified with hearing loss, it is important that the educational team knows what the severity of loss is, when the loss was identified, what interventions have been provided (e.g., amplification, speech–language therapy, educational programs), and what language mode the child uses to communicate (i.e., oral, manual, or total). The educational audiologist, SLP, and general and special educators should understand how the hearing loss impacts listening and learning in the classroom and collaborate on strategies that will help students succeed in school. Such strategies (discussed in Chapter 10) include environmental modifications (e.g., seating arrangement, acoustic considerations), teaching practices (e.g., increased visual input, high redundancy, oral and written language modes used together), speech–language therapy, and use of personal listening systems.

Summary

Hearing loss or deafness in children presents challenges for each child, the family members, and the school community because of its effects on communication and learning. Parents and educationists must be alert to signs of hearing loss in students so that assessment occurs quickly. The type of hearing loss and its severity must be considered for educationists to determine its effect on communication within the classroom. Thus, an audiologist, SLP, and teachers must work collaboratively not only to understand the problem, but to determine and implement appropriate classroom interventions.

Visual Impairment and Blindness

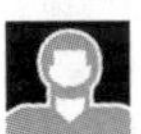

John

John is a 9-year-old third grader who was identified as having low vision during his first year. He has worn prescription lenses since his diagnosis. He has two older brothers and one younger sister who have normal vision. John's parents have been active and supportive in his development and education. John's speech and language development is within the average range and he is quite independent. However, his vision continues to deteriorate, making it more difficult to learn new tasks. He is learning to read and write using Braille and recently obtained a computer with scanning capability.

Definition and Characteristics

Any condition of the visual system that results in less than normal vision is considered a visual impairment. Severe visual impairment with some functional vision (as in John's case) is called *low vision*, and perception only to light is called *blindness* (Barraga, 1983; Faye, 1976). There is a higher incidence of vision problems in the deaf population (6%) than in the general school-age population (0.08%) (Wolff & Harkins, 1986), indicating that hearing and visual deficits can result from similar causal factors (e.g., genetic syndromes, substance abuse).

As is true of children with hearing problems, children who have low vision or blindness are at risk for developmental delays in cognition, speech, language, and social skills. The degree to which these areas are impacted depends on the age of onset, degree of impairment, presence of other handicapping conditions, and amount and quality of support from the environment (Ratner & Harris, 1994).

Infants' early interest in and exploration of the environment is motivated by the sight of moving or bright objects. They watch and reach out to grasp objects in the first few weeks of life. They rely on other senses, such as hearing and touch, to become aware of their body in relation to objects and people, but sound cues alone are not as effective for stimulating reaching. Sight, sound, and touch cues are needed for early explorations. Visual impairment can inhibit these early explorations and lead to delays in later cognitive and language functions, such as sensory integration of information, the use of imagery to store newly learned concepts, and the development of object permanence and symbolic play (Ratner & Harris, 1994). Children with low vision and visual-perceptual disabilities typically score poorly on the performance scales of intelligence tests, and when hearing impairment is also present, on verbal scales as well. Because visual and verbal information comprise most intelligence tests, professionals must use test results cautiously (Ratner & Harris, 1994).

Sighted infants engage in and even direct interactions through eye gazing and attention to the faces of caregivers during daily routines. The two-way visual and vocal communication patterns that develop early are mutually reinforcing and, therefore, foundational to future interaction patterns. Within the first 6 months, they make early requests and comments as they point and use gestures to indicate objects. Because children with visual impairments have limited awareness of objects in the immediate environment, their requests for and comments about objects through gestures are not common. Thus, meaningful connections about intentions and language can be delayed. Infants who are blind are also less directive in interactions and tend to rely on being recipients of interactions initiated by others (Landau & Gleitman, 1985).

Although infants who are visually impaired or blind do hear and respond to the vocal inflections of language, they do not see the accompanying facial expressions and body language. Landau and Gleitman (1985) reported that babies who are blind are quiet or even silent during interactions, perhaps because they are being attentive to the vocal information. However, family members and other caregivers may misinterpret the infant's interests and needs and, as a result, decrease the type and amount of interaction they engage in with the infant (Fraiberg, 1974; Ratner & Harris, 1994). In fact, family member interaction with blind babies tends to be heavy in directives, statements, and repetitive requests rather than requests for answers or comments (Landau & Gleitman, 1985). Children with visual impairments who are not guided in interactions can produce irrelevant or echolalic speech (Barraga, 1983). Social interaction also involves the awareness of cues that people use to convey emotion and affect. Youngsters with visual impairment need assistance in identifying their own as well as other people's emotions, and they need guidance in developing knowledge of verbal, vocal, and tactile cues to interpret emotion and affect in the absence of visual cues (e.g., facial expression, body posture).

When visual impairment or blindness occurs as the sole sensory problem, language acquisition tends to proceed along typical schedules and patterns, depending on the degree of visual functioning. However, linguistic deficits have been noted in the development of (a) action, directional, and relational words and concepts; (b) comprehension and use of personal pronouns; (c) syntactic complexity, including question forms, prepositions, adjectives, and complex sentence structures; (d) articulation precision for sounds that have visual information (/m, b, p, f, v, θ/); and (e) pragmatics, such as turn-taking, proxemics, and the use of questions and commands (Andersen, Dunlea, & Kekelis, 1993; Elstner, 1983; Erin, 1990; Hoff-Ginsberg, 1997; Nelson, 1993; Ratner & Harris, 1994). In addition to oral language deficits, these children may have difficulty acquiring reading and writing. Certainly, their learning of Braille and the use of computer technology depends on access to such instruction, which for some may not occur until school age (see Chapter 4 for a discussion of the importance of emergent literacy during the preschool years).

Implications for the Classroom

When particular students do poorly in school, many hypotheses and explanations can be offered. Referral for vision and hearing testing is a quick, decisive, and often definitive way to determine part or all of the problem. Vision screening is available at health fairs, through public health departments, and sometimes from school health professionals at the school. Parents need information about how visual problems can impact language development. They need information about how infants' and toddlers' vision problems can affect interactions within the family and how to provide more enriching language stimulation for such children (Paul, 1995).

In the classroom, general and special educators, as well as SLPs, can assist children in gaining access to and interpreting information, especially when it is presented visually. For example, during instruction in science about the atom, verbal descriptions and tactile experiences about the elements in the atom will enhance student understandings about new vocabulary (i.e., protons, neutrons, electrons). Students benefit from repetition of instructions when new content is being learned. Repetition is helpful because verbal information is often delivered rapidly, contains a large amount of detail, and is heard without benefit of gestures and other visual cues. Metacognitive strategies, such as comprehension monitoring, can be taught to students so that they become self-advocates when they do not understand information or when they need assistance. Finally, teachers must be open and accepting of augmentative and alternative systems for learning, such as Braille and computerized scanning devices, that enhance children's success in the classroom.

Summary

Although language development often occurs normally in children with visual impairments, it should be closely monitored as these children are at risk for delays. Of course, the impact that visual impairment has on language development depends on several factors within the child and the environment. Parents and educationists must stay alert to interactions that allow children complete access to verbal, nonverbal, and written language. When language delays are evident in preschool and school-age children, SLPs and teachers must determine and implement classroom interventions by analyzing the particular situations that cause difficulties and constructing plans that help remediate difficulties within such situations.

Motor Speech Disorders: Dysarthria and Developmental Apraxia of Speech

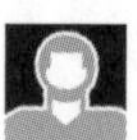

Cassandra

Cassandra is 7 years old and has had cerebral palsy from birth. Her motorized wheelchair provides independence at home and in her second-grade classroom. Cassie's expressive verbal speech and language are very limited due to severe oral-motor incoordination. Her receptive language is delayed about 1 year. One year ago, Cassie received a computer-based communication device that she operates with a joystick. She is able to form and express sentences through pictured icons. Cassie is very delayed in reading and writing.

Definitions and Characteristics

Dysarthria, one group of motor speech disorders, results when motor weakness, motor control and timing, or motor planning problems occur during the production of speech. This group of disorders is caused from neurological conditions such as cerebral palsy, degenerative muscular dystrophy, or paralysis of the upper trunk, head, and neck from spinal cord or traumatic brain injury. The dysarthric speech characteristics depend on the site and extent of the neurological damage, the age of onset, the degree of motor limitations, and the nature of the motor problem itself (e.g., weakness, control) (Bernthal & Bankson, 1998). For some individuals, severe motor problems preclude oral speech production. In such cases, augmentative or alternative communication (AAC) systems provide visual (communication picture or print boards, Bliss symbols) or verbal (computerized output devices) avenues for interaction, learning, and the development of reading and writing (Koppenhaver & Yoder, 1993; Pierce & McWilliam, 1993; Steelman, Pierce, & Koppenhaver, 1993). For others who can produce speech, it is characterized by slow, labored, and distorted articulation, reduced volume, and poor use of stress and intonation. Since the causal factors associated with neurological problems are numerous, other physical (e.g., sensory, respiratory) and developmental (e.g., cognition, language, social) impairments associated with such factors sometimes coexist with the oral-motor difficulties. Thus, children with dysarthria are at high risk for language, learning, social, and academic difficulties.

A second type of motor speech impairment is not caused by weakness or lack of control of the muscles controlling the speech mechanism. Rather, *developmental apraxia of speech* (DAS) occurs when motor planning and temporal sequencing problems of phonemes and syllables disrupt speech production (Hayden, 1994; Square, 1994). Some professionals have also considered it a language disability because of its temporal nature and its impact on learning the sounds and rules involved in sound production (Bridgeman & Snowling, 1988; Hall, 1992), yet speech perception, language comprehension, integration of information, and formulation of language are normal. Additionally, the speech mechanism is normal in structure, yet soft neurological signs such as fine motor coordination and gait clumsiness, drooling, and incoordination of speech mechanism structures (e.g., lips, tongue, soft palate) may exist in some children.

With DAS, children demonstrate several characteristics from among a group of characteristics described in the literature. These include (a) evidence of struggle and trial-and-error behaviors (e.g., "mata-bapa-potabo-potato"); (b) silent posturing, sound prolongations, and repetitions; (c) omissions of sounds in words; (d) immature use of phonological processes; and (e) transpositions of sounds and syllables (e.g., "aminal," "efelant"). Intelligibility during production of single words and short phrases is often better than in connected speech, and improvement in speech development is slow even with intervention (Square, 1994).

Implications for the Classroom

When students have severe expressive communication disorders, it is sometimes difficult to determine what they already know and the extent of their understanding of new information. It is tragic when a child is unable to express his or her wants, needs, feelings, knowledge, and opinions to others. Less severe expressive problems may improve these important interactions, yet distorted speech can limit social dialogue, cause misinterpretations, and result in isolation or ridicule from others. Thus, general education teachers, special educators, and SLPs have a special role in the education of children with motor speech disorders. They must collaborate to integrate effective instructional practice into the classroom.

First, they must understand the nature of the problem so that classroom and therapy practices are effective and are not contraindicated. For example, proper positioning of a child with spastic cerebral palsy will reduce overflow of muscle activity, allowing the child to reserve energy and concentrate on the learning task. For a child with DAS, practicing tongue twisters to improve articulation would be highly frustrating and not likely beneficial, but rate control techniques such as phrasing and pausing could be incorporated into classroom speaking situations (Rosenthal, 1994).

Second, educational team members must work together to determine the support that each student needs to participate expressively in the classroom. As mentioned earlier, the range of possibilities is great, depending on the severity of the problem, from low- to high-technology communication devices to monitoring speech production from a child. It is imperative that each child participate as fully as possible in dialogues, answer questions, construct language to express thoughts and feeling, and use language for social interactions.

Educationists play a role in informing others about communication problems and advocating for social acceptance. They should be watchful of verbal or physical abuse from other children, family members, or other school personnel. As advocates, they can make sure that the least restrictive environment and the educational rights of students are upheld.

Summary

Severe expressive speech (and language) problems are usually identified early in childhood or soon after a debilitating event occurs (e.g., head injury, stroke). Children who have dysarthria, who are nonverbal, or who have DAS face challenges in language development, social interactions, and academic learning. Educationists and parents must advocate for these children and work together systematically to remove barriers that impede progress in language, social, and academic development. They must fully understand the problem, provide appropriate technology and instruction, and educate others about the students' needs. Severe expressive speech problems are often conditions that persist into adulthood. Because the children's needs will change as they advance in years, SLPs and teachers must commit to ongoing assessment and intervention strategies within classrooms.

Cleft Lip and Palate

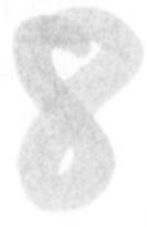

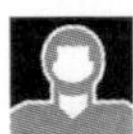

Jason

Jason is 6 years old and in the first grade. He was born in Korea and spent his first 3 years in an orphanage. Shortly after birth, Jason had surgery to close the cleft in his lip. At the time of his adoption, he had an unrepaired hard and soft palate, but these were repaired at age 4. He currently receives speech therapy for severe intelligibility problems. He has difficulty producing many sounds and has hypernasality and nasal air emission. The local cleft palate team recommends that further surgery (i.e., velopharyngeal flap) be scheduled within the next few months to provide him with the structure necessary for normal speech development to occur.

Definitions and Characteristics

A *cleft lip* or *palate* is "a lack of union of embryonic oral and facial elements" (Shprintzen & Bardach, 1995, p. 5). Clefts can be caused by chromosomal disorders; genetic diseases; environmentally induced (teratogenic) factors, including drugs and viruses; and mechanically induced abnormalities, such as intrauterine crowding, uterine tumor, and amniotic ruptures. Over 400 syndromes are associated with clefting (Shprintzen & Goldberg, 1995). Clefts can occur in the lip only, the lip and alveolus (bony ridge directly behind the front upper teeth), the hard and soft palate only, the soft palate, or all of these structures. They can be on one side (unilateral) or both sides (bilateral). The severity of the cleft depends on the type, its width, the position of the upper mouth (maxillary) segments, and the amount of hypoplasia (lack of plasticity) of the soft and hard tissues (Bardach & Salyer, 1995).

Early surgical repair of cleft lips and palates is typical. However, hard and soft palate closure, orthodontia (e.g., dental appliances, bone grafts), and facial surgeries may continue to be needed during elementary, middle, and high school years. The nature, size, and shape of appliances (e.g., maxillary expander), and the length of time they are in place, are among the factors that can impact speech articulation and resonation (LeBlanc & Cisneros, 1995). Dental braces are often required, along with continued speech therapy.

"All children born with a cleft of the lip and/or palate or a syndrome associated with clefting are at risk for communication impairment" (Witzel, 1995, p. 137). Such communication impairments are related to the specific abnormalities in the structure and function of the speech mechanism. The types of speech problems include articulation errors, phonological delay, resonance irregularities, voice problems, and overall reduced intelligibility. Some children, particularly those with syndromes, also have cognitive, hearing, and language impairments (Witzel, 1995).

The two most prevalent characteristics in cleft palate speech are articulation and resonance problems. These are due to the structural and functional irregularities of the oral cavity and its relationship to the nasal cavity. Children with hard and soft palate clefts have limited tissue in the back of the mouth (pharynx). This condition prevents *velopharyngeal closure*, which results when the soft palate rises and moves in a backward direction to make contact with the pharynx. Velopharyngeal closure makes it possible to direct the airflow from the lungs into the mouth without it escaping through the nose, and allows speakers to build up needed air pressure to make most of the consonant sounds for normal speech production. Difficulty with this function causes hypernasality and weak production of consonants. Surgical intervention or the fitting of a prosthetic device can significantly improve this problem. Specific sound errors vary with substitutions of one sound for another, compensatory sounds (non-English) made in unusual parts of the oral and pharyngeal mechanism (e.g., glottal stop), and errors in voicing (e.g., /b-p/, /d-t/).

Hypernasality exists when sound enters both the oral and the nasal cavities, causing both to resonate during speech. It is present during production of vowels and voiced consonants when velopharyngeal closure is poor. *Nasal air emission* occurs when there is silent or audible airflow during speech production. It accompanies consonants and can sound like snorting when severe. Sometimes the nostrils flare or the facial muscles around the nose contract (Witzel, 1995).

Implications for the Classroom

The habilitation and ongoing management needs of children with cleft lip and palate require cooperation of each child, the parents, members of the cleft palate team, and members of the educational team. The SLP has a primary role. He or she should provide information about speech and language development and describe the speech characteristics present in individual children. The SLP should also assist teachers in planning for absences when dental, orthodontic, or surgical interventions are needed. Teachers can minimize the impact of these periods by offering assignments for home completion. Speech production may be distorted due to swelling or the presence of new dental or oral appliances. Teachers can decrease speaking demands upon a student's return to the classroom until healing and comfort resumes. When language delays are also apparent, SLPs and teachers must work together to plan appropriate classroom-based interventions.

Summary

Infants born with clefts of the lip and palate face challenges as they acquire language and undergo surgeries or fittings of oral and dental appliances. Such children must be closely monitored for early feeding and for later delays in the development of speech. Speech and language intervention is an important part of the overall habilitation plans of children with oral clefts. As preschoolers become students, they may periodically have plastic or reconstructive surgery, dental interventions, and continued speech therapy. School-based SLPs should invite classroom teachers to develop interventions for such children, including home-based activities when necessary, modifications of speaking activities when appropriate, and speech production expectations in accord with each individual's abilities.

Phonological and Articulation Problems

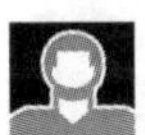

Denise

Denise is 10 and in the fifth grade at a rural school. She speaks readily, but her family members are the only ones who understand more than 60% of what she says. She leaves off sounds at the ends of words and rarely produces blends. In addition, her speech sounds immature due to distortions of /l/ and /r/. Denise has poor reading and writing abilities. Her word attack skills during reading are progressing at a slow rate, with greatest difficulty on vowels and ending sounds. She has difficulty remembering rules for long vowels and suffixes.

Definitions and Characteristics

Children in preschool and elementary grades can have significant delays in the development of the oral language systems or can have focal difficulties with the development of one or more systems. Such problems can result from many factors, from biological conditions to unknown causes. A *phonological disorder* exists when the simplification speaking patterns (phonological processes) that children use during the first 3 to 4 years persist beyond the point when these patterns are typical (Bernthal & Bankson, 1998; Lowe, 1997). Refer to Chapter 3 to review the phonological processes used during the first 4 years. A severe disorder will influence the development of other language systems, including morphological, syntactic, and written language development (Hodson, 1994). Perhaps the easiest way to determine the presence of a phonological problem is to compare the intelligibility of children in the same age range. Children with phonological problems often have difficulty communicating outside of their families because of poor intelligibility. Patterns such as fronting, stopping, final consonant deletion, gliding, and unstressed syllable deletion can dramatically affect intelligibility (see Chapter 3 for examples of simplification patterns).

Incomplete knowledge and use of phonological rules also lead to poor development of metalinguistics. When the sound system is not firmly established, awareness of sounds as they occur in spoken and printed words, rhymes, syllables, phonics activities, and word play typically lags as well. During preschool and early elementary grades, children appear slower in learning concepts related to print (e.g., sounds, letters, alphabet recitation). They often continue to learn literacy skills slowly, resulting in delayed reading and writing development (Clarke-Klein, 1994). (See Chapter 4 for discussion of the relationship between phonological awareness and literacy development.)

Articulation of speech occurs when the speaker manipulates the structures of the oral mechanism to produce rapid and precise speech sounds to form words. It requires that oral structures are present and in the correct positional relationship to other structures, and that the neurological system functions normally to allow controlled motor movements. Subtle delays in articulation can occur when fine motor coordination is not sufficiently developed or is hampered by mild motor impairments. Thus, sounds that require fine motor distinctions, such as fricatives (i.e., /s, ʃ, θ, tʃ/) (see Appendix 3.A in Chapter 3), or those requiring tongue blade modifications (i.e., /r, l, j/) are often distorted (Bernthal & Bankson, 1998).

Dental problems are usually not significant enough to cause severe speech errors. However, conditions such as a very high and narrow hard palate, or restricted tongue movement due to a short lingual frenulum (band of tissue connecting the tongue tip to the floor of the mouth) can cause sound distortions. *Lisping* is a term used to refer to the distortion of fricatives. When the tongue protrudes between the front teeth causing the /s/ to sound like /θ/, the error is called a frontal lisp. Lateral lisping occurs when the tongue is broadly positioned so that air escapes from the sides, creating a wet, sloppy sound (Smit, 1993). Lisping is often a sign of another condition known as *tongue thrust*, which is the habitual or frequent resting or pushing of the tongue against dentition in the front of the mouth (Hanson, 1994). A forward tongue carriage during speech, at rest, and when swallowing is normal in infancy through early childhood. However, a mature adult swallow should be present prior to age 9. In some children, tongue thrust is the result of an inadequate airway partially blocked by enlarged tonsils or adenoids. A persistent tongue thrust, therefore, may signal that upper respiratory problems need assessment and medical attention. Because tongue thrust also can result in dental malocclusion, it is important that the family dentist be involved in its management (Bernthal & Bankson, 1998).

Implications for the Classroom

Phonological and articulation problems have traditionally been assessed and then remediated through direct intervention by SLPs. Although this remains true to an extent today, SLPs are collaborating with general and special educators to implement programs within classrooms that heighten phonological awareness in all children and encourage correct articulation use in everyday interaction activities (see Chapter 10 for discussion). Because teachers are an important part of the remediation process, collaborative relationships are considered valuable and profitable for educators and children alike.

Some children need individual or small group sessions with the SLP during regular school hours for explicit teaching of sound production. SLPs should inform teachers when children need such services so that mutually convenient times are arranged that minimally disrupt academic learning or can be provided within the classroom. Flexibility in instructional schedules can allow for strong working relationships and less stress associated with interruptions in classroom participation.

The SLP should also share information about the progress of each child receiving direct service and provide teachers with specific ideas about how progress can be facilitated in the classroom environment. This transfer of learning to the classroom, or facilitation of learning within the classroom, affords each child greater responsibility to use learned information and provides teachers the opportunity to participate in the Individual Education Program and enhance student performance.

Summary

School-age children often exhibit phonological delays and difficulties involving sound precision. Whereas phonological delays can impact other developing systems of language, including reading and writing, articulatory delays affect intelligibility but not necessarily other systems. It is important, then, that the nature of each child's problem is fully understood by the SLP and teachers so that appropriate intervention occurs. The SLP not only plays a leading role in determining the nature of the problem, but also must involve teachers in the assessment process as well as in planning and implementing interventions both within and outside the classroom. For intervention to be maximally beneficial, educationists must collaborate in constructing expectations for each student and strategies for promoting expressive speaking competence. They must also determine when referrals to other professionals (e.g., dentist, otolaryngologist) are necessary and inform parents about their concerns and recommendations.

Fluency and Prosody Problems

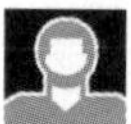

Brian

Brian is 16 and attends high school. He has stuttered since preschool. How-ever, during the past year he has been stuttering more often and has developed more noticeable characteristics. When Brian stutters, he struggles to produce the first words in a sentence, closes his eyes, and clenches his fists. Sometimes he just stops whatever he is trying to say and withdraws from the situation. He avoids speaking on the telephone and recently has seemed less interested in participating in social situations with his peers. Although some teasing occurs from peers and younger children, most students like him. However, they, as well as his teachers, do not know what to do or how to react when speaking with him. Brian received some private speech therapy during elementary school, but he does not want to leave his peers for speech class now that he is a high school student.

Definitions and Characteristics

Stuttering is easy to recognize because of its fragmentary nature. Verbal speech, which normally is easy, effortless, and smooth, is produced with part and whole word repetitions (e.g., "My-my-my name is B-B-B-Brian"), sound prolongations (e.g., "Let's go to the mo——vies"), and struggling behaviors involving visible tension. Stuttering can also be accompanied by unobservable characteristics, such as feelings of embarrassment and negative reactions and attitudes (Hillis, 1993). Most students experience disruptions in fluency for brief periods. Fortunately, a large proportion of them regain partial or complete fluency within months of its onset, and more than half of preschoolers who stutter regain fluent speech by age 7 (Yairi & Ambrose, 1992).

There are several contemporary ideas about why stuttering continues in a subset of children who experience it. Some professionals suggest that because language systems interact, difficulty in the development of one or more systems involved in language formulation (e.g., phonology, syntax) can lead to fluency difficulties (Neilson & Neilson, 1987; Starkweather, 1987). Others see the problem as one of motor planning and coordination difficulty (Perkins, Kent, & Curlee, 1991; Zimmerman, Smith, & Hanley, 1980) or reduction in speech motor flexibility (Caruso, Max, McClowry, & Chodzko-Zajko, 1998). Further, stuttering may relate to genetic predisposition, an underlying problem in the linguistic base, disruption of self-monitoring and feedback, and environmental demands exceeding the capacity to maintain fluency (Andrews et al., 1983; Postma & Kolk, 1993; Ratner, 1995; Starkweather, 1987). Parental behavior and emotional maladjustment in children *are not among the current theories* regarding the cause of stuttering, although some pediatricians and no doubt others still believe this to be the case (Yairi & Carrico, 1992). This belief may be perpetuated because of the variable nature of stuttering. When the speaking demands are high for communicating information (e.g., asking, commenting, explaining), stuttering can often increase, whereas when verbal messages contain rote and nonpropositional content (e.g., singing, reciting, reading), stuttering is often minimal.

Various language problems can co-occur with stuttering in children. Phonological and articulation delays have been noted (Louko, Edwards, & Conture, 1990), as well as increased fluency disruptions when complex grammatical structures are being formulated. Word-finding problems, naming difficulties, and fluency during conversations and narratives have also been observed (Hill, 1995).

Children who stutter are often teased (i.e., made fun of, called names) or even bullied (i.e., physical or verbal aggression, intimidated) by others and are considered at risk for victimization. Such a problem could go unnoticed, since children sometimes do not report incidences of teasing and bullying to parents or teachers (Langevin, Bortnick, Hammer, & Wiebe, 1998). The psychological consequences for bullied children include handicaps in psychosocial–emotional development, which can result in negative influences on cognitive, social, and language development (Gallagher, 1991; Hodge & Warkentin, 1994; Neary & Joseph, 1994), although further research is needed to determine how children who stutter are influenced by bullying.

Other disturbances in speech production are called *prosodic problems*. The interrelationships of the linguistic systems make it difficult to determine the precise causes of prosodic disturbance. Children who have autism, mental retardation, hearing impairment, motor speech impairment, or language impairment may have difficulty with prosody (Hargrove, 1997).

The suprasegmental aspects of speech, including pitch modulation, loudness levels, timing of speech and pauses, and stress on syllables, words, and phrases, allow for smooth transitions between words and sentences and provide the rhythm and cadence of oral speech and language (Hargrove, 1997). When prosodic features are impaired, the result is interference in intelligibility, word and sentence meanings, and communication of feelings and attitudes. Thus, not only is communication with others difficult, but the social nuances conveyed by the suprasegmentals are impacted, making the speaker appear unusual and conspicuous to others.

Implications for the Classroom

The SLP should be a resource to teachers and special educators when fluency or prosodic problems exist in children. The particular difficulties can be discussed in relation to academic performance and social interactions so that teachers and students understand the strengths and limitations of each child. Often, expressive speech disorders do not interfere with learning per se, although the verbal performance expectations of classrooms can make an impact on the student's attitudes about speaking and on the perception from teachers about what the student knows. Therefore, teachers and SLPs should be alert to each student's overall performance and sensitive to the particular expressive difficulties.

Just as normal speakers have periods of dysfluency, children who stutter or have prosodic difficulties have periods of fluency and normal prosody. Children should be encouraged to express themselves within their own capabilities. Accommodating them may require some adjustment in the verbal expectations of the classroom. For example, if narrative situations are particularly difficult, a question–answer format may promote more fluent speech and fulfill the expectations of the teacher. SLPs and teachers should jointly plan such modifications so that each student meets with success. Direct therapy services can provide the avenue where students learn and practice difficult expressive speech contexts within the classroom.

Summary

Many children exhibit fluency difficulties during speaking as preschoolers, yet a small subset of children continue to stutter in elementary, middle, and high school. Stuttering is characterized by disruptions in speech and often includes unusual facial and body movements. Further, speaking anxiety, social interaction difficulties, and the co-occurrence of language problems make stuttering a complex expressive speech disorder. Prosodic difficulties also cause speakers to be less intelligible and successful when conveying ideas, feelings, and attitudes. In most cases, prosodic difficulties occur as one of many characteristics associated with problems in cognition, hearing, motor abilities, and language development. SLPs should take the lead in collaborating with teachers to identify and remediate prosodic problems. The SLP should provide information about each child's problem and work together with teachers to determine an appropriate plan for intervention that fosters successful participation within classroom situations.

Fluency and prosody problems attract attention and can result in teasing and ridicule from others. Educators have the responsibility to teach respect for others to all children and act as advocates for their academic and social growth. Education about the problems and strict policies against verbal abuse and violence provide a safe and positive learning and social environment.

Voice Disorders

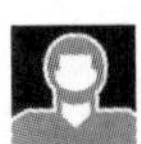 Molly

Molly is 13 and in the eighth grade. She is a good student who achieves high grades and is popular with the other students. She was accepted into the cheerleading squad after practicing for 6 months with her friends. Now that she is cheerleading at practice every day and during football and basketball games on weekends, her voice is hoarse and breathy. Her voice sounds very bad immediately after cheerleading, and it does not return to normal even after vocal rest or sleep. Some of her friends comment that they like the sound of her voice, but Molly does not like that she cannot sing or speak as well as she used to.

Definitions and Characteristics

Voice problems are often described by *pitch* (which refers to the musical tones of the voice), *loudness*, and *quality* (which refers to clarity and judgments of pleasantness). Voice disorders can occur in children, especially when they engage in vocally abusive practices. It is not uncommon to observe children on the playground or in the school gymnasium screaming, cheering, yelling, and imitating voices. They can develop swelling of the vocal cords or even callous-like growths called *vocal nodules* caused by trauma during vocal abuse. When the vocal cords are swollen or have nodules, they vibrate at a slower rate, causing low pitch and hoarseness. Nodules also result in breathiness caused by the escape of air between vocal cords that cannot close fully. Nodules can be difficult to eliminate, especially when the abusive behaviors are chronic. Other conditions of the vocal cords that affect the quality of the voice include laryngitis or growths such as polyps (fluid-filled sacs) (Colton & Casper, 1996; Wilson, 1987).

The interactions between breathing, voicing, and speech must be considered when the voice is not normal. Neurological conditions that cause irregularities in muscle strength and control (e.g., cerebral palsy, muscular dystrophy) may lead to weak volume, hoarseness, and difficulty coordinating voicing with speech. The status of a student's hearing can also relate to the loudness, pitch, and quality of the voice because of an imperfect feedback system to monitor these vocal parameters. Voice problems can occur when children try to compensate for structural problems that interfere with speech production. In the case of cleft palate, sounds are sometimes made in the pharynx so that the air is not directed through the nose. The increased tension to produce sounds lower in the vocal tract can lead to hoarseness of the voice. Finally, psychosocial factors have been related to problems in vocal use and abuse (Colton & Casper, 1996; Wilson, 1987).

Implications for the Classroom

Most voice disorders are preventable, but once they occur can be difficult to treat. Early identification of vocally abusive behaviors and education about the effects of such behaviors can prevent the occurrence of voice problems in children. Educationists should be alert to sudden changes in students' voices during or after prolonged illness, or after periods or single instances of vocal abuse. Parents should receive information when these changes are noted and be provided with referral information for assessment by an otolaryngologist and SLP. The physician will diagnose the physical condition of the vocal mechanism and will often recommend a period of voice therapy.

Education about abusive practices is the responsibility of all adults, but can be especially effective during health-related discussions in classrooms. Children can also benefit from information about lung, esophageal, and laryngeal cancer due to tobacco smoke.

Summary

Voice disorders in children occur as a result of vocal abuse, but can also occur from other factors (e.g., upper respiratory conditions, trauma to the larynx, neurological conditions). Since abusive practices can lead to growths or other changes in the vocal folds, educationists play an important role in prevention, referral, and intervention for voice problems in children. The SLP determines the characteristics of the voice and the otolaryngologist determines the physical state of the vocal mechanism and the cause of the problem. Once these professionals determine the presence of a voice problem, interventions should focus on eliminating abusive factors (or other health or environmental factors) and retraining the child's voice. Teachers and SLPs must work together to prevent children from developing voice disorders through education in classrooms, such as during health or science. Chapter 11 provides a number of suggestions for educating children and their families about proper voice use.

Summary and Conclusions

Speech disorders occur in school-age children and can be present through the high school grades and beyond. While phonological problems are most often seen in early grades, articulation, fluency, prosody, and voice problems influence the speaking abilities of children and adults. Just as with language problems (see Chapter 7), speech problems occur as a result of many factors intrinsic to the child or from outside influences. As such, careful assessment of the problems include thorough case histories, observation and testing, and team intervention planning.

Speech problems influence classroom participation, attitudes about school, and social development with peers. Therefore, educationists must work together (a) to find successful ways for children to participate fully, (b) to help children develop positive self-esteem and maintain personal pride, and (c) to educate other children in appropriate ways of interacting with peers who have speech problems.

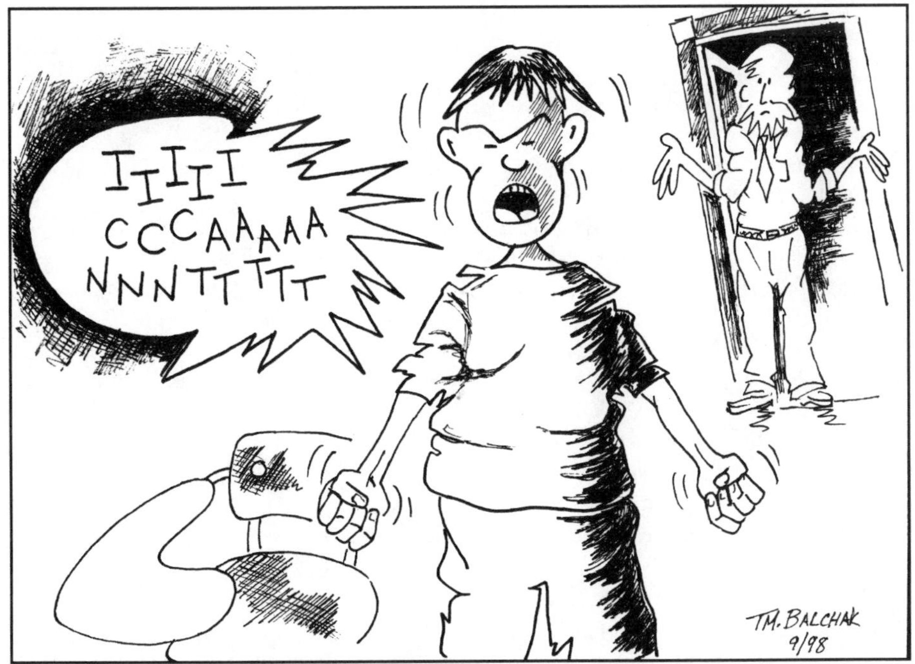

Just as normal speakers have periods of dysfluency, students who stutter or have prosodic difficulties have periods of fluency and normal prosody. Students should be encouraged to express themselves within their own capabilities.

References

Acredolo, L., & Goodwyn, S. (1985). Symbolic gesturing in language development: A case study. *Human Development, 28*, 40–49.

Andersen, E., Dunlea, A., & Kekelis, L. (1993). The impact of input: Language acquisition in the visually impaired. *First Language, 13*(19), 23–50.

Andrews, G., Craig, A., Feyer, A., Hoddinott, A., Howie, P., & Neilson, M. (1983). Stuttering: A review of research findings and theories circa 1982. *Journal of Speech and Hearing Disorders, 48*, 226–246.

Bardach, J., & Salyer, K. E. (1995). Cleft classification and cleft lip repair. In R. J. Shprintzen & J. Bardach (Eds.), *Cleft palate speech management: A multidisciplinary approach* (pp. 90–101). St. Louis, MO: Mosby.

Barraga, N. (1983). *Visual handicaps and learning*. Austin, TX: PRO-ED.

Bauman, M. (1993). An interview with Dr. Margaret Bauman. *Advocate: Autism Society of America, 24*(4), 1–14.

Bernstein Ratner, N. (1995). Language complexity and stuttering in children. *Topics in Language Disorders, 15*(3), 32–47.

Bernthal, J. E., & Bankson, N. W. (Eds.). (1994). *Child phonology: Characteristics, assessment, and intervention with special populations*. New York: Thieme Medical.

Bernthal, J. E., & Bankson, N. W. (1998). *Articulation and phonological disorders* (4th ed.). Boston: Allyn & Bacon.

Bridgeman, E., & Snowling, M. (1988). The perception of phoneme sequence: A comparison of dyspraxic and normal children. *British Journal of Disorders of Communication, 23*, 245–252.

Caruso, A. J., Max, L., McClowry, M. T., & Chodzko-Zajko, W. J. (1998). Cognitive stress and stuttering: An experimental paradigm for connected speech. *Contemporary Issues in Communication Science and Disorders, 25*, 65–75.

Clarke-Klein, S. M. (1994). Expressive phonological deficiencies: Impact on spelling development. *Topics in Language Disorders, 14*(2), 40–55.

Colton, R., & Casper, J. K. (1996). *Understanding voice problems: A physiological perspective for diagnosis and treatment* (2nd ed.). Baltimore: Williams & Wilkins.

Elstner, W. (1983). Abnormalities in the verbal communication of visually impaired children. In A. Mills (Ed.), *Language acquisition in the blind child: Normal and deficient* (pp. 18–41). San Diego: College-Hill.

Erin, J. (1990). Language samples from visually impaired four and five year olds. *Journal of Childhood Communication Disorders, 13*(2), 181–191.

Faye, E. (Ed.). (1976). *Clinical low vision*. New York: Little, Brown.

Gallagher, T. (1991). *Pragmatics of language: Clinical practice issues*. San Diego: Singular.

Gravel, J. S., & Wallace, I. F. (1995). Early otitis media, auditory abilities, and educational risk. *American Journal of Speech–Language Pathology, 4*(3), 89–94.

Hall, P. (1992). At the center of controversy: Developmental apraxia. *American Journal of Speech–Language Pathology, 1*(3), 23–25.

Hanson, M. L. (1994). Oral myofunctional disorders and articulatory patterns. In J. Bernthal & N. Bankson (Eds.), *Child phonology: Characteristics, assessment, and interventions with special populations* (pp. 29–53). New York: Thieme Medical.

Hargrove, P. M. (1997). Prosodic aspects of language impairment in children. *Topics in Language Disorders, 17*(4), 76–83.

Hayden, D. A. (1994). Differential diagnosis of motor speech dysfunction in children. *Clinics in Communication Disorders, 4*(2), 119–141.

Hill, D. G. (1995). Assessing the language of children who stutter. *Topics in Language Disorders, 15*(3), 60–79.

Hillis, J. W. (1993). Ongoing assessment in the management of stuttering: A clinical perspective. *American Journal of Speech–Language Pathology, 2*(1), 24–37.

Hodge, M., & Warkentin, C. (1994, October). *Management of children with bilateral facial paralysis*. Paper presented at the meeting of the Speech and Language Association of Alberta, Calgary.

Hodson, B. W. (1994). Helping individuals become intelligible, literate, and articulate: The role of phonology. *Topics in Language Disorders, 14*(2), 1–16.

Hoff-Ginsberg, E. (1997). *Language development*. Pacific Grove, CA: Brooks/Cole.

Holmes, K., & Holmes, D. (1980). Signed and spoken language development in a hearing child of hearing parents. *Sign Language Studies, 28*, 239–254.

Klein, S., & Rapin, I. (1992). Intermittent conductive hearing loss and language development. In D. Bishop & K. Mogford (Eds.), *Language development in exceptional circumstances* (pp. 96–109). Hillsdale, NJ: Erlbaum.

Koppenhaver, D. A., & Yoder, D. E. (1993). Classroom literacy instruction for children with severe speech and physical impairments (SSPI): What is and what might be. *Topics in Language Disorders, 12*(2), 1–15.

Lahey, M. (1988). *Language disorders and language development*. New York: Macmillan.

Landau, B., & Gleitman, L. (1985). *Language and experience: Evidence from the blind child*. Cambridge, MA: Harvard University Press.

Langevin, M., Bortnick, K., Hammer, T., & Wiebe, E. (1998). Teasing/bullying experienced by children who stutter: Toward development of a questionnaire. *Contemporary Issues in Communication Science and Disorders, 25*, 12–24.

LeBlanc, E. M., & Cisneros, G. J. (1995). The dynamics of speech and orthodontic management in cleft lip and palate. In R. J. Shprintzen & J. Bardach (Eds.), *Cleft palate speech management: A multidisciplinary approach* (pp. 305–326). St. Louis, MO: Mosby.

Louko, L., Edwards, M. L., & Conture, E. (1990). Phonological characteristics of young stutterers and their normally fluent peers: Preliminary observations. *Journal of Fluency Disorders, 15*, 191–210.

Lowe, R. J. (1997). *Phonology: Assessment and intervention applications in speech pathology*. Baltimore: Williams & Wilkins.

Neary, A., & Joseph, S. (1994). Peer victimization and its relationship to self-concept and depression among school girls. *Personality and Individual Differences, 16*(1), 183–186.

Neilson, M., & Neilson, P. (1987). Speech motor control and stuttering: A computational model of adaptive sensory-motor processing. *Speech Communication, 6*, 325–333.

Nelson, N. W. (1993). *Childhood language disorders in context: Infancy through adolescence*. New York: Merrill.

Northern, J. L., & Downs, M. P. (1984). *Hearing in children* (3rd ed.). Baltimore: Williams & Wilkins.

Orlansky, M., & Bonvillian, J. (1988). Early sign language acquisition. In M. Smith & J. Locke (Eds.), *The emergent lexicon: The child's development of linguistic vocabulary* (pp. 263–292). New York: Academic Press.

Paterson, M. M. (1994). Articulation and phonological disorders in hearing-impaired school-aged children with severe and profound sensorineural losses. In J. E. Bernthal & N. W.

Bankson (Eds.), *Child phonology: Characteristics, assessment, and intervention with special populations* (pp. 199–226). New York: Thieme Medical.

Paul, R. (1995). *Language disorders from infancy through adolescence: Assessment and intervention.* Boston: Mosby.

Perkins, W., Kent, R., & Curlee, R. (1991). A theory of neuropsycholinguistic function in stuttering. *Journal of Speech and Hearing Research, 34*, 734–752.

Pierce, P. L., & McWilliam, P. J. (1993). Emerging literacy and children with severe speech and physical impairments (SSPI): Issues and possible intervention strategies. *Topics in Language Disorders, 13*(2), 47–57.

Postma, A., & Kolk, H. (1993). The covert repair hypothesis: Prearticulatory repair processes in normal and stuttered disfluencies. *Journal of Speech and Hearing Research, 36*, 472–487.

Ratner, N. B. (1995). Language complexity and stuttering in children. *Topics in Language Disorders, 15*(3), 32–47.

Ratner, V. L., & Harris, L. R. (1994). *Understanding language disorders: The impact on learning.* Eau Claire, WI: Thinking Publications.

Roberts, J. E., & Clarke-Klein, S. (1994). Otitis media. In J. E. Bernthal & N. W. Bankson (Eds.), *Child phonology: Characteristics, assessment, and intervention with special populations* (pp. 182–198). New York: Thieme Medical.

Roberts, J. E., & Medley, L. (1995). Otitis media and speech–language sequelae in young children: Current issues in management. *American Journal of Speech–Language Pathology, 4*(1), 15–24.

Rosenthal, J. B. (1994, September). Rate control therapy for developmental apraxia of speech. *Clinics in Communication Disorders, 4*(3), 190–200.

Shprintzen, R. J., & Bardach, J. (1995). *Cleft palate speech management: A multidisciplinary approach.* St. Louis, MO: Mosby.

Shprintzen, R. J., & Goldberg, R. (1995). The genetics of clefting and associated syndromes. In R. J. Shprintzen & J. Bardach (Eds.), *Cleft palate speech management: A multidisciplinary approach* (pp. 16–43). St. Louis, MO: Mosby.

Smit, A. B. (1993). Phonological error distribution in the Iowa–Nebraska articulation norms project: Consonsant singletons. *Journal of Speech and Hearing Research, 36*, 533–547.

Spencer, P. (1993). The expressive communication of hearing mothers to deaf infants. *American Annals of the Deaf, 138*(3), 275–283.

Square, P. A. (1994, September). Treatment approaches for developmental apraxia of speech. *Clinics in Communication Disorders, 4*(3), 151–161.

Starkweather, C. W. (1987). *Fluency and stuttering.* Englewood Cliffs, NJ: Prentice-Hall.

Steelman, J. D., Pierce, P. L., & Koppenhaver, D. A. (1993). The role of computers in promoting literacy in children with severe speech and physical impairments (SSPI). *Topics in Language Disorders, 13*(2), 76–91.

Stoel-Gammon, C., & Kehoe, M. M. (1994). Hearing impairment in infants and toddlers: Identification, vocal development, and intervention. In J. E. Bernthal & N. W. Bankson (Eds.), *Child phonology: Characteristics, assessment, and intervention with special populations* (pp. 163–181). New York: Thieme Medical.

Wilson, D. K. (1987). *Voice problems of children* (3rd ed.). Baltimore: Williams & Wilkins.

Witzel, M. A. (1995). Communication impairment associated with clefting. In R. J. Shprintzen & J. Bardach (Eds.), *Cleft palate speech management: A multidisciplinary approach* (pp. 137–166). St. Louis, MO: Mosby.

Wolff, A., & Harkins, J. (1986). Multihandicapped students. In A. Schildroth & M. Karchmer (Eds.), *Deaf children in America* (pp. 55–81). Boston: College-Hill.

Yairi, E., & Ambrose, N. (1992). A longitudinal study of stuttering in children: A preliminary report. *Journal of Speech and Hearing Research, 35*, 755–760.

Yairi, E., & Carrico, D. M. (1992). Early childhood stuttering: Pediatricians' attitudes and practices. *American Journal of Speech–Language Pathology, 1*(3), 54–62.

Zimmerman, G., Smith, A., & Hanley, J. (1980). Stuttering: In need of a unifying conceptual framework. *Journal of Speech and Hearing Research, 25*, 25–31.

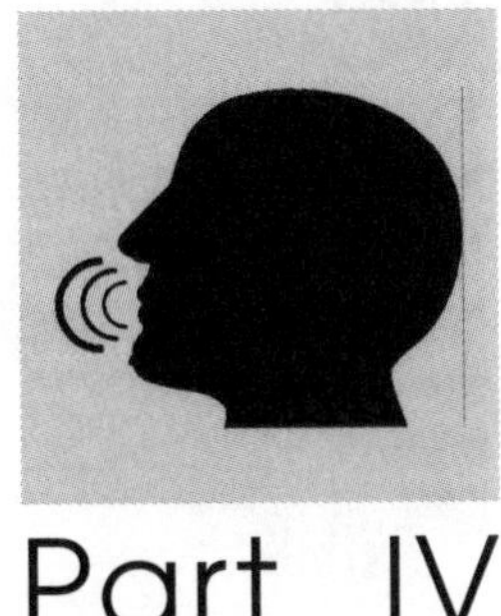

Part IV

Classroom-Based Language Interventions

Classroom Language Instruction: A Collaborative Approach

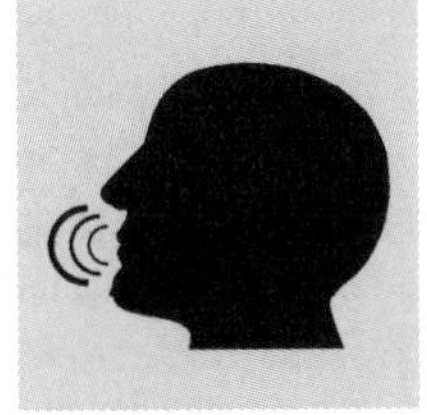

Chapter 9

D. Kim Reid, Molly McCarthy Leamon, and Kathleen R. Fahey

Collaboration is a shift . . . from advocacy to engagement, from confrontation to conversation, from debate to dialogue, and from separation to community.

(Chrislip & Larson, 1994, p. 4)

Between the passage of the Education for All Handicapped Children Act in 1975 and its reauthorizations under the Individuals with Disabilities Education Act (IDEA) in 1990 and again in 1997, significant changes occurred in the way schools defined and began to deal with students who are disabled, low achieving, or both. Where they were once uniformly isolated in self-contained schools, classes or resource rooms, students with special needs are now integrated into the least restrictive environment (LRE). Most schools still maintain a variety of service delivery options (see Table 9.1) that are used alone or in combination depending on the student's age, type of disability, level of communication competence, language and cultural background, academic performance, social skills, and attitudes about special services, as well as family and teacher concerns (American Speech-Language-Hearing Association [ASHA], 1996; Nelson, 1993). Nevertheless, the trend is increasingly toward interpreting LRE as providing services whenever possible within the general education classroom, especially for students with language learning disabilities (see ASHA's 1991 position paper) or language difference (Collier, 1995). ASHA (1998) defines classroom-based intervention as follows:

> This model is also known as integrated services, curriculum-based, transdisciplinary, interdisciplinary, or inclusive programming. There is an emphasis on the speech–language pathologist [or other specialist] providing direct service to students within the classroom and other natural environments.

Molly McCarthy Leamon is a special education teacher in the Denver Public Schools and an adjunct assistant professor at the University of Colorado, Denver. She received her doctorate from the University of Northern Colorado, Greeley, in 1997.

Table 9.1
Service Delivery Options for Addressing Students' Language Problems

1. *Collaboration*—Classroom teacher and special educator or speech–language pathologist (SLP) work directly in the classroom to provide assessment and interventions to students.
2. *Consultation*—Classroom teacher discusses student needs with special educator or SLP and then implements assessment and intervention strategies with students during regular classroom instruction.
3. *Combination of collaboration and consultation*
4. *Combination of collaboration and pull-out*—Classroom teacher and special educator or SLP work directly in the classroom for specific periods each week. The specialist takes individual children from the classroom to teach specific skills.
5. *Combination of consultation and pull-out*—Classroom teacher discusses student needs with special educator or SLP and then implements assessment and intervention strategies with students during regular classroom instruction. The specialist takes individual children from the classroom to teach specific skills.
6. *Pull-out services*—Special educator or SLP takes individual children from the classroom to assess or teach specific skills.
7. *Special education classrooms within regular education buildings*—Self-contained classroom for children with severe needs taught by special education teachers. Collaboration, consultation, and pull-out services may also occur. (This is a less desirable service option.)
8. *Special education classroom in special buildings*—Self-contained classroom within building with specialized equipment and teachers. Collaboration, consultation, and pull-out services may also occur. (This is the least desirable service option.)

> Team teaching by the speech–language pathologist and the regular and/or special education teacher(s) is frequent with this model. (p. 58)

Although it is not yet usual practice (Black, Meyer, Giugno, D'Aquanni, & Lowengard, 1996; Phillips & McCullough, 1990), there is widespread advocacy and mounting research support for the work of specialist teachers and speech–language pathologists (SLPs) to become increasingly collaborative and classroom based (Brandel, 1992; Christiansen & Luckett, 1990; Coufal, 1993; Elksnin, 1997; Merritt & Culatta, 1998; O'Shea & O'Shea, 1997; Paul, 1995). An important consequence is the expectation that general and special education teachers, SLPs, bilingual teachers, and teachers of English as a Second

Language (ESL) (sometimes with occupational therapists or other specialists) will learn to work together to deliver appropriate services to all students, often within the general education classroom, at the home, or in other natural contexts, rather than in isolated settings such as resource rooms and clinics.

Advocacy for classroom-based interventions stems in part from the problems associated with segregated intervention settings. To begin with, people with disabilities have the legal and moral right to be educated with their peers. When people are segregated, they are disempowered with respect to the larger society because they have no voice and no means to learn how to negotiate their place in it. An attempt at solving the problems of isolating students was to enroll them in mainstream classes, but to pull them out of those classes for a part of the day to instruct them in, usually, small, homogeneous groups. ASHA (1998) defines pull-out as follows:

> Services are provided to students individually and/or in small groups in the speech room [for special educators, in the resource room]. Some speech–language pathologists may prefer to provide individual or small group services within the physical space of the classroom. (p. 58)

As Allington and Johnston (1989) and Taylor (1991) discovered, however, this is not an acceptable solution: When students are pulled out for intervention, their days are often disjointed and confusing. Many students experience one type of instruction in the general education classroom and something different, sometimes even inconsistent, when working with the specialist in pull-out settings. One interventionist usually has little idea of what the others are doing. Moreover, difficulties generalizing skills taught in pull-out settings to the general classroom or the home are common. With different (and uncoordinated) approaches, different teachers, different topics, different procedures, and different locations, students seldom see any connections between their two sets of lessons. Furthermore, students are stigmatized and frequently miss valuable experiences in the general education classroom when they are singled out and pulled out (Reid & Button, 1995).

Consultation and Collaboration

Consultation and collaboration were the two major models that emerged during the 1980s for providing delivery of integrated services in general education classrooms (Cohen, Thomas, Sattler, & Morsink, 1997; Pugach & Johnson, 1995a), as well as in the home (Crais, 1993). Consultation was the first to dominate practice, because it was the easiest to implement. After almost 20 years of experience, however, there is a clear and decided shift toward a preference for collaboration models (ASHA, 1998; Elksnin, 1997; Ferguson, 1992; Merritt & Culatta, 1998; O'Shea & O'Shea, 1997; Pugach & Johnson, 1995b; Russell & Kaderavek, 1993; Ward & Landrum, 1994).

Consultation Versus Collaboration

Consultation refers to a problem-solving process in which two or more people work together to serve one or more other persons. In schools, it often takes two forms. The first is illustrated by the SLP who, having a thorough knowledge of a student's dialect, assists the general or special education teacher in taking that dialect into account in instruction (ASHA, 1998). A second form amounts to having specialists (in this case, the special education, ESL or bilingual teacher, or SLP) serve as *experts* who advise the consultee—that is, the general education teacher (who may also be a bilingual teacher) or parent. The purpose is for the expert to enable the consultee to conduct the intervention: therefore, the consultant serves the client indirectly. Coufal (1993) respectfully refers to consultees as "mediators," because they do not—indeed, because language is generative, *cannot*—mechanically perform interventions suggested by the consultant, whose role is to make suggestions, ensure they are carried out, and generally assist the mediator. The mediator, then, plays an active and dynamic role in the intervention process. Strategies used to provide the time necessary for consultation include bringing large groups of students together for specific activities (e.g., films, guest speakers, special programs) or in one place (e.g., the library) to allow classroom teachers and specialists to talk (West & Idol, 1990). The steps in a typical consultation, elaborated in Table 9.2, include forming relationships among the professionals, focusing on a problem, trying to solve it, and ending the relationship when the goal has been reached.

There are also problems, however, with consultation models. First and most obvious is its temporary and hierarchical nature. The "experts" coach general education teachers or parents about what to do, but, as Cohen et al. (1997) reported, the teachers often feel that the recommendations are unrealistic, unfair, or impossible to implement in the general education classroom. Crais (1993) reported similar reactions from parents about assessments and interventions that consultants recommend they carry out at home. Another problem with consultation is that the process is problem oriented—no attention is given to prevention—and many times assessment procedures or interventions begin before the specialist and general education teacher or parent

Table 9.2
Steps in a Typical Consultation Process

1. Establishing a relationship among the professionals.
2. Gathering information on the problem to be solved.
3. Defining the problem.
4. Deciding what specific behaviors to address.
5. Discussing options for intervention.
6. Selecting interventions to try.
7. Implementing the selected interventions and collecting data on their impact.
8. Determining whether the desired outcome(s) had occurred.
9. Modifying as necessary.
10. Ending the process when the goal is reached.

Note. Adapted from *Interactive Teaming: Consultation and Collaboration in Special Programs,* by C. V. Morsink, C. C. Thomas, and V. I. Correa, 1991, New York: Macmillan.

have had sufficient time to come to some kind of mutual understanding about what the problem is and how it should be solved. Finally, in consultation, the student benefits from the process but does not participate in the actual problem solving (Friend & Cook, 1996; Rhodes & Dudley-Marling, 1988). Students become the objects of instruction, rather than having opportunities to learn to be self-advocating agents who gain the skills and abilities they will need to negotiate their place in society. Consequently, a shift in emphasis from a consultation to a collaboration (sometimes also called collaborative-consultation) model promises to improve service delivery systems (Pugach & Johnson, 1995a).

We mention the consultation model because it is frequently used in combination with pull-out instruction: the specialist provides direct service in a pull-out setting and the general education teacher or parent supplies opportunities for practice and generalization in the classroom or home setting. In addition, there may be students for whom the general education classroom is not the LRE (see the National Joint Committee on Learning Disabilities' 1993 position paper). Furthermore, collaboration is a new and somewhat radical departure from the way schools have been operating (Skrtic, 1995). Many general education teachers, as well as SLPs and special education, bilingual, and ESL teachers, will need to be *taught* how to collaborate to ensure effectiveness (Voltz, Elliott, & Cobb, 1994). At least two additional obstacles to collaboration have surfaced in the relationships between general education teachers or parents and SLPs (Achilles, Yates, & Freese, 1991; Crais, 1993). The first is that each participant is not always willing to engage in collaboration and assume the shared responsibility that is necessary for a team relationship. The second is that not all teachers and parents believe it is important to extend language goals into the classroom or home, or they disagree with specialists about how it should be done. Proper instantiation requires team planning and the understanding of the connections between oral and written language, between language and the creation of the classroom and home environment, and between the linguistic environment and students' academic and social success. For collaboration to work, specialists need not only to be competent practitioners in their disciplines, but also to know how to educate others about individual and cultural language learning differences.

General education teachers (and there is an analogous new set of responsibilities for parents), on the other hand, may have to spend more time explaining what they are doing; assume greater accountability for students with special needs and language differences; present the curriculum differently; offer more time to certain students; modify learning environments; teach academic and social strategies, and study and interactional skills; and provide a relationship that nourishes and supports differences (Howard-Rose & Rose, 1994; Idol, 1997). Despite well-deserved enthusiasm about the potential of the collaboration model, many teachers and parents are not yet prepared to make such a commitment and many schools and clinics simply do not have the necessary time and training resources.

2 Models of Collaboration

Collaboration is an inclusive technique for building relationships among general educators, educational specialists, students and their parents, administrators, and community members. Chrislip and Larson (1994) defined collaboration as a

> mutually beneficial relationship between two or more parties who work toward common goals by sharing responsibility, authority, and accountability for achieving results. Collaboration is more than simply sharing knowledge and information (communication) and more than a relationship that helps each party achieve its own goals (cooperation and coordination). The purpose of collaboration is to create a shared vision and joint strategies to address concerns that go beyond the purview of any particular party. (p. 5)

There are any number of ways to engage in collaborative practices. As would be expected, they range from those that use collaboration as a means to ensure successful consultation (i.e., the "expert" collaborates, and not merely consults, with mediators to ensure that they carry out interventions successfully), to those that are joint ventures (e.g., a clinician and parent cooperate in the planning, evaluation, and implementation of interventions in a way that achieves the parental goals), to those that are truly collaborative (i.e., the specialist[s]— often there is an interdisciplinary team—and parents or general education teacher work together with the students as equals to prevent, understand, and solve problems).

Collaborative Consultation

Coufal (1993) identified the two primary goals of collaborative consultation: (1) to provide remedial services by relying upon people in the social environment of the target (i.e., the child who needs services) to act as effective change agents and (2) to enhance the change agent's problem-solving skills (assuming that they will be useful with other students in the future). Her focus is on collaboration between (a) SLPs, the experts or *consultants*, and (b) general education classroom teachers, the change agents—called consultees or *mediators*. Both, she argues, come to improve their understanding of the difficulties manifested by the target child through the communication involved in reaching the shared understandings necessary to carry out the collaboration.

For Coufal (1993), consultation and collaboration are independent concepts.[1] *Consultation* refers to the process of the expert's providing the remedial service through an intermediary. *Collaboration* defines the *style* of interacting: "collaboration includes working together in a supportive and mutually beneficial manner for the development of intervention plans derived through joint problem definition, planning, and provision of services, with shared responsibility for all outcomes" (p. 4). Collaboration, then, is not merely cooperation, but depends on the establishment of mutual goals; reciprocity of influence; shared participation, resources, and accountability; and voluntariness—administrators

---

[1]ASHA (1998, p. 58) does not make this distinction. The association defines collaborative consultation as follows: "The speech–language pathologist, regular and/or special education teacher(s), and parents work together to facilitate a student's communication and learning in educational environments. It is essential that the administrator allow the speech–language pathologist and the collaborator(s) to have regularly scheduled planning time throughout the duration of service. This is an indirect model in which the speech–language pathologist does not provide direct service to the student."

cannot legislate successful collaboration. Collaborative consultation, then, requires more highly developed interpersonal skills than consultation. West and Cannon (1988) included among these skills the ability to establish and maintain rapport and mutual respect; effective listening, interviewing, questioning, brainstorming, and responding skills; and flexible application of assessment, planning, and management knowledge.

As the consultant, the SLP identifies a mediator who can influence the target student (see Figure 9.1) for a considerable amount of time within a natural setting (some direct service by the SLP may also be part of the plan). Coufal's (1993) approach to language intervention, especially for older students, is from a generative perspective that requires determining what language the target students are self-generating, how well it is working, and whether there is a discrepancy between their language performance and their language needs. This generative approach obviously suggests that intervention be carried out in functional and natural contexts. By working through a mediator, the SLP is able to change the instructional discourse patterns within classrooms or the students' homes. However, soliciting the willing participation of already busy teachers and parents necessitates that they understand the importance of changing the communicative contexts in which the target students participate.

In schools especially, complete understanding of the language problem is often hampered by a tendency for "context stripping," that is, treating problems as if they exist within the target students and ignoring the impact that the demands of various communicative contexts place upon them. In addition to analyzing communication issues per se, however, it is important to understanding the problem to take into account the target's behavior, feelings, attitudes, expectations, knowledge, and so forth. Coufal (1993) suggested that SLPs model data gathering strategies for teachers (and parents) and also engage them in the processes of evaluating evidence to define the problem and to set goals for its amelioration. Once the problem has been defined and the goals set, the consultant and mediator can turn their attention to generating alternatives for intervention. Because the work of problem definition and goal setting is

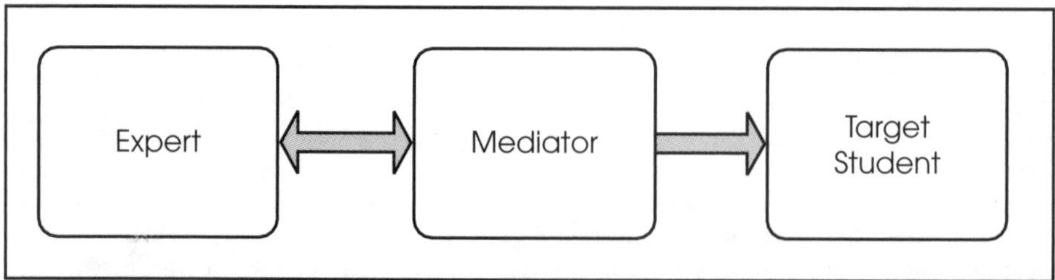

Figure 9.1. Collaborative consultation model.

done jointly, this approach eliminates many of the conflicts inherent in consultation practices that are not collaborative.

One strategy for generating alternative interventions is brainstorming—generating as many alternatives as possible without judging them for their quality. The purpose is to list so many alternatives that the participants feel assured that the best solution is among them. Only after the possible alternatives have been exhausted should participants discuss their relative merit and select one (or more) that addresses the outcomes desired, seems feasible, and meets whatever other criteria are important to the consultant and mediator.

The final step in collaborative consultation is objective verification that the intervention is being carried out and is effective. Coufal (1993) used the example of a teacher's trying to prompt a target student with poor expressive language skills to give topic-relevant, multiword responses by modeling and then asking open-ended questions (e.g., "I see a big billy goat in this picture. What else do you see?"). Verification would then include observations (perhaps 15 minutes a couple of times a week) by the SLP to count the frequency with which the intervention occurs and to determine whether the target student replies with topic-relevant, multiword responses. These observations then serve as data for periodic reviews in which the SLP and teacher decide together whether to continue or modify the intervention.

Finally, Coufal (1993) noted that collaborative consultation can occur with an SLP and a teacher or among members of a multidisciplinary team. The team might select a single mediator or several, working with the child in a variety of times and settings. In the case of a team, depending on the nature of the target behavior, any member of the team could serve as consultant or mediator.

Notice that in this model there is little emphasis on prevention. The idea is that the "expert" delivers services through the collaboration of an intermediary who can influence the target student for a longer time and in a more natural situation than would be possible in pull-out or even classroom-based direct intervention by the SLP. The entire collaboration is focused on a problem that needs solving and the student who manifests it. The overriding goal is for the SLP to develop more efficient and effective interventions by enlisting the support of the mediator. What differentiates this model from consultation is its insistence on mutual understandings, joint planning, and shared accountability—which change the nature of the interaction substantially.

Families as Collaborators

Crais's (1993) model for collaborating with parents is one step closer to a pure collaboration model, because it carefully specifies options, asks parents to make many of the important decisions, and reverses the power structure by putting the "expert" at the service of the parents and family (but it could just as easily be the classroom teacher and the students) (see Figure 9.2). Crais argued the need for collaboration on the basis that, traditionally, specialists have focused more on the outcomes of intervention than on the processes through which those outcomes have been achieved. The result has been that those receiving services (what in Coufal's, 1993, model are called the mediators), such as the families of young children being assessed for apparent language difficulties, have often expressed dismay and dissatisfaction. Crais suggested that the situation could be improved by considering (a) the balance of power, (b) the choices available, and (c) the sequence of services.

By actively and explicitly negotiating the director's role in language assessment, the family (or classroom teacher) can make decisions about when they would like to take the lead and when it might be better for the specialist to do so. Simply by negotiating the role, however, the professionals indicate that they are there to serve the needs of the family (teacher); they are collaborators in the process and not the primary decision makers.

As collaborators, specialists need to be certain that their clients make as many of the important decisions as possible. For example, if there is to be an assessment, do the clients have input with respect to the "location, types of activities performed, people present, roles taken by different people (including family members), interpretations of results, recommendations made, and

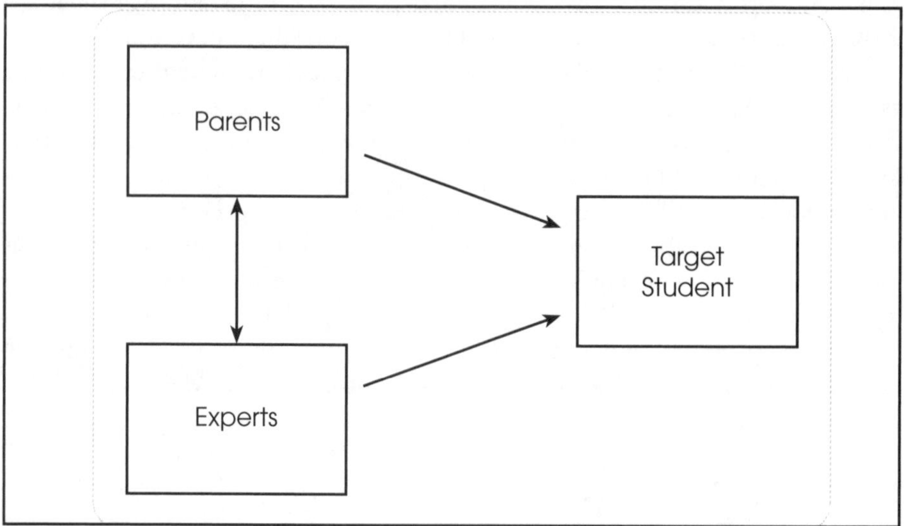

Figure 9.2. Collaboration with families model.

outcomes planned?" (Crais, 1993, p. 32). For example, many specialists typically use standardized tests, which are often important for their needs. Knowing the position of the target child in the national ranking of students seldom, however, is useful information for parents. What they want to know is how their children accomplish a variety of tasks, what they can and cannot do well, and how the information gathered can be used to help their children. Specialists clearly must share their own needs with respect to legal mandates, school and district policies, and so forth, but, according to Crais, they also need to identify the concerns and priorities of the family and then respond as directly to those concerns and priorities as is possible in planning and follow-up. Often, this goal of collaboration can be achieved by including parents (teachers) in the assessment process itself, rather than having the specialist conduct the assessment and then present the client with the results and a list of recommendations.

Finally, parents (teachers) can take an active role in deciding the sequence of activities to be performed. Should the target child be observed for a period of time before testing, or vice versa? Can some intervention services be begun while the assessment process is in progress? Can assessment and intervention strategies be redefined to better meet the needs and expectations of the family? For example, could the child be enrolled in services while the evaluation is carried out at home by the parents and in the school setting by the teacher before a diagnosis is made?

According to Crais (1993), what choices the consultees make about their needs and roles is less important than the fact that they have those choices. In current practice, clients are seldom in the driver's seat, probably because setting priorities and schedules at the specialist's convenience is more efficient. However, the costs are also significant with respect to the level of cooperation engaged in and the satisfaction experienced by the families and teachers whom specialists serve.

Note that this model incorporates the expertise of the specialist within a different power dynamic than the previous one. It allows the client to set goals and priorities that the consultant–collaborator attempts to meet, but nevertheless within a context of support and collaboration in which a shared perspective drives the work. Although the relationship among the participants who serve the target student is less hierarchical, the process is still problem oriented. There is little or no concern for prevention and the target child is not included in the decision-making process. These limitations, however, may be due to the very nature of the problem—a preschool child still at home or too young to participate in a reasonable and productive way in setting goals and making decisions.

Full Collaboration

Full collaboration is typically classroom based. Prelock, Miller, and Reed (1995) described how this transdisciplinary model, in which team members share responsibility for student learning, works. Because they are working together, team members naturally learn about each others' roles and realms. Their shared knowledge releases them from their roles, so that each may engage in effective interactions with students without concern for expectations associated with a specified set of obligations. Each participant can provide the others with information, insights, and strategies regarding assessment and intervention, and the use of time and material resources. The adage that two (or more) heads are better than one applies here, as in the previous models, but there are some distinctions.

Typically, collaboration begins with classroom teachers sharing with collaborating specialists the curricular objectives for all students in their classrooms, and these then serve as the foundation for the discussion, development, implementation, and assessment of interventions. The specialist (i.e., special education teacher, bilingual or ESL teacher, or SLP) can discuss the strengths and needs of particular students in relation to the class's curricular objectives. Strategies for student stimulation and support as well as curricular adaptations can then be jointly planned and implemented. Through this process, individualized instructional interventions can be effectively matched to the overall objectives of the classroom. Each participant has a critical role in determining the course of action for particular students. Lunday (1996) described the model used to empower students and teachers to improve their communication abilities in vocational, academic, alternative, and Job Corps classrooms (see Table 9.3). This model is especially pertinent to our purpose here, because it specifically addresses language issues.

Table 9.3
Characteristics of a Typical Collaboration

1. Goals are long term and aim at providing in-depth services.
2. The systems approach includes the family and the environment.
3. Decision making is based on judgment and consensus.
4. Collaborators consider interacting with community and other agencies, as needed.
5. Planning is proactive and designed to avert future problems.

Note. Adapted from *Interactions: Collaboration Skills for School Professionals* (2nd ed.), by M. Friend and L. Cook, 1996, White Plains, NY: Longman.

This ideal model is something to strive for (see Figure 9.3), but it would certainly be more difficult to carry out in schools where the SLP or other specialist has a substantial caseload of students with presenting problems competing for time and attention. In full collaboration, the collaborative activity includes the full range of behaviors engaged in in the classroom, and is carried out by the full range of participants, including the target students, in the context in which the shared activities will be implemented and with a considerable emphasis on prevention (e.g., teaching listening and test-taking skills, preteaching vocabulary). It includes coaching, modeling, and team teaching in which participants often change or cross roles (e.g., students doing strategy demonstrations).

This basic model (e.g., Table 9.4), then, solves many of the problems associated with consultation. In full collaboration, general education teachers and specialists come together with other interested parties, including the student, as equals contributing their own perspectives and expertise. From the outset, the goal is to engage in *long-term problem solving and prevention*, as well as joint planning and implementation. Because it involves a shared vision, it does not leave students feeling disoriented and fragmented during their educational day. Also, because students are engaged in the collaboration, they are able to learn both to cooperate and to self-advocate, important skills for their upcoming years in the workplace. Full collaboration may be school or community based. The latter addresses communication goals within the home, social settings, and

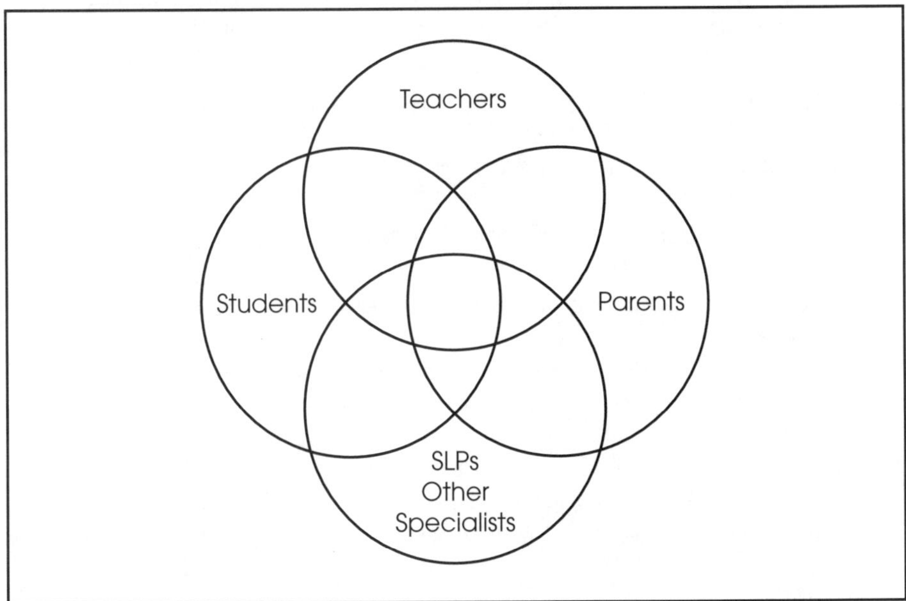

Figure 9.3. Full collaboration model.

Table 9.4
Prototype Collaborative Communication Model

1. *Cooperative planning*—working together to plan modifications to meet the students' needs. Specific communication and language skills may need to be included either in coordination with or in addition to content area objectives.
2. *Coaching*—working side-by-side to encourage and facilitate successful communication skills during structured or naturalistic interactions. Simultaneously, teachers learn through observation of the coaching done by specialists.
3. *Strategy demonstration*—students or specialists assuming the role of the teacher for a short time to model an approach, technique, or strategy.
4. *Adapting classroom materials*—working together to find modifications in materials or material presentations that will help students become more successful or work sooner without the adaptations. Many students with depressed communication skills benefit by hands-on presentations or demonstrations instead of verbal-only presentations.
5. *Team teaching*—providing an opportunity for professionals to focus on their areas of expertise. The objectives may include enhancing a lesson using communication-based materials or organizational objectives necessary for study skills, test taking, or development of social skills.
6. *Small group intervention within the classroom*—specialists working with an individual or small group of students in one area of the classroom while the teacher works with the rest of the class. This intervention has several foci:
   a. Paying attention to the language weaknesses of each student and providing direct feedback to enhance communication.
   b. Giving students naturalistic opportunities to practice communication skills with peers.
   c. Assessing each student's understanding of the content and determining when further instruction is required.
   d. Providing opportunities for students to put new concepts into practice.
7. *Preteaching vocabulary, concepts, or skills*—anticipating possible problems and preteaching specific students before the information is presented in the classroom. (The most frequent breakdown of communication in Job Corps training has been due to vocabulary.)
8. *Mini-lessons*—providing brief, informative lessons to the entire class or a small group as problems arise on language skills needed to complete the activity.

(*continues*)

Table 9.4 *Continued.*

9. *Classroom rules*—using face-to-face interactions to help students learn appropriate communication behaviors for classrooms, including how to determine when and with whom they are allowed to communicate and what they are allowed to say. Make teacher expectations explicit.
10. *Test preparation and test-taking skills*—working with students individually or in small groups to help them understand terminology used in directions, how to study for the kind of test expected (essay, true or false, fill in the blank), and how to identify the information to be covered in a test.
11. *Prelistening, listening, postlistening*—preparing students for listening by teaching them to attend to key words, vocal inflections, and pauses and to interpret directions into common vocabulary and use mnemonic devices. Help students learn strategies to be mentally and physically prepared to listen (i.e., to listen for terminology indicating a speaker is presenting a key point and to review or skim notes and add the information they remember but did not have a chance to write during the presentation).
12. *Writing*—recognizing limitations in students' reading and writing skills, assigning activities to ameliorate them or substituting alternative modes of expression.

Note. Adapted from "A Collaborative Communication Skills Program for Job Corps Centers," by A. M. Lunday, 1996, *Topics in Language Disorders, 16*(3), pp. 23–36. Adapted with permission.

work environments. High school intervention teams, for example, sometimes help students make the transition into the community while the student is completing high school or even after graduation (ASHA, 1996). Much of the impetus for full collaboration is resulting from the availability of technology, increasing numbers of diverse family communities (Friend and Cook, 1996), and economic scarcities (O'Shea & O'Shea, 1997).

Benefits of Collaboration

Various collaborative models, such as the three explicated in this chapter, have been successful for a wide range of communicative and educational applications. These applications include (a) teaching students with normal language abilities (Damico, 1987; Dudley-Marling, 1987); (b) facilitating language acquisition and development in students with language and learning disabilities (Bunker, McBurnett, & Fenimore, 1987; Catts & Kamhi, 1987); (c) ameliorating attention problems (Westby & Cutler, 1994); (d) engaging in family-centered intervention after TBI (DePompei & Williams, 1994; Szekeres & Meserve, 1994); (e) promoting hearing conservation in schools (Chermak, Curtis, & Seikel, 1996); (f) correcting stuttering (Cooper, 1997); (g) improving voice (Pindzola, 1993); (h) developing accurate phonological concepts (Masterson, 1993); (i) advancing literacy (Dudley-Marling, 1987); (j) teaching English as a second language (Bohn, Langville, Samples, & Sandt, 1991); (k) lessening the impact of behavior disorders in adolescents (Monast & Smith, 1987); and (l) preparing legal testimony after TBI, abuse, or neglect (Snyder, Nathanson, & Shaywitz, 1993; Ylvisaker, Kolpan, & Rosenthal, 1994). In collaborative settings, it is also possible to try environmental modifications or strategies to improve students' communication behaviors before they are referred or instead of referring them for special services.

Teachers and specialists who collaborate with each other and their students are less isolated and, as a consequence, better able to expand their ideas, materials, and methods. Specialists have some input into the instruction of students with whom they are concerned and, therefore, can participate in the planning and carrying out of instruction that is meaningful in the larger educational context. Shared vision also provides coherence and vitality to the curriculum and, often, higher quality solutions to problems. The collaborative interchange, because it is interactive, can lead to the co-construction of transformative knowledge and the process of continuous, active learning rather than highlighting only changes in behavioral outcomes and knowledge products. The negotiation of meaningful learning opportunities empowers all participants through the construction of an intellectual and cultural democracy in the classroom (Reid & Leamon, 1996; Reid, Robinson, & Bunsen, 1995). As Goodman and Goodman lamented, "It ought to be easier to learn in school than out of school because there are professional teachers to mediate the learning. But instead of adjusting school to the learners we require them to adjust to the school" (cited in Moll, 1990, p. 234). Collaboration is designed specifically to ameliorate that problem.

Walther-Thomas (1997) asked teachers and principals about the benefits of collaborative teaching. They reported that students who are engaged in collaboration benefit not only from positive feelings about themselves as learners and self-advocates, but also from improved social skills and stronger peer relationships. The general education students benefit from improved academic performance, time and attention from the specialists, increased emphasis on cognitive strategies and study skills, increased emphasis on social skills, and improved classroom communities. The benefits for general educators and the specialists with whom they collaborate include increased professional satisfaction, opportunities for professional growth, and personal support. Other benefits (Lambert,

Collay, Dietz, Kent, & Richert, 1996) also accrue. Teachers see themselves as powerful in the creation of curriculum and in relation to districts, unions, and outside agencies. With collaboration also comes a redefinition of roles and responsibilities for general education teachers, specialists, and the school administration. Finally, mutual trust and joint accountability often lead to the active solicitation of feedback and coaching and, through them, to better outcomes for students.

Benefits from collaboration also have been reported by classroom teachers, SLPs, and students who are in special education. For example, in a survey conducted by Elksnin and Capilouto (1994), classroom teachers reported increased support; growth in knowledge about the relationships among speech, language, and academic success; better carryover of language skills in the classroom; less disruption from pull-out services; and smaller student–teacher ratios. SLPs reported that services provided in natural settings promoted the integration of learning objectives into everyday tasks. This integration led to better generalization, more efficient service delivery, more time with students, and increased awareness of language goals by teachers. Students responded positively to remaining in the classroom, not being labeled, receiving coordinated instruction, working in groups with other students, and having opportunities to use their new abilities in the classroom.

Competencies Needed Among Collaborators

Language is not only the goal of collaboration (i.e., the content of instruction), it is also the vehicle for it. In addition to the competencies suggested by West and Cannon (1988) noted earlier, participants must be able to listen, communicate verbally and nonverbally in an effective manner, ask appropriate questions, provide helpful feedback, conduct interviews, and deal positively with conflict and resistance (Friend & Cook, 1996). These are competencies that many school personnel as well as students with special needs or language differences need to develop. Everyone involved, therefore, potentially can develop more effective communication skills from efforts to collaborate. Some principles for improving communication are highlighted in Table 9.5 (see also Friend & Cook, 1996; Pugach & Johnson, 1995). Communication is most effective when it is meaningful and focused to the goal or task that is being addressed.

For any collaborative system to work, however, both the general education teachers and the specialists (i.e., SLPs, special education teachers, bilingual teachers, ESL teachers) must be willing to reflect critically on their practice

Table 9.5
Communication for Successful Collaboration

1. Strive for consistency between the verbal and nonverbal messages being communicated.
2. Give concrete and specific instances/evidence to support points or illustrate questions.
3. Recognize that comments are from one point of view: use "I" messages.
4. Listen well and be open and supportive of others in your interactions.
5. Use purposive statements and ask appropriate questions.
6. Solicit and offer constructive feedback that is direct, well timed, descriptive, and directed.
7. Understand your own and others' conflict management style.
8. Learn how and when to use silence, when to understand contextual meanings as opposed to literal meanings, when to offer support, and when to challenge.

and be willing to share with and learn from others. Very importantly, time must be provided for discussion (Fullan, 1993), and the participants' concerns (i.e., awareness, information, management, personal and interpersonal relationships, collaboration, and refocusing) need, at least to some extent, to be addressed, perhaps as the basis for inservice training (Hord, Rutherford, Huling-Austin, & Hall, 1987). Collaborative models make the most sense if they are possible, because general educators and specialists alike are beginning to recognize that the capacity for renewal is rooted within *community* and not in programs or individuals (Chrislip & Larson, 1994). Consequently, the emphasis in this handbook is on classroom-based collaborative interventions for students with language differences and disorders.

Systemic Practitioner Discourses

One seldom-acknowledged problem that causes conflicts between and among the student, family members, and professionals attempting to engage in collaboration is the difference between language usage and the mostly unarticulated values and goals that it reflects. Harry (1992), for example, commented that differences in communication styles between school personnel and parents continue to preclude genuine collaboration. The meeting in which parents and professionals develop and agree to the Individualized Education Program (IEP) is a good example. Frequently, the professionals use labels, jargon, or references to tests and norms that are unfamiliar to parents and often difficult to understand even when they are explained (e.g., the concept of standard error of measurement). Much of the tension that such communication difficulties cause can be avoided if the professional team makes a concerted effort to do so and plans in advance explanations that it will provide for students and their families.

Davenport, Reid, and Fortner (1999) addressed another source of communication conflict: differences in language usage among professionals. We seldom note these differences, because we seem always to assume that we are all in the business of educating students. Beneath the surface assumptions, however, are significantly different values and goals. When we attempt to work collaboratively, such differences come to the fore, often causing open conflicts of the kinds noted throughout previous sections of this chapter and possibly a slowing or even failure of operations within a school (Henley, Ramsey, & Algozzine, 1996).

Although educational jargon is apparently unified—that is, we all use many of the same terms and concepts in talking about our work with students—there are discourses used by subgroups of educationists that reflect real differences. General education teachers, for example, emphasize academic growth and rigor, and curriculum mastery. Special educators, on the other hand, stress the target student's individual development as it is articulated in the IEP. Their goals, then, are less curriculum based and more child specific. As another example, while general education teachers tend to look to teacher-to-teacher (or specialist) collaboration to support students with special learning needs, teachers of special education tend to promote peer tutoring or students' self-advocacy (Davenport et al., 1999). School administrators, bilingual education teachers, teachers of ESL, SLPs, school psychologists, and parents all have their own specific values and accompanying discourses.

However, the problem goes well beyond language and values. According to Davenport et al. (1999), the interactions among various groups are frequently hegemonic and hierarchical. One example of hierarchical structuring was revealed in the second consultation model, in which a specialist cooperates with a mediator for the purpose of carrying out professional goals more efficiently. Consultants, therefore, often feel the need to *convince* general educators of the need for and viability of their carrying out interventions in the general education classroom.

One example of a hegemonic assumption is the expectation that schools revolve around the needs of general education and that it is the system of general education that constitutes the norm against which other instructional interventions are compared and evaluated. Although this expectation often works, there are situations in which it does not. For example, one does not need research evidence to realize that students with social skills difficulties cannot improve those skills in isolation or within groups whose other members manifest social difficulties as well. Nevertheless, students with poor social skills are frequently withdrawn from the general education classroom. Additionally, research (see Gartner & Lipsky, 1987; Stainback & Stainback, 1984, 1987a, 1987b) has shown that students with moderate to relatively severe disabilities typically exhibit improved social interactions and language usage when they are included in general education classrooms. Still, many general education teachers object to their presence in the classroom and feel uncomfortable about teaching them, because they cannot meet the demands of the general education curriculum.

If collaboration in any form is to work—and it has become increasingly clear that there cannot be effective consultation without some level of collaboration (Davenport et al., 1999)—participants must become aware of and sensitive to these discourse differences, acknowledge them, share them, and negotiate compromises. Recognizing the differences as systemic enables practitioners to treat them as such, rather than interpreting resulting conflicts as personal. Recognizing them as hierarchical and hegemonic can help to level the playing field. General educators can learn to value specialists for their unique points of view. Specialists can come to appreciate the pressures on teachers of general education classes. Professionals and families, especially nonmainstream families, can also improve relations through a mutually informing, two-way dialogue that seeks to eliminate jargon and to address values and goals as well as issues related to the policies of schooling (Crago, 1992).

Lee (1997) noted accurately that much of what we need to do to improve collaboration with adults is to engage in more of the behaviors that we use with students—and students, of course, may also be included in collaborative meetings. She pointed out, for example, that when we work with children, we make certain to generate the rules together, or at least to explain them. In adult meetings, we tend to assume that everyone knows the rules and that meetings should be conducted in ways that they have always been conducted. When teaching, we prepare and rehearse what to say. In meetings, we tend to say the first thing that comes to mind. While teaching, we recognize that different students have different interests, skills, and achievement levels. In meetings, we behave as if everyone were the same, as if they never had a bad day, and as if emotional states did not affect productivity. Lee explained that when students have a tough time, we ask about it and express empathy. Often, when adult collaborators experience problems, we avoid the subject and expect them to leave their problems at home. This differential treatment often leads to confusion, conflict, and hurt feelings that make trust difficult. Effective collaboration, then, requires better knowledge of one another, more tolerance and caring, and some significant changes in the ways that schools are organized.

Problems Related to Bureaucracy

Skrtic (1995) argued that in many ways schools are products of the time in which they were created and that a lot of the expectations that govern education today are the result of trying to prepare passive students for roles in an industrial economy that no longer exists. School curricula and practices reflect the idea that teaching can be segmented into bits that accumulate into learnings and that different people can be assigned different responsibilities to help students in an assembly-line fashion. Referring to Dewey's idea that the function of schooling should be to prepare citizens for participation in democracy rather than as workers in a factory, Skrtic questioned whether schools the way they are now constituted can accomplish that goal. Instead, he remarked (p. 218) that, "By design, there is no need for collaboration or mutual adjustment in schools because specialization and professionalization locate virtually all of the necessary coordination within the role of individual specialists."

What Skrtic (1995) advocated instead of our current types of bureaucratic structures is problem-solving *adhocracies* whose main reason for being is to invent new practices for work that is ambiguous—as teaching is when students do not fit easily into the general education mold. In such adhocracies, full collaboration would exist. Instead of limiting ourselves as teachers and specialists to the repertoire of skills and curricula we currently have, we would work together to both prevent and address problems by considering each case individually and, when typical practices do not work, inventing others. Instead of explaining disability as some pathology in the student and context stripping (i.e., failing to examine the contributions the dynamics of the environment make to the problem), educators would assume responsibility for instructing all students by jointly inventing and reinventing solutions. Because there would not be expectations for dividing the labor, time and procedures for collaborating would be built into the school day.

Although we have not made significant inroads into the bureaucratic structuring of schools, we have begun to recognize and value the importance of collaboration among the target students, families, and teachers and specialists who have the expertise to serve them. There is more pressure on schools for accountability and more pressure on school administrations to support collaborative enterprises by professionals who work within them, by university faculty who educate those professionals, and by professional organizations. Even the reauthorization of IDEA maintains its focus on shared assessment, planning, and delivery of services. We need to move slowly, finding feasible and effective ways to work together, doing what we can and tailoring our collaborations to fit the needs of our clients. Keeping full collaboration in mind will help us move in the right direction.

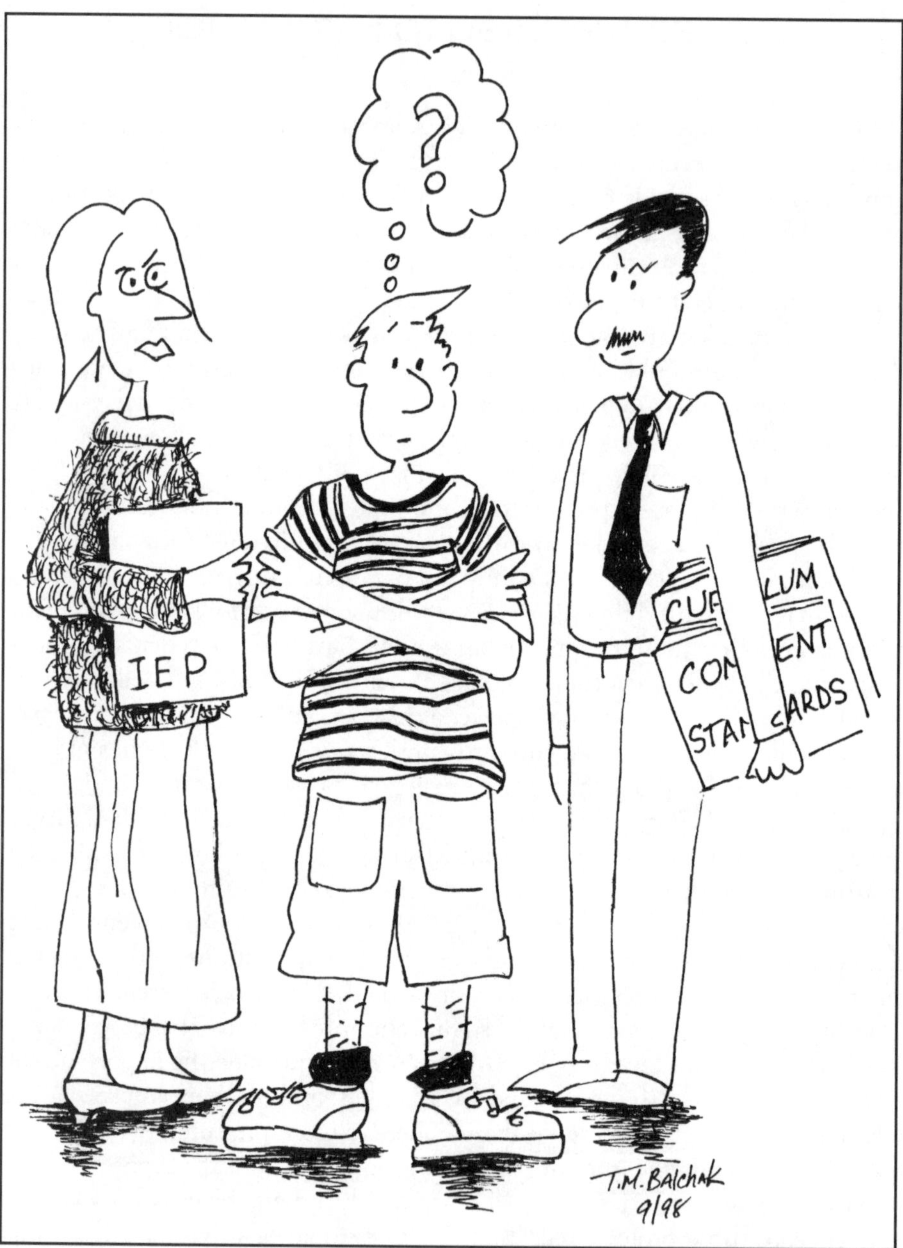

An important consequence of research support for collaboration is the expectation that general and special education teachers, speech-language pathologists, and others will learn to work together to deliver appropriate services to all students.

References

Achilles, J., Yates, R. R., & Freese, J. M. (1991). Perspectives from the field: Collaborative consultation in speech and language program of the Dallas Independent School District. *Language, Speech, and Hearing Services in Schools, 22*, 154–155.

Allington, R. L., & Johnston, P. (1989). Coordination, collaboration, and consistency: The redesign of compensatory special education interventions. In R. Slavin, N. Madden, & N. Karweit (Eds.), *Preventing school failure: Effective programs for students at risk* (pp. 320–354). Boston: Allyn & Bacon.

American Speech-Language-Hearing Association. (1991). A model for collaborative service delivery for students with language-learning disorders in public schools. *Asha, 33*(Suppl.5), 44–50.

American Speech-Language-Hearing Association. (1996). Helping children communicate: Speech–language pathologists and audiologists in schools. *Asha, 38*.

American Speech-Language-Hearing Association Ad Hoc Committee on the Roles and Responsibilities of the School-Based Speech–Language Pathologist. (1999). *Guidelines for the roles and responsibilities of the school-based speech–language pathologist*. Rockville, MD: Author.

Black, J., Meyer, L., Giugno, M., D'Aquanni, M., & Lowengard, D. (1996, October). *A process for restructuring service delivery models for inclusion in New York State*. Paper presented at the annual meeting of the Association for Supervision and Curriculum Development, New Orleans.

Bohn, L., Langville, N., Samples, M., & Sandt, S. V. (1991). Creating a language program: A cooperative approach. *Journal of Childhood Communication Disorders, 11*, 193–198.

Brandel, D. (1992). Implementing collaborative consultation: Full steam ahead with no prior experience! *Language, Speech, and Hearing Services in Schools, 23*, 367–368.

Bunker, V. J., McBurnett, W. M., & Fenimore, D. L. (1987). Integrating language intervention throughout the school community. *Journal of Childhood Communication Disorders, 11*, 185–192.

Catts, H. W., & Kamhi, A. G. (1987). Intervention for reading disabilities. *Journal of Childhood Communication Disorders, 11*, 67–80.

Chermak, G. D., Curtis, L., & Seikel, J. A. (1996). The effectiveness of an interactive hearing conservation program for elementary school children. *Language, Speech, and Hearing Services in Schools, 27*, 29–39.

Chrislip, D. D., & Larson, C. E. (1994). *Collaborative leadership: How citizens and civic leaders can make a difference*. San Francisco: Jossey-Bass.

Christiansen, S. S., & Luckett, C. H. (1990). Getting into the classroom and making it work! *Language, Speech, and Hearing Services in Schools, 20*, 110–113.

Cohen, S. S., Thomas, C. C., Sattler, R. O., & Morsink, C. V. (1997). Meeting the challenge of consultation and collaboration: Developing interactive teams. *Journal of Learning Disabilities, 30*(4), 427–432.

Collier, V. P. (1995). Acquiring a second language for school. *Directions in language and education*. National Clearinghouse for Bilingual Education. Washington, DC: The George Washington University.

Cooper, C. S. (1997). Using collaborative/consultative service delivery models for fluency intervention and carryover. *Language, Speech, and Hearing Services in Schools, 22*, 152–153.

Coufal, K. L. (1993). Collaborative consultation for speech–language pathologists. *Topics in Language Disorders, 14*(1), 1–14.

Crago, M. B. (1992). Ethnography and language socialization: A cross-cultural perspective. *Topics in Language Disorders*, 12(3), 28–39.

Crais, E. R. (1993). Families and professionals as collaborators in assessment. *Topics in Language Disorders*, *14*(1), 29–40.

Damico, J. (1987). Addressing language concerns in the schools: The SLP as a consultant. *Journal of Childhood Communication Disorders*, *11*, 17–40.

Davenport, J., Reid, D. K., & Fortner, A. K. (1999). Systemic practitioner discourses: Implications for collaborative consultation between general and special educators. *Journal of Educational and Psychological Consultation*, *10*, 25–50.

Davenport, J., Reid, D. K., & Fortner, A. K. (1999). Systemic practitioner discourses: Implications for collaborative consultation between general and special educators. *Journal of Educational and Psychological Consultation*, *10*, 25–50.

DePompei, R., & Williams, J. (1994). Working with families after TBI: A family-centered approach. *Topics in Language Disorders*, *15*(1), 68–81.

Dudley-Marling, C. (1987). The role of SLPs in literacy learning. *Journal of Communication Disorders*, *11*, 81–90.

Education for All Handicapped Children Act of 1975, 20 U.S.C. §1400 *et seq*.

Elksnin, L. K. (1997). Collaborative speech and language services for students with learning disabilities. *Journal of Learning Disabilities*, *30*(4), 414–426.

Elksnin, L. K., & Capilouto, G. J. (1994). Speech–language pathologists' perceptions of integrated service delivery in school settings. *Language, Speech, and Hearing Services in Schools*, *25*,258–267.

Ferguson, M. (1992). The transition to collaborative teaching. *Language, Speech, and Hearing Services in Schools*, *23*, 371–372.

Friend, M., & Cook, L. (1996). *Interactions: Collaboration skills for school professionals* (2nd ed.). White Plains, NY: Longman.

Fullan, M. (1993). *Change forces*. Bristol, PA: Falmer Press.

Gartner, A., & Lipsky, D. K. (1987). Beyond special education: Toward a quality system for all students. *Harvard Educational Review*, *57*(4), 367–390.

Harry, B. (1992). *Cultural diversity, families, and the special education system: Communication and empowerment*. New York: Teachers College Press.

Henley, M., Ramsey, R., & Algozzine, R. (1996). *Characteristics and strategies for teaching students with mild disabilities*. Needham Heights, MA: Allyn & Bacon.

Hord, S. M., Rutherford, W. L., Huling-Austin, L., & Hall, G. E. (1987). *Taking charge of change*. Alexandria, VA: Association for Supervision and Curriculum Development.

Howard-Rose, D., & Rose, C. (1994). Students' adaptation to task environments in resource room and regular class settings. *The Journal of Special Education*, *28*(1), 393–425.

Idol, L. (1997). Key questions related to building collaborative and inclusive schools. *Journal of Learning Disabilities*, *30*(4), 384–394.

Individuals with Disabilities Education Act of 1990, 20 U.S.C. § 1400 *et seq*.

Individuals with Disabilities Education Act Amendments of 1997, 20 U.S.C. § 1400 *et seq*.

Lambert, L., Collay, M., Dietz, M. E., Kent, K., & Richert, A. E. (1996). *Who will save our schools? Teachers as constructivist leaders*. Thousand Oaks, CA: Corwin Press.

Lee, P. (1997). *Collaborative practices for educators: Strategies for effective communication*. Minnetonka, MN: Peytral.

Lunday, A. M. (1996). A collaborative communication skills program for Job Corps centers. *Topics in Language Disorders, 16*(3), 23–36.

Masterson, J. J. (1993). Classroom-based phonological intervention. *American Journal of Speech–Language Pathology, 2*(1), 5–9.

Merritt, D. D., & Culatta, B. (1998). *Language intervention in the classroom*. San Diego: Singular.

Moll, L. (1990). *Vygotsky and education: Instructional implications and applications of sociohistorical psychology*. New York: Cambridge University Press.

Monast, S., & Smith, E. (1987). Identifying and expressing emotions: A language therapy program for behavior disordered adolescents. *Journal of Childhood Communication Disorders, 11*, 217–224.

Morsink, C. V., Thomas, C. C., & Correa, V. I. (1991). *Interactive teaming: Consultation and collaboration in special programs*. New York: Macmillan.

National Joint Committee on Learning Disabilities. (1993). Providing appropriate education for students with learning disabilities in regular education classes. *Journal of Learning Disabilities, 26*(5), 330–332.

Nelson, N. W. (1993). *Childhood language disorders in context: Infancy through adolescence*. New York: Macmillan.

O'Shea, L., & O'Shea, D. (1997). Collaboration and school reform: A twenty-first century perspective. *Journal of Learning Disabilities, 30*(4), 449–462.

Paul, R. (1995). *Language disorders from infancy through adolescence: Assessment and intervention*. St. Louis, MO: Mosby.

Phillips, V., & McCullough, L. (1990). Consultation based programming: Instituting the collaborative ethic in schools. *Exceptional Children, 56*(4), 291–304.

Pindzola, R. H. (1993). Materials for use in vocal hygiene programs for children. *Language, Speech, and Hearing Services in Schools, 24*, 174–176.

Prelock, P., Miller, B., & Reed, N. (1995). Collaborative partnerships in a language program in the classroom. *Language, Speech, and Hearing Services in Schools, 22*, 148–149.

Pugach, M., & Johnson, L. (1995a). *Collaborative practitioners, collaborative schools*. Denver, CO: Love.

Pugach, M., & Johnson, L. (1995b). Unlocking expertise among classroom teachers through structured dialogue: Extending research on peer collaboration. *Exceptional Children, 62*(2), 101–110.

Reid, D. K., & Button, L. (1995). Anna's story: Narratives of personal experience about being labeled learning disabled. *Journal of Learning Disabilities, 28*, 602–614.

Reid, D. K., & Leamon, M. M. (1996). The cognitive curriculum. In D. K. Reid, W. P. Hresko, & H. L. Swanson (Eds.), *Cognitive approaches to learning disabilities* (pp. 401–432). Austin: TX: PRO-ED.

Reid, D. K., Robinson, S. J., & Bunsen, T. D. (1995). Empiricism and beyond: Expanding the boundaries of special education. *Remedial and Special Education, 16*(3), 131–141.

Rhodes, L. K., & Dudley-Marling, C. (1988). *Readers and writers with a difference: A holistic approach to teaching learning disabled and remedial students*. Portsmouth, NH: Heinemann.

Russell, S., & Kaderavek, J. (1993). Alternative models for collaboration. *Language, Speech, and Hearing Services in Schools, 24*, 76–78.

Skrtic, T. M. (1995). *Disability democracy: Reconstructing (special) education for postmodernity*. New York: Teachers College, Columbia University.

Snyder, L. S., Nathanson, R., & Shaywitz, K. J. (1993). Children in court: The role of discourse processing and production. *Topics in Language Disorders, 13*(4), 39–58.

Stainback, S., & Stainback, W. (1984). A rationale for the merger of special and regular education. *Exceptional Children, 51*(2), 102–111.

Stainback, S., & Stainback, W. (1987a). Facilitating merger through personnel preparation. *Teacher Education and Special Education, 10*(4), 185–190.

Stainback, S., & Stainback, W. (1987b). Integration versus cooperation: A commentary of educating children with learning problems: A shared responsibility. *Exceptional Children, 54*(1), 66–68.

Szekeres, S. F., & Meserve, N. F. (1994). Collaborative intervention in schools after traumatic brain injury. *Topics in Language Disorders, 15*(1), 21–36.

Taylor, D. (1991). *Learning denied.* Portsmouth, NH: Heinemann.

Voltz, D. L., Elliott, R. N., Jr., & Cobb, H. B. (1994). Collaborative teacher roles: Special and general educators. *Journal of Learning Disabilities, 27*(8), 527–535.

Walther-Thomas, C. S. (1997). Co-teaching experiences: The benefits and problems that teachers and principals report over time. *Journal of Learning Disabilities, 30*(4), 395–407.

Ward, S., & Landrum, M. (1994). Resource consultation: An alternative service delivery model for gifted children. *Roeper Review, 16*(4), 276–279.

West, J., & Cannon, G. (1988). Essential collaborative consultation competencies for regular and special educators. *Journal of Learning Disabilities, 21*(1), 456–505.

West, J. F., & Idol, L. (1990). Collaborative consultation in the education of mildly handicapped and at-risk students. *Remedial and Special Education, 11*(1), 22–31.

Westby, C. E., & Cutler, S. K. (1994). Language and ADHD: Understanding the basis and treatment of self-regulatory deficits. *Topics in Language Disorders, 14*(4), 58–76.

Ylvisaker, M., Kolpan, K. I., & Rosenthal, M. (1994). Collaboration in preparing for personal injury suits after TBI. *Topics in Language Disorders, 15*(1), 1–20.

Classroom-Based Interventions for Language Problems

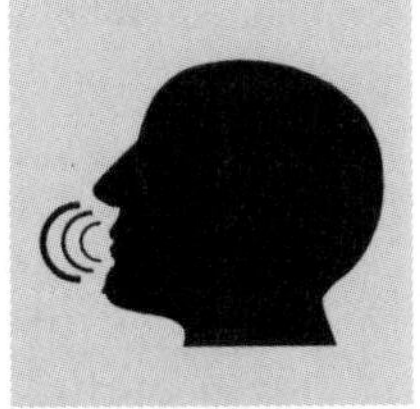

Chapter 10

Kathleen R. Fahey

Chapters 7 and 8 describe the nature and characteristics of eight types of language and speech problems. Some types are clearly labeled by cause (e.g., traumatic brain injury) and others by their behavioral characteristics (e.g., language learning disability). These descriptions are based on traditional perspectives from fields such as medicine, psychology, education, special education, and communication disorders. They explicate the delays and abnormalities common to various conditions.

Traditional approaches to intervention, in providing better health, personality adjustment, education, and communication, focus on identifying the problems in each area, and then working to decrease deficits. Remediation of this nature is often done in isolation from the daily environments in which the person ultimately must function (e.g., home, school, work, community) and without an integration of approaches from various disciplines. Such a reductionist perspective has left many professionals and their clients dismayed that progress is slow and not very relevant for functional settings (Duchan, 1997; Owens, 1999).

This chapter presents more contemporary views of intervention, which focus on whole people in the context of the environments in which they are situated. Such holistic views recognize the need for cross-disciplinary integration so that each system (e.g., cognition, language, personality) is considered as a part of the whole. Regarding language, Norris (1997) stated,

> Functioning cannot be predicted from any one language component; or from the language domain in isolation from cognitive, social, or physical domains; or from the child outside of the social and physical context where the communication takes place. Every part of the communicative situation contributes to the total dynamics. (p. vi)

Thus, *diagnostic labels cannot be used to prescribe interventions*. They are helpful only in noting common characteristics that others with the same label share. Each child or adult has a different set of characteristics with respect to the developmental systems (see Chapters 2, 3, and 4), but even more important has different situations in which to function. The goal of this chapter is to discuss ways in which classroom teachers, special educators, and speech–language pathologists (SLPs) collaborate to support children with language problems in classrooms. The next chapter addresses classroom-based interventions for speech problems, including those that result from hearing and vision difficulties.

Functional Intervention Within Classrooms

Families recognize early on when one of their members has physical or developmental disabilities. Even when the problem has not been formally identified, they seem able to adjust physical care and communication to the functional level of the individual. A ramp may be built for accessibility to and from the home. A series of questions may be asked to determine what the individual would like for breakfast. Routines may be set up to allow primary caregivers respite from daily responsibilities. In fact, participants in the family find ways to make the environment responsive to the needs of the person as well as to the entire family unit. Although special treatments may occur (e.g., medications, surgeries, physical therapy), these are often for long-term benefits rather than daily life concerns.

Duchan (1997) used the term *situated pragmatics* to discuss ways that educators and specialists can "consider whether everyday situations are accessible to their clients, and if not, to remove the barriers that limit their accessibility" (p. 4). In the schools, this concept involves the students themselves in a problem-solving discourse that seeks to build consensus among participants—educators, specialists, and family members—so that appropriate support contexts are designed for the target students. Beukelman and Mirenda (1992) show how their communication participation model for children requiring alternative and augmentative communication (AAC) focuses support on meaningful, everyday activities. They analyze situations for the degree of involvement the student has and for existing barriers to more independent involvement. Interventions occur to overcome the identified barriers.

As another example, language and learning disabilities occur within social and educational contexts. It makes sense, then, that interventions should occur within these same contexts so that individuals with such problems can function more effectively. For interventions to occur within classrooms, it is imperative that a team approach be adopted (see Chapter 9) in which roles and responsibilities of professionals and families merge into a plan that results in the full and meaningful participation of each child in the classroom. Both short- and long-term goals increase opportunities for each child to participate more fully in classroom activities. For example, consider a third-grade girl who has difficulty with understanding directions, new concepts, and classroom rules of order. One way to increase her success during activities and decrease unwanted behaviors is to use peer coaching techniques, in which other students show her how to complete activities, help her directly, or inform the teacher when she needs assistance. A long-term goal for this girl might be to increase her own self-advocacy skills so she can monitor her understanding and ask for assistance when needed.

Teams can select among six types of support when creating an intervention plan. These include social, emotional, functional, physical, event, and discourse supports (Duchan, 1995, 1997). The types and amount of support in each area will depend on the needs of each student within the social and educational contexts of the school and classroom. Decisions about friends, transportation to and from school, mobility within the classroom, and the ability to participate in classroom activities are only a few of the areas that professionals, parents, and students need to address. In a functional approach to intervention, progress is measured by looking at changes in the support provisions and how such changes have improved the student's participation in various real-life situations (Duchan, 1997).

Classroom settings involve a complex set of language functions. Norris's (1997) functional model of language (Figure 10.1) reminds us that students draw on several types of language, often simultaneously, to engage in classroom activities. Students with language problems face numerous situations in which functional use of language is difficult. The SLP's and special educator's roles are to act as collaborative consultants and to provide direct service when needed. For example, note-taking requires being able to listen to oral language and understand its meanings, extract relevant ideas as information is presented sequentially, translate the ideas into written language, organize the information into supraordinate and subordinate categories, and relate new knowledge with prior knowledge. A student having difficulty with note-taking could describe the problem or might be observed to determine what aspects of this task pose difficulty. Once the problem has been understood, the intervention focus is toward removing the barriers. If a student has difficulty remembering details, he might choose to tape-record lectures, and then listen to short segments, writing down details as they are spoken. Or perhaps the student might use an outline guide or graphic organizer to increase success in organizing and categorizing information. The goal of such interventions is to modify the language of the classroom to be consistent with the student's ability to learn (Norris, 1997).

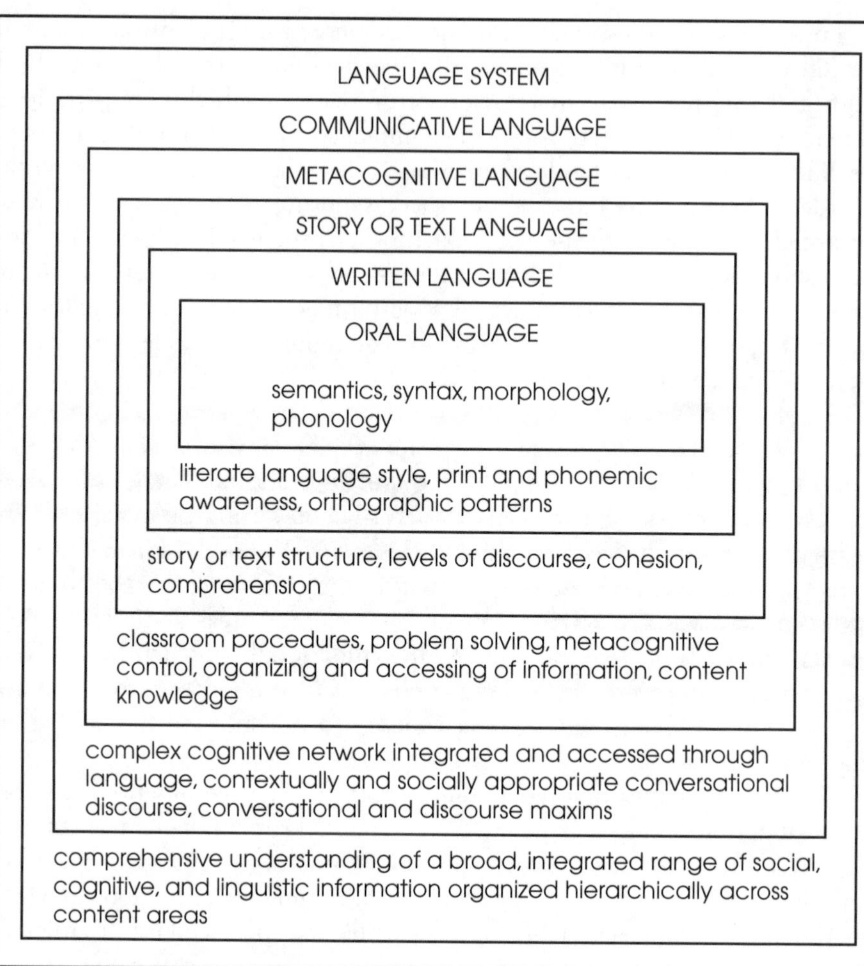

Figure 10.1. Embedded levels of language operating interactively within a functional model of language. From "Functional Language Intervention in the Classroom: Avoiding the Tutoring Trap," by J. A. Norris, 1997, *Topics in Language Disorders, 17*(2), p. 51. Copyright 1997 by Aspen. Reprinted with permission.

Classrooms that foster functional language and learning goals tend to be integrated and holistic (Chaney, 1990; Kamhi, 1994; King & Goodman, 1990; Larson, McKinley, & Boley, 1993; Norris, 1994; Norris & Damico, 1990; Norris & Hoffman, 1990; Poplin, 1988; Schneider & Watkins, 1996; Westby, 1990). The philosophies about language, learning, and teaching in such classrooms (Table 10.1) contrast with traditional views. Learning and teaching are seen as active and constructive processes involving motivation, self-actualization, and decision making. Although the content areas of holistic classrooms are the same

Table 10.1
Tenets of Language and Learning in Integrated, Holistic Classrooms

Language

- Language exists for the formulation, comprehension, and transmission of meaning.
- Language use always occurs in a context or situation that is critical to the creation of meaning for the participants.
- Language learning is a process involving cognitive, linguistic and nonlinguistic, and social development.
- Language and culture are inseparable.
- Oral and written language have parallel but not equal components.
- Language processes (listening, speaking, reading, writing) are integrated across the curriculum with a focus on communication.
- Language processes are interrelated systems that develop through complex interactions from early childhood.

Learning/Teaching

- Learning is an active constructive process involving the integration of prior knowledge with new learning.
- Learners make choices, because they are competent decision makers capable of knowing what they need to know.
- Learners develop self-regulation, self-organization, and self-evaluation of their knowledge.
- Learners learn best from experiences about which they are passionately interested and motivated.
- Errors are critical to learning.
- Teachers and speech–language pathologists (SLPs) strive to make education fit the learner, not to make learners fit a preconceived education model.
- Teachers and SLPs provide guided instruction, materials selection, evaluation, and transactions to facilitate integration of all language processes.
- Teachers and SLPs advocate for multicultural acceptance.
- Teachers and SLPs use information about student's interests, abilities, and needs to increase oral pragmatic, semantic, and phonemic knowledge.
- Teachers and SLPs use whole texts, stories, and conversations as phenomena that occur naturally in life to structure learning opportunities.

(*continues*)

Table 10.1 *Continued.*

Learning/Teaching *Continued.*

- Teachers and SLPs view all students as having *abilities* in language and learning, including those students with language and learning disorders and students with language differences.
- Teachers and SLPs engage in direct observation, evaluation, and teaching as determined by the needs of specific children rather than by external curricula.
- Teachers and SLPs emphasize literacy in all forms and respond to the personal and social needs of student.
- Teachers and SLPs work to expand and guide student learning through a process of negotiated shared meanings.

as traditional ones, in holistic classrooms there are more opportunities to use all the modes of language (i.e., listening, speaking, reading, writing) and all the functions (see Figure 10.1) to help learners construct meaning and communicate effectively.

Teachers who use an integrated framework foster students' participation and lead them to become self-directed and self-sustaining in their learning efforts. Teachers guide instruction to respond directly to what each student is ready to learn (i.e., within the zone of proximal development; Vygotsky, 1978) so that information is relevant, useful, and builds on prior knowledge. Teachers and SLPs provide as much support as needed to allow students to succeed at their developing edge of competence (Nelson, 1998), and then they increase expectations for students' self-regulation as learning occurs. Students learn to regulate, organize, and evaluate their learning in an ongoing fashion. Some students, especially those who have language and learning difficulties, require more help than their peers in developing these internal aspects of control. They require focused instruction that guides learning and assistance in regulating, organizing, and evaluating their learning attempts.

In summary, classroom-based interventions are grounded in a holistic and functional view of learning and teaching. That is, they tend to use all modes of language in active and constructive processes that maintain student motivation, self-actualization, and decision making. The members of the education team work collaboratively to determine the obstacles each student faces within classrooms and selects strategies that remove barriers so that students engage in meaningful participation. Educationists provide guidance and support while increasing expectations as students meet with success. Progress within a functional framework is measured by looking at the adaptations made relative to the students' participation.

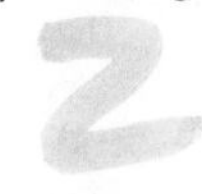

Classroom-Based Assessments

During each school day, teachers and SLPs make observations about student learning. They check with students about whether they understand new concepts and directions, whether background knowledge is sufficient to support new information, how much information students remember from previous instruction, and so forth. Teachers and SLPs use oral and written assignments to strengthen learning and to determine how individual students are progressing with tasks across the variety of content areas. They listen to students speak and read what they write. Assessment of student progress happens throughout all of these daily classroom interactions.

For students with language and learning problems, further assessment strategies help teachers and specialists clarify the nature and extent of problems and strengths as they relate to classroom learning. Whereas norm-referenced testing is often accomplished by specialists during private testing sessions, classroom-based assessments are conducted within the classroom by one or several professionals involved in the educational team. Because classroom-based assessments view the student within the functional environment, they are an important addition to delineating the descriptions of strengths and weaknesses a student has, and they have direct interpretive value for designing appropriate classroom interventions. Their qualitative rather than quantitative nature is useful for focusing on family and team goals, the outcomes of previous interventions, the student's strengths, and environmental considerations (Westby, Stevens-Dominguez, & Oetter, 1996). Assessment strategies include checklists, criterion-referenced tests, naturalistic assessment, and dynamic assessment. Some additional assessment and planning strategies that teachers and specialists find useful include journaling and focus teams. Assessment and planning strategies can be used for students from preschool through high school.

Checklists

Checklists are useful for observing particular aspects of communication, content-area knowledge, skill competencies, and virtually any other set of observable characteristics. They are used for identification of students who need further assessment, for keeping track of progress when new information or skills are being learned, for documenting areas of emphasis for children with special needs, and to plan future interventions. Checklists can be developed by the assessment team or any of its members to focus on language or learning problems or strengths exhibited by students within their classrooms.

Criterion-Referenced Tests

Teachers and specialists create criterion-referenced tests to explore specific knowledge or behavior in depth. They construct them to sample information that has been taught in order to determine the extent to which students have learned and remembered it (posttest) or to determine students' prior knowledge about a concept or skill (pretest). These tests help determine when most students are ready to move on and which students need more intensive instruction. They can be given to the entire class or group (e.g., math or science unit test), but can also be individualized and conducted in an informal and naturalistic manner (Paul, 1995). For instance, a special education teacher who wants to determine whether a student comprehends key vocabulary for an upcoming social studies lesson presents a teacher-made story to the student with the key vocabulary embedded. The student retells the story or responds to direct questions, allowing the teacher to assess the student's understanding of the key concepts. When criterion-referenced testing is curriculum based, outcomes can inform teachers and other team members about the status of each student and assist them in planning and implementing instruction. In the case above, the teacher would be informed about the vocabulary the student does and does not understand, thereby facilitating preteaching of the necessary concepts prior to the social studies lesson.

Naturalistic Assessment

During naturalistic assessment, the teacher or specialist observes children in natural contexts (e.g., lunchroom, playground, group project meetings) for the purpose of determining the relevant goals for the students within the situation itself (Lund & Duchan, 1993). For example, a student with severe communication problems might socialize and make his needs known to others through nonverbal means, such as with gestures, head nods, voicing, and facial expressions. In this case, the nonverbal strengths offset the degree of the verbal production problem. Goals for this student would be different from those of a student whose verbal and nonverbal communication skills are both poor. Only within naturally occurring contexts can such observations be made. This type of assessment is especially valuable for specifying how individual students function within and across situations. These observations inform educationists about the supports necessary to enable students to participate effectively.

Dynamic Assessment

Sometimes it is difficult to determine how much and what kind of support is necessary for individual students. An effective way to discover this information is for teachers and SLPs to engage in dynamic assessment. This type of assessment occurs interactively with students as teachers employ structured teaching activities that utilize pretests and posttests to determine appropriate content (Campione & Brown, 1987). Trial teaching of daily lessons serves as the assessment framework to determine the amount and type of prompts needed for successful learning. Teachers see whether the support they provide is sufficient, excessive, or insufficient to promote learning and can immediately adjust the support to facilitate learning and self-regulation (Campione & Brown, 1987). Thus, the dynamic nature of these assessments provides useful feedback about supports that can be generalized to similar classroom activities.

Journaling

Journaling is a valuable practice because it enables teachers and specialists to note changes in student competence and performance across time. This practice involves engaging in routine written reflections about students who present challenges in classrooms. During a recent elementary school and university partnership on language diversity (UNC–Dos Rios Partnership on Language Related Learning Problems) (Reid, 1996; Reid & Fahey, 1997a, 1997b), teachers used journaling as one technique of gathering information during case studies. Some of the six collaborating teachers made journal entries daily, whereas others found that weekly (or even monthly) entries were most beneficial in describing changes or reflecting on problems. Teachers found journaling to be particularly useful during the assessment and intervention phases of the project. Some direct comments taken from interview transcripts about this technique (Fahey & Helwick, 2000) are included here.

- The journaling was important for several reasons. I think the first thing is that it was a written record that we can keep and refer back to. But also that reflecting piece as the time goes on is what the research is all about. It's through the reflections that we get the ah-ha moments. We can see what is taking place. (G.W., Kindergarten–1st grade teacher)

- I'm sure what I've gone through knowing and writing about him, the journaling was helpful. I had to make myself do it, but I could really see the changes over time. In fact, every time I'd journal I'd look back a couple pages and read it and go "Oh, look at that." I would surprise myself and think "Oh, you did pick up some interesting details." If we did it routinely can you imagine what kind of information we'd have on kids? (R.T., Kindergarten–1st grade teacher)
- The writing down has an accountability feature to it and it's something I can go back to and reflect on. The journaling allowed me to write down different periods or aspects of his life at school. And then go back and read them, to look for patterns, things that were happening over time. It held you accountable for things you were thinking and feeling. (P.B., 4th–5th grade teacher)

Journaling is a technique that teachers and SLPs might use to communicate with each other as they observe students responding to interventions provided in classrooms. Trading journals can provide each with the other's perspective, thereby broadening the observations and allowing for written dialogues when verbal dialogues are difficult to schedule.

Focus Teams

In collaborative models of service delivery to students with special education needs, it is important that team members confer regularly about the status of assessment and intervention. Regular meetings, especially during the initial stages of assessment and intervention provide multiple perspectives on student needs as well as mutual participation by all team members. However, some assessment teams are quite large and members do not share similar schedules, philosophies, or responsibilities regarding intervention. In such instances, a small subgroup whose responsibility is to construct and implement the intervention plan can be effective. An example of a small focus group occurred during the UNC–Dos Rios Partnership on Language Related Learning Problems (Reid, 1996; Reid & Fahey, 1997a, 1997b). The focus team (called a triad) was composed of the classroom teacher, a doctoral student in special education, and a university faculty member from a discipline applicable to curricular issues (i.e., communication disorders, English, bilingual education or English as a Second Language, reading, special education). The three members interacted regularly to design interventions, implement interventions in the classroom during instruction, and use dynamic assessment to modify interventions for improving student learning. Specific comments from interview transcripts (Fahey & Helwick, 2000) about triads reveal the value they had in collaborative problem solving and intervention planning.

- The triads were really the heart and soul of it as far as support for individual teachers. When I couldn't see things, she (the SLP) saw many, many things. And when I didn't understand things like language assessment and what you're looking for, she spent time talking to me and explaining how we were checking for variety and sentence length and all that kind of thing, which was new material for me. When we met in the triad, she could verify ideas or thoughts I might have about what was going on. (G.W., Kindergarten–1st Grade Teacher)
- I think the most beneficial part was our triad. We worked together to really focus in on the strategies that need to be taught. I think I learned the most with my group and working on things together, seeing if our interventions work and then talking with each other. Seeing that sometimes the things you're doing are OK. (F.D., 4th–5th Grade Teacher)
- From the dialogues we had together we came up with data that helped us plan things we could do to help him learn better and more efficiently. (P.B., 4th–5th Grade Teacher)

Summary

Classroom-based assessments are those practices that help teachers, specialists, and SLPs determine student strengths and weaknesses during the activities of the daily classroom environment. Their descriptive nature helps team members to work with students and parents in designing appropriate interventions. Assessment strategies include checklists, criterion-referenced tests, naturalistic assessment, and dynamic assessment. Regular journaling about student participation and focus group meetings are valuable practices for team members to reflect on student outcomes and to communicate among team members, including parents and students.

Teaching Practices That Support Students with Language and Learning Problems

In keeping with the concept of situated learning, teachers and specialists must determine the most appropriate changes necessary in the classroom environment that will result in successful education for students with language and learning problems. Instructional flexibility is important in producing positive learning outcomes for students. "Instructional modifications and accommodations consist of purposeful adaptations made by the teacher [or other team members] to improve the child's opportunity to learn" (Colorado Department of Education, 1997). *Accommodations* (e.g., note taker, visual supplements, study guides, oral vs. written tests) provide students with access to information and an equal opportunity to demonstrate knowledge and skills. *Modifications* are changes made in the instructional level, content, or performance criteria (e.g., reducing difficulty, shortening assignments, alternative assignments) that allow students participation and success. For most students with language and learning problems, accommodations are appropriate and reasonable changes. A few students whose needs are great require a combination of accommodations and modifications. Such instructional flexibility helps teachers and SLPs address the specific needs of each student and encourage all students to participate and become successful in classrooms.

It is the team's challenge to determine the changes necessary for each student and to monitor how the changes benefit the student in the classroom and other related environments (e.g., lunchroom, playground). Of course, the types and degrees of support will vary across students. The intervention team must carefully study assessment information and the contexts in which the student is expected to function to determine the supports needed. Referring to Duchan's (1997) six types of support mentioned earlier (i.e., social, emotional, functional, physical, event, discourse), team members construct the intervention plan to provide accommodations or modifications across the needed support areas. For example, one student may need access to small group participation through the use of an alternative or augmentative communication system. Another student may need increased mobility for optimal accessibility to other children and specific activities. Techniques such as modeling, scaffolding, and dialoguing may assist a student in interpreting information and intentions during ongoing interactions.

Intervention teams should also consider how changes made in the classroom environment minimize interferences and distractions, such as noise from ventilation systems, open windows and doors, sounds and voices from other rooms, and student movement. Rearrangement of furniture, carpeting of bare floors, and specifying interaction guidelines during small group activities can reduce distractions that decrease attention and concentration during classroom learning.

Language intervention can exist in many forms. Unfortunately, consistent, well-planned services for students do not always occur. Gibbs and Cooper (1989) found that only 6% of 242 students with documented language learning disabilities between the ages of 9 and 11 years received language intervention. When interventions did occur, they were behavioral, decontextualized, and drill oriented, and resulted in decreased interaction with other students. Lessons proceeded at a slower pace and resulted in outcomes well behind what other students were accomplishing in the classroom. Allington and Walmsley (1995) directed educationists to provide a curriculum to students with language and learning problems that is *more intense* and provides maximum exposure to the kinds of rich, multifaceted instructional environments available to other learners. With proper levels of assistance, students with LLD can acquire knowledge and knowledge acquisition strategies, increase motivation and persistence, and engage in the personal construction of meaning (Wansart, 1990, 1995).

In summary, teachers, specialists, and SLPs who ascribe to an integrated language philosophy adopt teaching practices that are flexible and functional. Instructional flexibility involves making purposeful adaptations in functional situations for students with language or learning problems that provide access to information, equal opportunity to demonstrate knowledge and abilities, and successful participation in meaningful activities. Intervention teams must carefully study assessment information within functional contexts to determine appropriate supports for individual students. Students with language and learning problems need more intense instruction with maximum exposure to the kinds of rich, multifaceted instructional environments available to other learners.

Strategies for Teaching and Learning

The processes involved in teaching and learning information are numerous and complex. Teachers, parents, and specialists need to decide what information is to be learned, when it should be learned, how it can be learned in the most efficient and thorough manner, and for what purposes it should be learned. These questions can guide decision making regarding the methods to be used during instruction and learning. For some teams, these questions are routinely addressed, whereas for others they are rarely asked. Team members who regard learning as an interactive process select from a variety of instructional strategies to accomplish educational goals.

Teaching strategies are the techniques and methods employed by teachers and SLPs to guide students to organize, interpret, and integrate information. Strategic teaching involves helping students discover information, develop independent thinking and reasoning, expand interests, and evolve in the ability to use all modes of language and cognitive processes to learn. As specialists in content areas and instructional techniques, team members make decisions, together with the learner, about objectives, materials appropriate for learning levels, expected outcomes for students, and accommodations or modifications for students who need them. Teachers and specialists also carefully observe and listen to their students so that student goals and desires are addressed. Teachers and SLPs who are highly attuned to their own strategies for learning can use these understandings to inform their own instructional practices.

Learning strategies are cognitive processes that help students maintain motivation and focus attention, organize information for understanding and remembering, and assist in monitoring the learning process (Wisconsin Department of Public Instruction, 1989). They involve conscious thinking and reasoning before, during, and after learning activities, and enable students to activate background knowledge, focus their attention, select and organize information, and integrate new information with prior knowledge. Strategic learners use thinking processes along with prior knowledge to construct meaning, to understand through all mediums of language, to solve problems, and to become independent in learning.

Strategic learners actively and purposefully take charge of information (Torgesen, 1982; Wong, 1993). For example, with regard to reading (see also Chapter 4), students set purposes for reading, identify and use strategies involving the manipulation of content, integrate new information into existing information schemes, demonstrate confidence and positive self-concept, and use self-monitoring and self-instruction (Routman, 1991; Swanson, 1993; Wisconsin Department of Public Instruction, 1989). Turner (1995) demonstrated that when students learn to use strategies, their motivation during tasks also improves. In addition, when strategies were available to students, tasks were more varied and students engaged in planning, organizing, monitoring, and collaborating with peers.

Teaching and learning strategies become difficult to differentiate in classrooms because they interact and complement each other. In the following sections I discuss six strategies useful for teachers and students: dialogue, cooperative learning, verbal mediation, scaffolding, reciprocal teaching, and self-monitoring. All six strategies involve metacognition and, with the exception of self-monitoring, involve interaction with others.

Dialogue

Reid and Leamon (1996) discussed two key elements in the instructional environment for students with language learning disabilities. The first key element is dialogue, which serves to foster growth of self, enables the sharing of different discourses, and promotes the learning of critical reflection (Burbules & Rice, 1991; Nieto, 1994; Perl, 1994).

> Students learn from participating in events and activities with others, from comparing their own thoughts and solutions with those of others, from hearing arguments and perspectives that are new to them, from having to explain or defend their own thinking, and from gradually adopting the ideas and strategies to which they are exposed. (Reid & Leamon, 1996, p. 406).

Dialogue also allows negotiation to occur in learning situations as teachers, SLPs, and students determine the levels of support needed for successful learning outcomes.

Because students with language learning disabilities evidence difficulties in conversational skills, they will likely need assistance in using dialogue during classroom interactions. They may require modeling and practice within situational contexts to make their dialogic interactions relevant to the topic, accurate, appropriately stated, and concise. In addition, knowing when and how to request explanations, examples, and repetitions when comprehension problems occur, as well as appropriate use of turn-taking cues, will be important for students as they advance through the grades (Nelson, 1998).

Peer conversations are an important aspect of language use during the school years for social growth and peer acceptance. Students with language and learning problems benefit from peer modeling of dialogue in social situations (Bryan, 1986), increased opportunities within social contexts to learn slang (Donahue & Bryan, 1984), and structured modeling programs for those students needing explicit and focused instruction (Hess & Fairchild, 1988).

Cooperative Learning

The second key element in instructional programs for students with language learning problems is cooperative learning (Reid & Leamon, 1996), which involves interdependent relationships between participants in a learning situation. Group participation allows students to share the responsibility for socializing and learning, with each member contributing to the full extent of his or her capabilities. Cooperative learning situations allow opportunities for multiple student models, natural social interaction, variation in discourses, and a variety of levels of knowledge and insight. The learning and the products generated through cooperative efforts often surpass those of individual students

(Doise, Mugny, & Perret-Clermont, 1975; Reid, 1989; Shachar & Sharan, 1994). Heterogeneous groups with varied skills, ability levels, interests, and motivations make strong cooperative learning groups because they build on the unique contributions of each member. Students who have higher levels of understanding provide scaffolding and modeling to those at less sophisticated levels. Thus, students with low achievement learn from students with higher levels of achievement, and students with high achievement test and expand their knowledge through discussion and consensus building with other group members. Cooperative learning can be guided by the classroom teacher or specialist, and strategies for assisting students with language and learning problems are modeled so that peers begin to use them in their interactions. The amount of coaching done by the adult (or a peer) depends on the makeup of the cooperative group. Coaching can be increased or decreased as the need arises (Nelson, 1998).

Cooperative learning can foster creativity and fun, as well as take the pressure off individual students to compete with more able peers. This type of learning environment has been shown to increase social interaction, especially among students with severe learning impairments (Eichinger, 1990).

Verbal Mediation

Mediated learning occurs when an adult (or more experienced student) acts as a co-participant in a learning situation to use naturally occurring opportunities intentionally to focus a student's attention on specific information. Verbal mediation can involve modeling a self-talk strategy so that students eventually (typically after third grade) use it as an independent learning strategy. Self-talk consists of inner speech (or talking aloud) that expresses what is being thought about as the learner engages in a task. For instance, a student writing a story about a horse might think about the general theme of a favorite story such as *Black Beauty* (Sewell, 1982) as she decides on her title and theme. She might think and talk about what her horse looks like, a plot involving adventure, the other characters, and an ending based on her prior experience with similar stories.

The teacher, SLP, or peer can model think-aloud strategies to help students work through curricular tasks. For example, the mediator can direct the student's attention to the written directions for a science experiment, helping the student understand and organize the steps and materials necessary to complete it correctly. The use of self-questioning (e.g., What do I need to prepare first? What does it mean to dissolve something? How many cups are in a quart?) directs the student to gain meaning and to think through the components of the task (Wong & Jones, 1982).

Teachers, specialists, and peers can also use questioning strategies to guide student thinking about topics. Fact-oriented questions show students what information is important from a lecture or reading. Questions (e.g., What did the astronauts do to get ready for their walk? What dangers did they know about? What precautions did they take to avoid these dangers?) cue students to discuss relevant details.

In addition to fact-oriented questions to check comprehension, teachers and SLPs use process-oriented questions to stimulate thinking about how the student learned the information. A student focusing on subtraction of two- and three-digit numbers, for example, might correctly identify the answer from three choices. The teacher or SLP might want to know, however, whether the student understands the concept and method behind borrowing in the numerator. Questions (e.g., How did you subtract this larger number from the smaller number in this column? What happens to the number when you borrow from this column?) provide opportunities for the student to think about the process and to express it verbally to the teacher. When the student has difficulty, the teacher can provide a verbal explanation as well as a verbal model for expressing the answers to these types of questions.

Teachers and SLPs also use questions to probe into students' thinking about problems. Questions that direct students to focus on how they solve problems and how they knew answers to other questions help students recognize their metacognitive and metalinguistic processes and the extent of prior knowledge.

Verbal mediation strategies, including self-talk, think-alouds, and questioning, can be geared toward any level of language; thus they are highly recommended strategies for classroom learning and are particularly useful strategies for students with language and learning problems.

Scaffolding

Another technique used by teachers and specialists that supports and guides student learning is known as scaffolding (see also Chapter 1). It is an interactional strategy between learners and teachers or SLPs that occurs in contextually based situations. The participants use dialogue to share insights and discuss information for the purpose of extending understandings.

The strategic use of scaffolding occurs when teachers and specialists have specific goals in mind during an interaction, but assume the role of a participant so that students arrive at their own solutions to problems (Nelson, 1998; Reid & Leamon, 1996). When engaging in scaffolding, teachers and SLPs follow the students' lead and provide verbal and nonverbal prompts to assist students in their dialogue, sometimes with teachers or SLPs and sometimes with peers. Prompting within naturally occurring interactions results in expanded messages, which in turn lead to more dialogue (Norris & Hoffman, 1990). Teachers and SLPs enter dialogues with students not to evaluate them, but to facilitate a variety of opinions, acknowledge all student contributions, help students organize information, and pull information together into a cohesive summary. Teachers should keep in mind that not all of their students participate in the classroom discourse in the same way. Furthermore, an awareness of discourse from a sociocultural perspective is important if scaffolding is to be effective (Reid, 1996, 1998).

Systematic scaffolding can be useful in facilitating language development. As shown in Table 10.2, thoughtful planning is required to provide opportunities for scaffolding, maximize active participation, attend to content and form, and interact at an appropriate level (Norris & Damico, 1990).

More structured learning opportunities using scaffolding are recommended when specific interventions for language problems are being addressed. For instance, Wallach (1989) focused on the use of scaffolding to develop increasingly more complex narrative structures. Norris and Hoffman (1990) suggested the use of scaffolding within a three-part process of intervention that provides appropriate organization of the environment, communicative opportunity, and feedback that confirms, expands, expatiates, or extends students' messages.

Reciprocal Teaching

A classroom instructional method that takes advantage of dialogue and cooperative learning is called reciprocal teaching. The students and teacher(s) jointly problem solve to arrive at the task solutions through consensus seeking (Brown, Campione, Reeve, Ferrara, & Palincsar, 1991; Palincsar, 1986). A set of procedures govern this approach to interactive learning, which involves repeated predicting, questioning, clarifying, and summarizing (Table 10.3). A verbal instructional format provides general guidelines (domain independent), but the participants engage in interactions that occur within the particular problem to be solved, such as during math or science (domain-specific) activities.

Reciprocal teaching engages students in social dialogue and makes the learning process more observable and accessible. This is critical for students with language and learning problems who have difficulty judging the accuracy of their assumptions and answers (Berger & Reid, 1989). The goal is for all students to apply the procedures independently in classroom contexts and to generalize them to other contexts. Competence in various educational tasks should be viewed according to each student's ability to use problem-solving strategies and to develop knowledge and abilities to solve more complex problems. Reciprocal

Table 10.2
Systematic Scaffolding To Facilitate Language

Provide Opportunities for Scaffolding

- Engage students as active participants in classrooms
- Facilitate leadership and decision making
- Provide invitations for students to give directions, directives, and explanations to peers, while providing support to ensure successful communication

Maximize Active Participation

- Talk with students rather than at them
- Provide new information to existing materials
- Ask progressively more abstract questions to help students integrate information
- Provide relevant cues to help students achieve success during discussion
- Help students relate ideas to their own experiences

Attend to Content and Form

- Build opportunities to make content and form explicit
- Focus on student self-monitoring by asking for repairs when communication breakdowns occur
- Prompt for elaboration and summarize statements
- Extend student vocabulary, sentence length, and complexity

Interact at an Appropriate Level

- Use demonstration and sensory experiences (touch, taste, seeing) to support language
- Gain students' interest through engaging activities
- Accept all communication attempts and assist students in using higher levels of competence
- Allow students to experiment with language freely and without evaluation and correction
- Use consistent and repeatable experiences so that information becomes familiar

Note. Adapted from "Whole Language in Theory and Practice: Implications for Language Intervention," by J. A. Norris and J. S. Damico, 1990, *Language, Speech, and Hearing Services in Schools, 21,* pp. 212–220.

Table 10.3
Strategies Within Reciprocal Teaching

Predicting

Students engage in dialogue about a topic. They discuss what they know based on prior experiences and study. They talk about what they will learn next from text, a lesson, demonstration, or film. Students determine purposes for reading, watching, or listening. Text can be scanned for headings, subheadings, boldface, and graphs.

Questioning

Students ask questions of each other after reading, watching, or listening. They listen to each other's answers and generate more questions.

Clarifying

Students identify what they understand after reading, watching, or listening. They discuss how they can restore meanings such as by using additional resources (e.g., dictionaries, encyclopedias, adults).

Summarizing

Students engage in dialogue about the important information in the lesson. They paraphrase information and integrate it for review and deeper understandings.

Note. Adapted from "Reciprocal Teaching: Can Students' Discussions Boost Comprehension?" by A. S. Palincsar, 1987, *Instructor, 96*(5), pp. 56–60

teaching allows for ongoing dynamic assessment of each student's progress during interactions within specific contexts, so that decisions about instruction can be adjusted according to each student's needs.

Self-Monitoring

Effective learners use self-monitoring strategies, including searching and self-questioning, which require assessment and evaluation of learning attempts. Searching strategies enable learners to gather cues within the context of the information. For example, cues gathered during reading include print (graphophonemic), grammatical structure (syntactic), and meaning (semantic). During speaking, learners use cues such as communicative intent, the formality of the situation, background knowledge about the topic, and the selection of vocabulary, sentence structure, and sounds for the production of words. Such cues allow the learner to adjust how information is accessed and used appropriately to the situation (Polloway & Patton, 1993; Prater, Joy, Chilman, Temple, & Miller, 1991; Swanson, 1996).

Self-questioning involves self-evaluation of what is being learned. Students ask themselves whether their attempts at a task are successful. When tasks are not successful, self-correction is an important strategy students must learn to employ. Students can be guided to ask questions and use self-correction strategies, such as rereading or employing problem-solving techniques.

Teachers and specialists, along with their students, determine the types of self-monitoring strategies students use in the classroom. They jointly observe the degree to which each student uses available cues in the environment and self-questioning and self-correction to learn. Self-monitoring is often lacking in students who have language and learning problems. These learners do not effectively construct and use these strategies without assistance (Swanson, 1996).

Teachers and SLPs can facilitate the development of self-monitoring in children with language and learning problems. They can provide models of searching strategies and evaluation strategies through self-talk and think-aloud methods. They can provide opportunities to use strategies and to practice them in learning tasks as they occur during typical school activities. Through teacher, SLP, and peer modeling, students can observe and engage in self-monitoring behaviors.

Consider a student who decodes text accurately but does not understand much of what is read. After reading a short story or chapter about dinosaurs, a small group discusses not only the relevant facts presented in print, but also the strategies used to comprehend the meanings. The following are some questions that promote conscious awareness of such strategies:

- Does the author give some information in the first paragraph to alert us about what will be included in the chapter?
- What is the main idea conveyed in the first paragraph?
- Why does the author talk about the setting early in the text?

Small group discussion can bring the use of cues to the forefront for all students and help students who have difficulty with self-questioning to use the questions posed by others as a model for their own questioning.

Summary

Both teaching and learning strategies are important in implementing classroom language intervention. Teaching strategies guide students to organize, interpret, and integrate information. Learning strategies help students to develop and maintain cognitive and metacognitive processes to increase attention, motivation, organization of information, understanding and remembering, and monitoring of learning. These strategies involve conscious planning and the employment of thinking and reasoning before, during, and after learning activities. Six strategies that educationists and students use involve interaction with others as well as interaction with self: dialogue, cooperative learning, verbal mediation, reciprocal teaching, scaffolding, and self-monitoring. Students with language and learning problems need more exposure to these strategies, through modeling, practice, and cueing from others, than do their peers.

Targeting Language Components in Classrooms

Classroom-based intervention strategies for specific components of language and learning are numerous. Some examples include teaching of analogical reasoning (Masterson & Perry, 1994), teaching narratives (Hoggan & Strong, 1994), metapragmatic awareness of explanation adequacy (Kaufman, Prelock, Weiler, Creaghead, & Donnelly, 1994), lexical acquisition in early language intervention (Wilcox, Kouri, & Caswell, 1991), concept instruction (Ellis, Schlaudecker, & Regimbal, 1995; Seifert & Schwarz, 1991), remediating humor comprehension deficits (Spector, 1992), social skills training (Dodge & Mallard, 1992), and enhancing idiom comprehension (Nippold, 1991). Such specific interventions have the common thread of helping children to see and hear the particular forms of language, providing practice so that the form is developed, and becoming independent in the comprehension and production of the forms as they occur in classroom interactions. Another common thread in these interventions is the collaborative relationship between the student, parents, teacher, and specialist(s).

All of the areas noted above can be considered within a larger framework of the components of language as outlined in Chapter 3. Paul (1995) and others (Nelson, 1998; Owens, 1999; Simon, 1991) discuss a variety of ideas related to classroom-based language intervention for school-age students and adolescents. The components they focus on include syntax, semantics, metalinguistics, and pragmatics. Paul's ideas are summarized in separate tables (Tables 10.4, 10.5, 10.6, 10.7). One example from each table is provided here to show practical application in classrooms. Teachers, the SLP, and other specialists on the intervention team determine which aspects are relevant for particular students so that classroom-based intervention can occur.

Syntax

The understanding and expressing of grammatical structures during listening, speaking, reading, and writing contribute greatly to competent interactions. When syntax is delayed, communication can be ineffective for learning and social interaction within the classroom. Focus areas for improving syntax may include the integration of comprehension and expression, development of advanced morphology, elaboration of sentences to include complex forms, and increasing syntactic maturity in written language contexts (Table 10.4). Each of these focus areas can be accomplished at the elementary level or in middle and high schools.

Students who have language and learning problems tend to use simple, nonelaborative sentences during speaking and writing. How, then, might elementary teachers and specialists *promote noun phrase elaboration through activities involving adjectives, prepositional phrases, pronouns, and articles?* Paul (1995) suggests the use of printed cards (or pictured cards for younger children) that include modifiers, prepositional phrases, and so on. Students can manipulate the cards to create and elaborate sentences. Figure 10.2 is an example of some possible syntactic manipulations. Students can work together to build on simple sentences and make changes by substituting different elaborative forms. This exercise should be done in the context of an ongoing activity such as writing short stories. Students can engage in self-monitoring by judging whether elaborations make sense or cause syntactic or semantic conflict (e.g., "The tall, two-foot-high tree is in the forest next to Grandma's house"). Students in middle or high school can work cooperatively to expand the use of elaboration through editing paragraphs, rewriting narrative or expository papers, or verbally discussing the use of expanded forms.

Semantics

In Chapter 3, semantics was defined as a system of meaning comprising word knowledge and relationships among concepts. Students with language and learning problems struggle with vocabulary development; accessing words during thinking, speaking, or writing; integrating and relating ideas; and using known information to infer missing information. Semantic knowledge is also important for the development of figurative language forms, such as metaphors and humor. When students have underdeveloped semantic systems, they require lots of opportunities to hear new information and time to practice the new information in appropriate contexts, benefiting from interactions that involve dialogue and collaboration discussed earlier (e.g., verbal mediation, scaffolding, cooperative learning). Table 10.5

Table 10.4

Classroom Suggestions for Improving Syntax

Integrating Comprehension and Expression

Elementary School

- Focus on production to teach both production and comprehension of grammar and sentence structure
- Use production tasks to check for understandings
- Break up sentences with left, right, and center embedding and engage students in discussion of meanings of the clauses
- Manipulate grammatical forms in sentences, such as changing tense, word order, and number of modifiers
- Encourage student modeling and independent manipulation of grammatical forms

Middle and High School

- Check student comprehension by encouraging students to explain their interpretations of new information
- Encourage students to explain and discuss new information with peers
- Involve students in listening, speaking, reading, and writing of new information
- Ask students to independently find supportive information on topic

Advanced Morphology

Elementary School

- Help students understand root words, prefixes, suffixes, and derivation
- Discuss the meaning relationships of derivational words to their root words
- Make explicit the relationships between spellings and morphological changes

Middle and High School

- Require students to use examples of words with inflections and derivations in oral and written language activities
- Check comprehension of inflections and derivations through word definition exercises as related to the meaning of the text

(*continues*)

Table 10.4 *Continued.*

Complex Sentences

Elementary School

- Expose students to many examples of complex sentences in literature-based activities
- Increase opportunities for students to analyze propositions within complex sentences
- Encourage students to write complex sentences with models and independently
- Ask students to paraphrase sentences from stories or texts
- Manipulate clauses and ask students to discuss changes in meanings
- Ask students to arrange pictures according to the ideas presented in complex sentences

Middle School

- Require students to edit for the inclusion of complex sentences in written stories or expositions
- Encourage students to rewrite paragraphs focusing on using a variety of conjunctions and clausal structures
- Teach students to use codes during editing of their own and peers' written paragraphs

Syntax and Literate Language

Elementary School

- Promote noun phrase elaboration through activities involving adjectives, prepositional phrases, pronouns, and articles
- Introduce and practice the use of relative clauses in sentences and stories
- Combine simple sentences with relative clauses in sentences and stories
- Manipulate the position of relative clauses and ask students to compare meanings
- Promote verb phrase elaboration through activities involving adverbs
- Use varied and combined auxiliary verbs to modulate meaning
- Discuss meaning changes when verb tense changes occur
- Encourage students to retell short stories in different tenses

(*continues*)

Table 10.4 *Continued.*

Middle and High School

- Analyze literature for the use of tense and voice (active or passive)
- Discuss the role of tense and voice to suit the author's purpose
- Increase opportunities for students to experiment with tense and voice in oral and written narratives and expositions
- Practice reducing the complexity of texts into outlines with a focus on meanings conveyed through paragraph structure

Note. Adapted from *Language Disorders from Infancy Through Adolescence: Assessment and Intervention*, by R. Paul, 1995, St. Louis: Mosby.

contains a summary of ideas that teachers and specialists can use to focus on vocabulary, word finding, and semantic integration and inferencing.

For instance, consider a student in fourth grade who has difficulty accessing words during oral and written tasks. How can this student *expand and elaborate word knowledge and meanings to develop a broader semantic network?* One technique that can make meaningful links between words is known as semantic mapping (see also Chapter 2). A topic that has immediate relevance for classroom participation is selected. If students are studying about zoo animals, the

	Adjectives	Nouns	Prepositional Phrases	Pronouns	Articles
Color:	red	car	in the tree	I	a
	green	boat	at the zoo	you	an
	blue	fence	around the corner	he, she	the
	yellow	dog	over the fence	it	
		fish	across the street	they	
Size:	big, large	banana	beside the chair		
	small, little				
	tall, short				
Shape:	round				
	square				
	triangular				
	skinny				
	fat				

Examples:

He put the big round pumpkin beside a chair.

They put the large blue cover over the fence.

I have a green and red kite stuck in the tree.

Figure 10.2. Sentence manipulation to promote noun phrase elaboration.

Table 10.5
Classroom Suggestions for Improving Semantics

Vocabulary

Elementary School

- Activate what students already know through discussion of personal experiences, then relate this knowledge to the new words
- Make connections among words and topics
- Use both spoken and written contexts to focus on word meanings
- Refine and reformulate meanings of words through discussion and comparison
- Use newly learned words in writings and readings

Middle and High School

- Use root words, suffixes, and affixes to broaden lexical understandings
- Use dictionaries and create dictionaries to look for relationships among words
- Help students to use semantic cues to determine unknown words
- Promote understanding of words with multiple meanings (homonyms) and word meaning changes in context (e.g., "*Pick up* the pencil," "*Pick up* your room")
- Teach word relationships such as analogies, idioms, metaphors, and similes

Word Finding

Elementary School

- Expand and elaborate word knowledge and meanings to develop broader semantic networks
- Use visual maps to increase semantic associations between words and word categories
- Use familiar event scripts as a basis for visual mapping and encourage discussion using specific vocabulary
- Increase phonological awareness in listening and speaking activities to gain access to the words from memory
- Use oral and written cloze activities to promote the use of syntactic and semantic cues for word retrieval
- Allow students to repeat words under timed conditions for practice in retrieving new words

(*continues*)

Table 10.5 *Continued.*

Middle School

- Have students guess words from phonological or semantic cues
- Encourage students to self-cue when word retrieval is difficult using grapheme cues, imagery, gestures, associations, and synonyms
- Increase reflective pausing to allow students to wait and think about the word

Semantic Integration and Inferencing

Elementary School

- Use literacy-based activities to promote prediction of character motives, internal states, events, solutions to problems, and conclusions
- Encourage oral and written stories around classroom themes
- Increase student sharing of stories and provide opportunities to create new endings, beginnings, or middles
- Help students discuss how they know information that is not directly stated
- Present sentences and then questions requiring inferences

Middle and High School

- Involve students in using more than one source of information in retelling stories or in written compositions
- Allow group discussions about what is not directly in stories
- Use poetry as a basis for discussing figurative forms of language

Note. Adapted from *Language Disorders from Infancy Through Adolescence: Assessment and Intervention,* by R. Paul, 1995, St. Louis: Mosby.

semantic map could include types of animals according to classification (e.g., reptiles, pachyderms, cats, mammals) and some examples of each class. Figure 10.3 is an example of a semantic map. The students cooperatively work to organize the information so that ideas are linked meaningfully in a hierarchical fashion. For students with word finding problems, the semantic map provides cues to word retrieval and an organizational strategy for information which helps them engage effectively in discussion. Older students who have learned self-cueing strategies may need some reminders to reflect about and then use the strategies as needed. For instance, a student may be directed to construct a

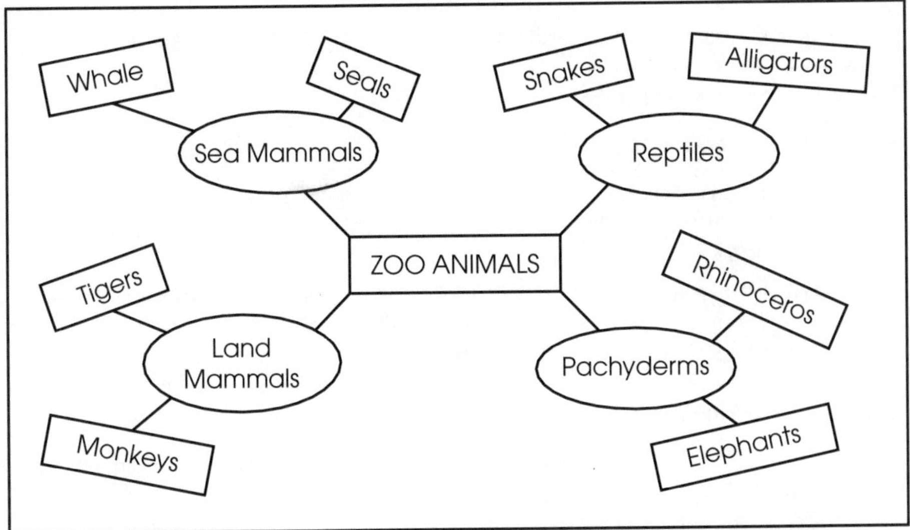

Figure 10.3. Semantic map for strengthening word relationships and word finding abilities.

semantic map, to visualize the information in his or her mind, or to use mental associations to trigger information.

Metalinguistics

The knowledge students have about how the other components of language work separately and together is called *metalinguistics*. The awareness and understanding of phonology and suprasegmentals is referred to as phonological awareness, whereas knowledge about syntax, semantics, and pragmatics is included under the broad umbrella of metalinguistics. Students also have knowledge about how they think, which is known as *metacognition*. Table 10.6 summarizes these areas and potential targets for elementary and older students who have language and learning problems.

One metacognitive strategy for elementary students is to *teach them to recognize when messages are inadequate*. Imagine that a teacher provides verbal directions but does not specify important details, as in this example: "You are to read the chapter on mechanical inventions and answer the questions in the back." Students must determine when to read, which book contains the chapter, whether answers should be written or simply thought about, and the due date or hour for completion of the assignment. Teachers and SLPs can facilitate discussions about these details as a strategy for getting students to think

Table 10.6
Classroom Suggestions for Improving Metalinguistics

Phonological Awareness

Elementary School

- Increase phonological awareness through rhyming, word segmentation, identification of sounds within words, and manipulation of sounds in words
- Point out the relationships of spoken language to written language through sound–symbol associations, syllable structures and stress patterns, alphabetizing, and spelling rules

Middle and High School

- Point out the differences in pronunciations of words when derivations occur, as for the vowel shift rule in *divide–division and manager–managerial*
- Help students recognize the relationship between English words and their origins such as Latin forms

Metalinguistics

Elementary School

- Increase student awareness of the suprasegmental aspects of spoken language, such as syllable and word stress, pauses, intonation, and rate of speech
- Promote reflection and discussion of word order as students create sentences using word cards
- Encourage students to think about meaning and then paraphrase sentences
- Engage students to rewrite selections from textbooks and stories
- Increase opportunities for students to transform written or oral information into drawings, diagrams, or maps
- Allow students to edit their own and others' work to detect errors in syntax, word choice, conveyed intent, use of conjunctions, pronoun use, spelling, and mechanics

Middle and High School

- Focus on comprehension monitoring to help students detect gaps in their understanding
- Assist students in reflection on the structure of texts (e.g., headings, subheadings, questions at the beginning or end of chapters)

(*continues*)

Table 10.6 *Continued.*

- Focus student attention to the purpose of the listening, speaking, reading, or writing activity

Metacognition

Elementary School

- Teach students to recognize when messages are inadequate
- Promote use of comprehension monitoring by encouraging clarification or repetition
- Help students activate background knowledge using discussion of personal experiences and prediction activities when new information is being presented
- Teach students to ask themselves questions to guide their own learning

Middle and High School

- Teach strategies that facilitate the acquisition of information such as verbal mediation, paraphrasing, and outlining
- Teach strategies that facilitate the retention and access of information, such as rehearsal, visual imagery, use of systematic questions, and acronyms

Note. Adapted from *Language Disorders from Infancy Through Adolescence: Assessment and Intervention*, by R. Paul, 1995, St. Louis: Mosby.

about them. Older students might ask questions directly of the teacher, SLP, or other students. They should be more independent in generating questions and seeking solutions to problems when information is inadequate or ambiguous. Peer coaching can be an effective strategy for students who lack independence in this area and can alleviate embarrassment and misunderstanding for the student.

Pragmatics

The ability to use language appropriately in a variety of situations involves both understanding of social communication rules and the ability to construct language for engaging in discourse (see Chapters 1 and 2 for discussions of discourse). Pragmatic development is necessary for participation in conversational and classroom discourse, narrative discourse, and exposition. Therefore, it is an important component for successful interactions in school.

Table 10.7 provides many suggestions for working on pragmatics with students during elementary school and in the middle and high school years. Conversational discourse objectives include providing opportunities for students to develop and practice conveying thoughts and intentions clearly and appropriately in situational contexts, whereas classroom discourse objectives help students maneuver within the social and academic expectations of school environments. Because literacy is so important to academic learning, narrative development encompasses a broad range of objectives that build knowledge and application of oral and written narrative structures. In addition, the use of cohesive devices can be targeted to expand students' semantic and syntactic sophistication during speaking and writing.

Consider an example from the suggestions regarding narrative development. How can teachers and specialists *involve students in comprehension activities that promote literal interpretation, personal responses, and deep understandings?* Middle and high school students might be asked to reflect on and talk about word meanings from the story *Kon-Tiki* (Heyerdahl, 1973). Sailing vocabulary can be discussed, as well as the feelings and thoughts of the men on the vessel. The personal experiences of students who have sailed or seen movies about sailing can be shared to broaden and deepen the discussion of this topic. Table 10.8 provides a passage from the book and questions that could facilitate the discussion. Younger children could engage in a similar discussion after a story has been read aloud.

Summary

Classroom-based interventions for students with language and learning problems are not only possible, but also preferable to individualized interventions. They provide rich and contextualized opportunities for learning and using strategies that impact social interaction and academic growth. Teachers and specialists must work together with the students, families, and team members to discover the particular teaching, learning, and language objectives appropriate for each student's maximum participation in the classroom. A decision tree (Figure 10.4) is included to assist team members in developing classroom-based interventions.

Language intervention in classrooms requires collaboration among teachers, specialists, SLPs, parents, and students. The particular focus of such intervention depends on the needs of each student. Activities for improving syntax, semantics, metalinguistics, and pragmatics should focus on improvement of these components of language within the context of daily interactions and content areas. Educationists should use the teaching and learning cognitive

(*text continues on page 390*)

Table 10.7
Classroom Suggestions for Improving Pragmatics

Conversational Discourse

Elementary School

- Create conversational opportunities whereby students practice semantic and syntactic forms
- Provide opportunities for more advanced communicative intentions through think-aloud strategies, pretend activities, and scaffolding
- Use barrier games to facilitate the use of explanations and clarifications
- Discuss common rules of conversations such as turn-taking, eye contact, appropriate physical distance, and use of body language

Middle and High School

- Teach discourse intentions, such as persuasion, negotiation, presenting adequate information, and appropriate speech register
- Promote discussion of the situations where discourse intentions can be used
- Increase opportunities for students to construct meaningful intentions and to practice them with peers
- Use scripts from plays or movies to help students identify discourse intentions
- Encourage the use of conscious planning, self-cueing, and self-monitoring as students practice discourse intentions

Classroom Discourse

Elementary School

- Make explicit the rules in the hidden curriculum through discussion and practice of common routines
- Identify rules not being used consistently and model appropriate use of each rule
- Use role-playing to demonstrate and practice rules and routines
- Encourage students to discuss the similarities of social and classroom discourse

Middle and High School

- Use supportive prompts, including verbal cues or choices (dialogic mentoring), to assist students in solving a problem

(*continues*)

Table 10.7 *Continued.*

Middle and High School Continued.

- Encourage students to self-cue as a strategy for solving problems
- Use reciprocal teaching to help students engage in self-regulated learning
- Provide accepting but corrected versions of student comments, identify areas of misunderstanding, provide direct instruction when skill development is needed, and expand on student comments at a higher cognitive level (postscript modeling)

Narrative Development

Elementary School

- Use preparatory activities such as discussion of title, concepts related to the topic, and predictions about the story to activate student background knowledge
- Ask questions after a story is read to focus on specific meanings
- Increase the difficulty of questions asked of students to correspond to the level of narrative read by the students
- Allow students to work cooperatively to map story grammar elements using visual aids
- Engage students in writing a group book report that focuses on the story grammar elements
- Focus on particular aspects of the narratives such as character traits and feelings
- Involve students in comprehension activities that promote literal interpretations and in activities that promote personal responses and deep understandings
- Encourage students to compose oral and written narratives by modifying existing narratives
- Help students create semantic webs to facilitate new ideas for narratives
- Introduce and discuss story grammar elements as a basis for writing stories in groups or individually
- Use word processing software to enable students to create texts
- Use computer graphics software to illustrate stories and to rearrange story elements

(*continues*)

Table 10.7 *Continued.*

Middle and High School

- Continue assisting students in the development of narrative texts through oral and written practice with narrative story grammar elements
- Engage students in outlining of narratives according to the story grammar elements (i.e., setting, problem, internal response, plan or attempt, response, additional plan or attempt, additional response, resolution or consequence)
- Help students identify macrostructures of expository texts as a tool to organizing information
- Use learning strategies such as SQ3R (Survey, Question, Read, Recite, Review) to improve student comprehension of expository texts
- Guide students in developing written compositions through steps that foster organization and expansions of ideas
- Encourage planning and editing in written compositions

Cohesive Devices

Elementary School

- Help students identify pronouns and referents in sentences
- Provide oral and written opportunities for students to use pronouns
- Use the ambiguity of pronouns to encourage discussion about meanings and usefulness in sentences
- Provide a list of conjunctions and discuss their roles in sentences
- Practice combining two or more sentences by using conjunctions
- Substitute conjunctions in sentences and discuss the changes in meaning
- Incorporate conjunctions in writing activities

Middle and High School

- Help students identify cohesive devices such as anaphoric reference (the noun is referred to before the pronoun is used) and the use of conjunctions
- Engage students in rewriting narrative and expository text where cohesive devices are weak
- Require students to use cohesive devices in paragraphs and within entire compositions

Note. Adapted from *Language Disorders from Infancy Through Adolescence: Assessment and Intervention,* by R. Paul, 1995, St. Louis: Mosby.

Table 10.8
Comprehension for Literal Interpretations and Deeper Understandings

On the third night the sea went down a bit, although it was still blowing hard. About four o'clock an unexpected deluge came foaming through the darkness and knocked the raft right round before the steersman realized what was happening. The sail thrashed against the bamboo cabin and threatened to tear both the cabin and itself to pieces. All hands had to go on deck to secure the cargo and haul on sheets and stays in the hope of getting the raft on her right course again, so that the sail might fill and curve forward peacefully. But the raft would not right herself. She would go stern foremost, and that was all. The only result of all our hauling and pushing and rowing was that two men nearly went overboard in a sea when the sail caught them in the dark. (Heyerdahl, 1973, p. 88)

1. What do you think is meant by "the sea went down a bit, although it was still blowing hard"?
2. Does a sea blow?
3. What was the author referring to?
4. What is a deluge and why does the author say it was foaming?
5. Which words in the third sentence tell us that this storm was very violent?
6. How do you think the men felt during the storm?
7. What were they thinking when the raft would not get back on course?

and metacognitive strategies discussed earlier to make interventions functional and meaningful.

Classroom Interventions for Special Populations

Several conditions that coexist with or cause language and learning problems were described in Chapters 7 and 8. The basic principles of classroom-based language intervention presented thus far in this chapter are appropriate for all of these problems. However, three problems in particular (i.e., attention-deficit/hyperactivity disorder [ADHD], traumatic brain injury [TBI], and autism) require additional intervention considerations.

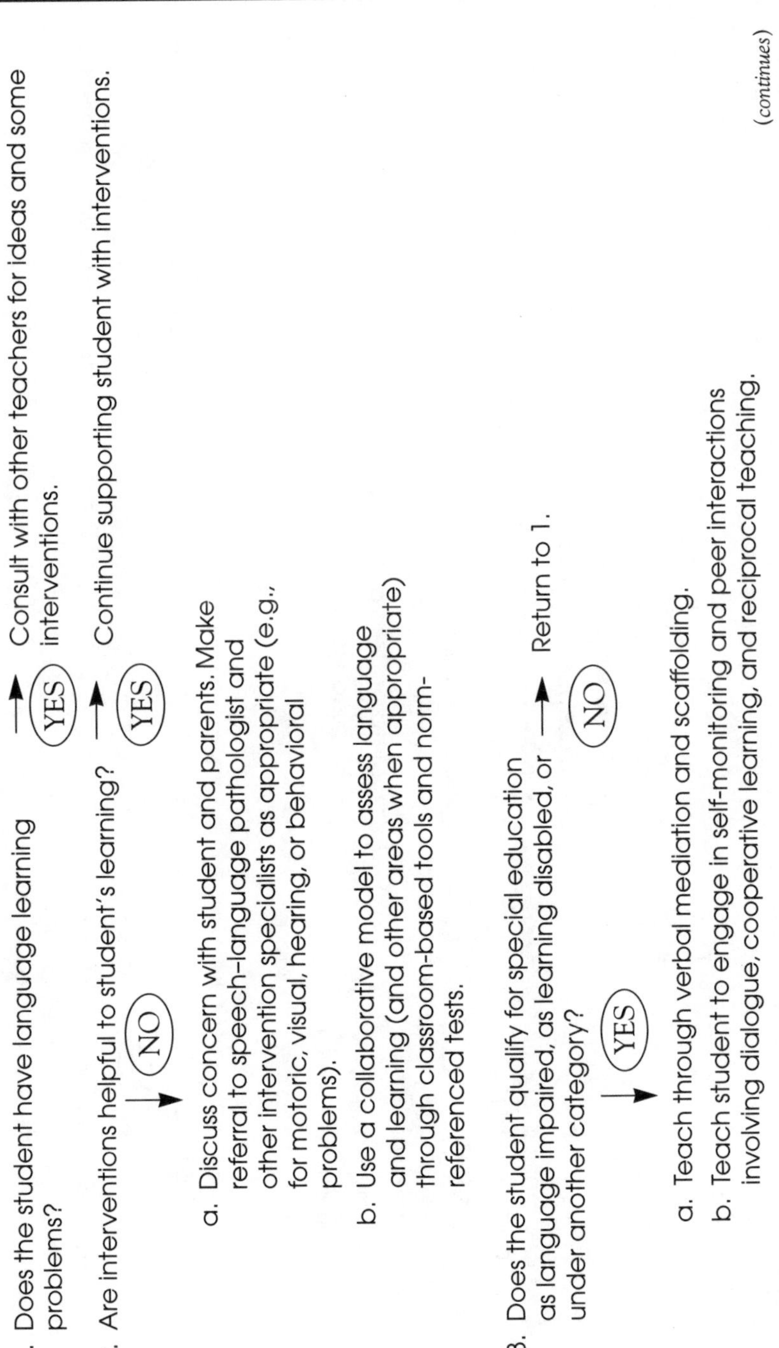

Figure 10.4. Decision tree for language intervention in classrooms: language and learning problems.

4. Does the student have specific problems in semantics, syntax, pragmatics, or metalinguistics?

→ 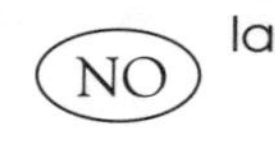

Use Strategies 3a and 3b to facilitate continued language growth.

↓ YES

a. Teach semantics
   - Vocabulary
   - Word finding
   - Semantic integration and inferencing
b. Teach syntax
   - Integrate comprehension and expression
   - Advanced morphology
   - Complex sentences
   - Syntax and literate language
c. Teach pragmatics
   - Conversational discourse
   - Classroom discourse
   - Narrative development
   - Cohesive devices
d. Teach metalinguistics
   - Phonological awareness
   - Metalinguistic concepts
   - Metacognition

5. Has the student improved in language learning in the classroom?

→ NO

See Strategy 2b.

Use assessment information to explore the specific needs of the students. Discuss other service delivery models with team members (e.g., combination collaboration and pull-out, special classrooms).

↓ 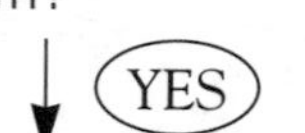

Continue using teaching and learning Strategies 3a and 3b and relevant aspects of language in Strategies 4a through 4d.

Figure 10.4. *Continued.*

Interventions for ADHD

As discussed in Chapter 7, attention problems can either be a single area of concern or coexist with language and learning problems. In either case, a student with ADHD poses a challenge to classroom-based interventionists. Two intervention paths are typically used with students who have ADHD. The traditional path involves use of stimulant medication and a behavioral management approach. The contemporary path involves cognitive-behavioral management techniques (Weaver, 1993; Westby & Cutler, 1994), with or without the use of stimulant medication. Each approach is aimed to improve the regulation of behavior by rules, consequences, and awareness training.

Behavioral approaches were popular in past years for students with ADHD, based on the belief that these students require more frequent and more direct use of feedback than do students without ADHD. Such approaches stressed clear rules and consequences that were listed for appropriate and inappropriate behavior. The lists were explicit, well defined, and contained powerful consequences delivered immediately (Barkley, 1990). Rich incentives and motivational reinforcements served to accentuate the positive, while negative feedback served to change inappropriate behavior. Because students with ADHD have changing needs, the rules and consequences were regularly adjusted so that motivation for appropriate behaviors remained high and the likelihood of inappropriate behaviors remained low. Although behavioral approaches have some effectiveness in highly controlled environments and in some situations, teachers and specialists find them difficult to implement in classrooms. They are cumbersome to administer, they isolate and draw attention to the student, they limit social interaction, and they do not generalize easily to other situations.

Increasingly, evidence indicates that children with ADHD have problems with self-regulation of behavior rather than inattention per se (Barkley, 1990). Thus, in classrooms, students demonstrate pragmatic and metacognitive deficits. Approaches that favor cognitive-behavioral interventions focus on enabling students to increase metacognitive strategies to regulate behavior during social interactions and academic learning. Westby and Cutler (1994) outlined three essential components to such interventions, which are similar to those discussed earlier in this chapter: cognitive modeling, verbal mediation, and problem-solving techniques. These components involve adult and peer models demonstrating the thinking and reasoning processes used during tasks (e.g., think alouds, self-talk), rephrasing by students to check understandings, and self-questioning during problem solving and evaluation of learning. Weaver (1993) also supported a metacognitive approach, along with medication when needed. (The use of medications for ADHD is discussed in Chapter 7.) She suggested that classrooms provide "a curriculum that keeps language and learning whole and meaningful, that offers students choice and ownership of learning and supports learners in taking more responsibility for their own learning and behavior" (p. 84).

For students with ADHD, classroom interventions should be aimed at increasing metacognitive strategies to improve self-regulation, supporting the use of medication when it is determined appropriate, and providing instructional support in language and learning. Other factors that are important for successful intervention include adequate time for program implementation, motivation of the student and cooperation of parents, and the team's ability to integrate social and academic planning (Westby & Cutler, 1994).

Interventions for TBI

Students with TBI require educational planning from knowledgeable team members within the school and rehabilitation agencies. The SLP often serves as team leader and resource person regarding the complex issues such as organic brain dysfunction, memory deficits, emotional unpredictability, and neurological instability (Russell, 1993). However, it is important to note that many school-based SLPs do not have direct experience with TBI and, therefore, will require continuing education and supportive team members who may take the lead as assessment and intervention strategies are determined for individual students (Hux, Walker, & Sanger, 1996). A collaborative model for treatment within classrooms is essential so that information is learned within meaningful contexts. Students with TBI require assistance with reasoning, problem solving, storing and accessing information in long-term memory, organizing oral and written language, and using language appropriately in social interactions (Russell, 1993).

Cognitive-communication approaches for students with TBI have been the focus in educational settings (Szekeres & Meserve, 1994). This perspective of intervention is an outgrowth of the belief that TBI results in an enduring educational disability with cumulative effects. Classroom-based interventions, then, "must allow for flexible assessment, management, and delivery of curriculum and instruction in a variety of school settings and include a strong family service component" (p. 23).

The accommodations and modifications that are necessary in classrooms for children with TBI involve redesigning how information is provided and received. Szekeres and Meserve (1994) recommended several ways in which this can occur. To increase success and decrease frustration in written language, teachers (a) use large print with reduced amounts of information; (b) reduce the number of practice items in assignments; (c) provide organizational tools such as checklists, flowcharts, or step-by-step instructions; and (d) allow additional time and use of a word processor for tests and assignments. Teachers also modify their oral language to assist students who have memory and comprehension problems. They use short, simple sentence structures; repeat information or provide it in a highly redundant manner; and use simpler vocabulary.

Students with TBI often have difficulty recognizing when and how to use strategies for learning. They benefit from a verbal mediation strategy called cognitive-communication coaching (Szekeres & Meserve, 1994). This technique requires a teacher, SLP, or peer to provide models and prompt behaviors. Modeling and prompting can occur during individual or group work during the school day so that the student is assisted in thinking and reasoning, maintaining attention, employing searching strategies, enhancing memory, creating and using learning strategies, promoting independence and self-esteem, identifying problems and seeking solutions, and using planning, self-monitoring, and reflection.

An example from Szekeres and Meserve (1994) shows how a cognitive goal is facilitated through coaching. A goal such as promoting self-reflection involves engaging the student to think about and perhaps talk about what was learned from an experience. The coach might ask the following questions.

> What did you do? How did you do it? Would you do it differently next time? What did you learn about yourself? What did you learn about this task? What did you learn about strategies? Were you too demanding of yourself or not demanding enough? (p. 32)

The motor, physical, and cognitive demands of classrooms can be adjusted within tasks, as well as within the structure of the school day. For example, materials should be readily available for students, especially those with motor limitations. Interferences such as noise, high activity from others, and poor lighting should be minimized and preferential seating should be provided. Student helpers can provide quick and effective changes in the physical environment for students needing these changes.

It is important that students with TBI receive respect and appropriate social support from the school community as a whole and in individual interactions. Teachers and specialists must carefully monitor classroom and school environments so that verbal and physical abuse of any form is not tolerated. They can reduce the social penalties imposed by others by involving students with TBI in small groups where dialogue, cooperative learning, and other interactive techniques can be used to facilitate social and academic participation.

Interventions for Autism

In Chapter 7, autism was described as a disorder affecting the biological system, development of the linguistic system and social interaction, and cognitive and information processing abilities. In recent years, the behaviors that characterize autism have been thought to result from motor planning problems (Maurer & Damasio, 1982) or difficulty in coping with and extracting meaning from sensory information (Greenspan & Wieder, 1998).

Traditional intervention programs for children with autism focused on the reduction or elimination of unusual physical or verbal behaviors that were perceived as bizarre and inappropriate to social interactions. Behavior modification programs sought to impose rules for the types of behaviors children were allowed and not allowed to engage in. These approaches tended to be quite frustrating for both the individual with autism and the interventionist, and they have not produced positive results, especially regarding classroom functioning.

More recent views of autism as a sensory processing problem have led to the realization that the behaviors students demonstrate may be attempts at communication (Caruso & Caruso, 1998; Quill, 1995). The behaviors, when viewed from this perspective, should be considered as starting points for intervention rather than as requiring elimination. Caruso and Caruso (1998) outlined an approach to facilitate communication abilities in students with autism. The approach uses a student's verbal and nonverbal behaviors as starting points to more appropriate communication, and it teaches others within the environment to understand the student's intentions and to facilitate communication through modifications in language. The underlying philosophy of the approach recognizes that student-directed intervention involve active participation from the student. Teachers, specialists, and family members build on the student's natural inclinations and interests in accordance with his or her strengths and skill levels. In addition, the opportunities available to the student provide choice regarding the nature and structure of the interactions. Communication partners follow the lead of the student so that he or she learns to express intentions.

Both sensory considerations and the communication environment are considered when designing intervention for students with autism. The assessment team must carefully determine how each student reacts to various sensory inputs. For example, students may overreact or underreact to sound, light, touch, and movement (Fisher, Murray, & Bundy, 1991). Observation of sensory input in classroom situations as well as other school and home situations is important for determining the adjustments necessary within each setting.

Children with autism seek out sensory input by swinging, spinning, hand flapping, and so on, in order to increase neural organization. Caruso and

Caruso (1998) advocated the use of play equipment so that students can obtain sensory input. During sensory stimulation, communication partners should provide verbal or gestural descriptions of what the student is doing. This pairing of sensory and verbal or nonverbal information enhances the student's understanding and eventual use of language. Another modification of sensory information is to regulate it by adjusting the amount, length, and intensity level of verbal or nonverbal messages. Systematic alterations of these variables within functional communication settings help communicative partners determine the combinations of sensory input that are most conducive for communication.

Specific interactional techniques for enhancing communication with students with autism include (a) use of a metascript such as pause, wait, watch, and listen; (b) lengthening of response time latency (RTL); (c) emphasizing key words and keeping words concrete and specific; (d) imitating nonspeech behaviors and vocalizations, then shaping them into words; (e) decreasing question asking and increasing describing and commenting; and (f) using rhythmic patterns and music (Caruso & Caruso, 1998). These techniques are student centered and allow the student a structure in which his or her needs are given priority. For example, when the adult watches what the student does in a situation and waits for him or her to adjust, the adult can determine what the student is trying to communicate. If a question is asked, the student should be given a much longer interval of time to respond than is typical in communicative exchanges. Caruso and Caruso recommended that a full 10 seconds elapse before additional input is given. Short, telegraphic speech (content words only) reduces the amount of information provided, whereas direct imitation of behaviors allows the adult to gradually shape the behaviors into more recognizable and meaningful behaviors or words. Students learn language through interacting with other language users in natural contexts. Thus, descriptions and comments provide a natural avenue for meaningful input of language, including vocabulary and grammar. Direct questioning should be used judiciously as it puts children in a situation where complex language processing and production are required. Finally, music appears to be helpful in motor and sensory integration for individuals with autism. It can be used in combination with language to facilitate receptive and expressive language development.

It is especially important that consistent, well-planned interventions for students with autism include environments beyond the classroom. Parents and other family members must be included in the intervention team and receive counseling and training in the techniques listed previously. Parents and family members need up-to-date information about autism. Meetings should be planned to allow sufficient time and provide a supportive environment so that questions can be answered. Parents should be invited to engage in direct participation in the intervention process. Practice with live observations of the techniques being used in the classroom, therapy sessions, and the home, along with role plays and direct interaction with their child, helps parents and family members provide consistent and complementary intervention (Caruso & Caruso, 1998).

Other interventions for children with autism (or those with emotional and severe behavioral disorders) target functional interactions with peers and adults in home and classroom situations. Specific areas of focus should include (a) expanding vocabulary to enhance expression of personal feelings, empathic reactions, and emotional responses of others; (b) teaching rules within classrooms, such as recognizing routines, asking for clarification, and appropriately gaining the teacher's attention; (c) teaching acceptable ways of engaging in play, dialogue, and conflict resolution; and (d) improving attention and listening through direct teaching of the use of cues to select and store information (Giddan, 1991). Giddan also recommended that teachers use concrete social reinforcers (e.g., verbal praise, positive facial expressions) for small accomplishments, use highly structured tasks that are likely to result in success, and focus on planning and organizational skills.

Team involvement in monitoring the progress of children with autism or severe emotional or behavioral problems is essential. The goal is to help these children understand and communicate feelings and intentions in appropriate ways, which can significantly enhance success in school and home situations (Giddan, Bade, Rickenberg, & Ryley, 1995). Teachers and specialists should dialogue with family members and physicians so that monitoring occurs regarding the effect of medication on behavior and learning. Routine sharing of information helps the team to stay current regarding the needs of the child and promotes positive and supportive interactions.

Summary

Some students have educational challenges that coexist with language problems. Classroom-based interventions for ADHD, TBI, and autism require strategies that take into account the unique characteristics of these problems. Such strategies include those that increase self-regulation, organization, and thinking and reasoning. Environments and activities may also require accommodations and modifications that remove barriers to success, such as decreasing distracting noise, light, or movement; decreasing verbal input to prevent linguistic overload; allowing more time for students to complete assignments; decreasing obstacles when motor limitations exist; and providing student-directed opportunities for learning.

Summary

Students with language and learning problems present challenges for educators, peers, and families in educational and social settings. In the past, students were evaluated and interventions were determined based on their weaknesses in communicating, learning, and social competence. Today, students are being described according to strengths as well as weaknesses, and intervention programs seek to include students as active participants in all settings. Rather than fixing deficits, teachers, specialists, and parents are collaborating to provide appropriate accommodations and modifications in the environments in which students are required to function. Teaching and learning strategies are aimed at increasing interactions, providing support to enhance language and learning opportunities, and teaching students to recognize and monitor their own learning. The degree and type of interventions depend on each student's needs. Some students require more direct instruction in the use of language and metacognitive strategies, whereas others with disorders such as ADHD, TBI, and autism require additional and more intense intervention strategies. All students who have language and learning problems require careful observation, specific intervention goals, and selection and implementation of teaching and learning strategies. It is important that team members monitor the progress of each student and make adjustments in the intervention plan as changes are needed to maximize success in both academic learning and social interactions.

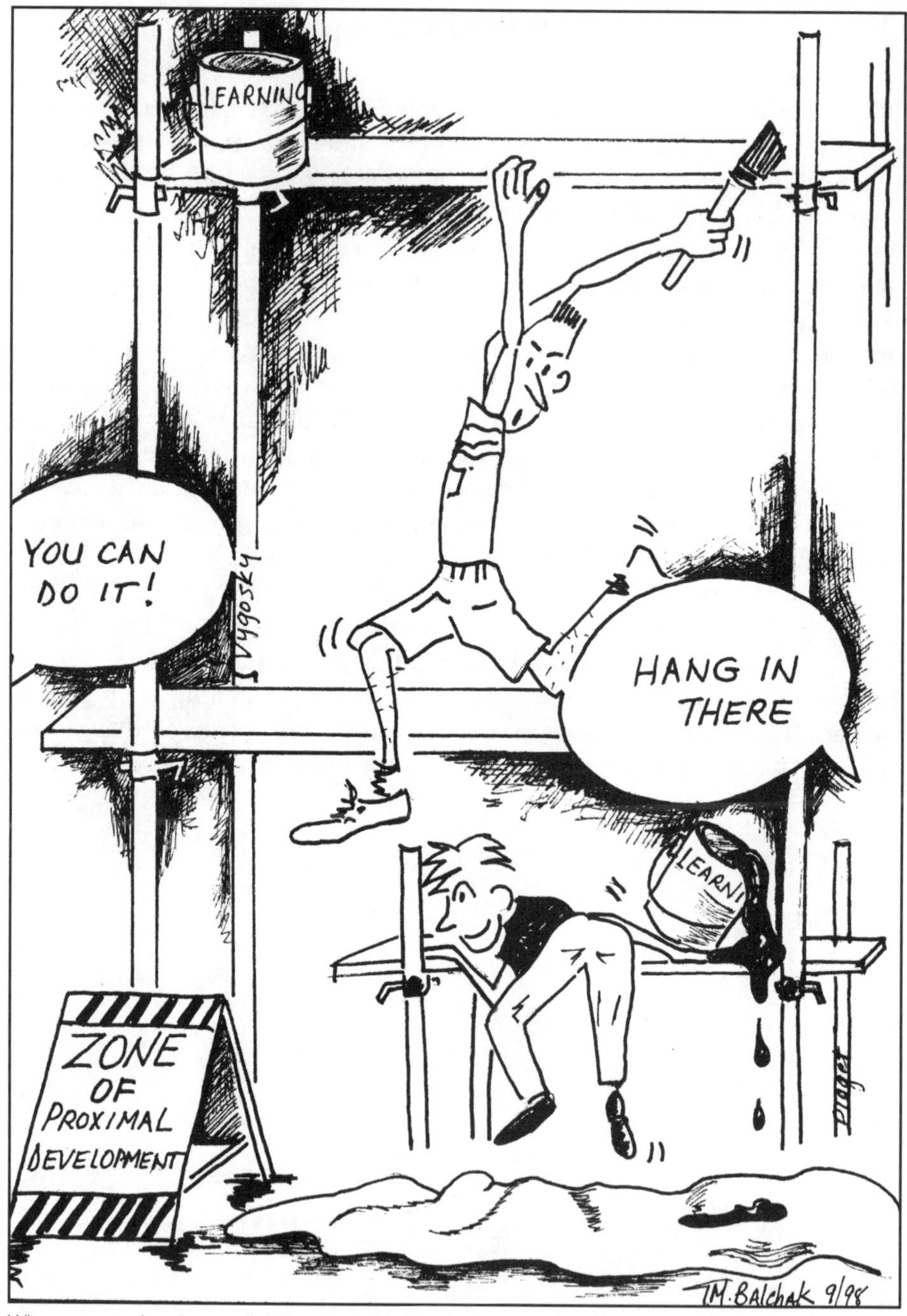

When engaging in scaffolding, teachers and speech–language pathologists follow the student's lead and provide verbal and nonverbal prompts to assist students in dialogue.

References

Allington, R. L., & Walmsley, S. A. (1995). *No quick fix: Rethinking literacy programs in America's elementary schools*. New York: Teachers College Press.

Barkley, R. A. (1990). *Attention deficit hyperactivity disorder: A handbook for diagnosis and treatment*. New York: Guilford Press.

Berger, R. S., & Reid, D. K. (1989). Differences that make a difference: Comparisons of metacomponential functioning and knowledge base among groups of high and low IQ learning disabled, mildly mentally retarded and normally achieving adults. *Journal of Learning Disabilities, 22*, 422–429.

Beukelman, D. R., & Mirenda, P. (1992). *Augmentative and alternative communication: Management of severe communication disorders in children and adults*. Baltimore: Brookes.

Brown, A. L., Campione, J. C., Reeve, R. A., Ferrara, R. A., & Palincsar, A. S. (1991). Interactive learning, individual understanding: The case of reading and mathematics. In L. T. Landsman (Ed.), *Culture, schooling and psychological development* (pp. 136–170).

Bryan, T. (1986). A review of studies on learning-disabled children's communicative competence. In R. L. Schiefelbusch (Ed.), *Language competence: Assessment and intervention* (pp. 227–259). Austin, TX: PRO-ED.

Burbules, N. C., & Rice, S. (1991). Dialogue across differences: Continuing the conversation. *Harvard Educational Review, 61*(4), 393–416.

Campione, J. C., & Brown, A. L. (1987). Linking dynamic assessment with school achievement. In C. Lidz (Ed.), *Dynamic assessment* (pp. 82–115). New York: Guilford.

Caruso, D. S., & Caruso, A. J. (1998). Children with autism spectrum disorder: Strategies for communication intervention. *Contemporary Issues in Communication Science and Disorders, 25*, 32–38.

Chaney, C. (1990). Evaluating the whole language approach to language arts: The pros and cons. *Language, Speech, and Hearing Services in Schools, 21*, 244–249.

Colorado Department of Education, Task Force on Central Auditory Processing. (1997). *Central auditory processing disorders: A team approach to screening, assessment and intervention practices*. Denver: Author.

Dodge, E. P., & Mallard, A. R. (1992). Social skills training using a collaborative service delivery model. *Language, Speech, and Hearing Services in Schools, 23*, 130–135.

Doise, W., Mugny, G., & Perret-Clermont, A. N. (1975). Social interaction and the development of cognitive operations. *European Journal of Social Psychology, 5*, 367–383.

Donahue, M., & Bryan, T. (1984). Communication skills and peer relations of learning disabled adolescents. *Topics in Language Disorders, 4*(2), 10–21.

Duchan, J. (1995). *Supporting language learning in everyday life*. San Diego: Singular.

Duchan, J. (1997). *Evaluation reports are more negative than they need to be: A viewpoint based on some preliminary analyses*. Manuscript submitted for publication.

Eichinger, J. (1990). Goal structure effects on social interaction: Nondisabled and disabled elementary students. *Exceptional Children, 56*, 408–416.

Ellis, L., Schlaudecker, C., & Regimbal, C. (1995). Effectiveness of a collaborative consultation approach to basic concept instruction with kindergarten children. *Language, Speech, and Hearing Services in Schools, 26*, 69–73.

Fahey, K. R., & Helwick, G. (2000). *Qualitative evaluation of the UNC/Dos Rios Partnership on Language Diversity*. Manuscript in preparation.

Fisher, A., Murray, E., & Bundy, A. (1991). *Sensory integration: Theory and practice*. Philadelphia: F. A. Davis.

Gibbs, D. P., & Cooper, E. (1989). Prevalence of communication disorders in students with learning disabilities. *Journal of Learning Disabilities*, *22*, 60–63.

Giddan, J. J. (1991). School children with emotional problems and communication deficits: Implications for speech–language pathologists. *Language, Speech, and Hearing Services in Schools*, *22*, 291–295.

Giddan, J. J., Bade, K. M., Rickenberg, D., & Ryley, A. T. (1995). Teaching the language of feelings to students with severe emotional and behavioral handicaps. *Language, Speech, and Hearing Services in Schools*, *26*, 3–10.

Greenspan, S. I., & Wieder, S. (1998). *The child with special needs*. Reading, MA: Addison-Wesley.

Hess, L. J., & Fairchild, J. L. (1988). Model, analyse, practice (MAP): A language therapy model for learning-disabled adolescents. *Child Language Teaching and Therapy*, *4*, 325–338.

Hoggan, K. C., & Strong, C. J. (1994). The magic of "once upon a time": Narrative teaching strategies. *Language, Speech, and Hearing Services in Schools*, *25*, 76–89.

Heyerdahl, T. (1973). *Kon-Tiki*. New York: Ballantine Books.

Hux, K., Walker, M., & Sanger, D. D. (1996). Traumatic brain injury: Knowledge and self-perceptions of school speech–language pathologists. *Language, Speech, and Hearing Services in Schools*, *27*, 171–184.

Kamhi, A. G. (1994). Paradigms of teaching and learning: Is one view the best? *Language, Speech, and Hearing Services in Schools*, *25*, 194–198.

Kaufman, S. S., Prelock, P. A., Weiler, E. M., Creaghead, N. A., & Donnelly, C. A. (1994). Metapragmatic awareness of explanation adequacy: Developing skills for academic success from a collaborative communication skills unit. *Language, Speech, and Hearing Services in Schools*, *25*, 174–180.

King, D. F., & Goodman, K. S. (1990). Whole language: Cherishing learners and their language. *Language, Speech, and Hearing Services in Schools*, *21*, 221–227.

Larson, V. L., McKinley, N. L., & Boley, D. (1993). Service delivery models for adolescents with language disorders. *Language, Speech, and Hearing Services in Schools*, *24*, 36–42.

Lund, N., & Duchan, J. (1993). *Assessing children's language in natural contexts* (3rd ed.). Englewood Cliffs, NJ: Prentice-Hall.

Maurer, R., & Damasio, A. (1982). Childhood autism from the point of view of behavioral neurology. *Journal of Autism and Developmental Disorders*, *12*(2), 195–205.

Masterson, J. J., & Perry, C. D. (1994). A program for training analogical reasoning skills in children with language disorders. *Language, Speech, and Hearing Services in Schools*, *25*, 268–270.

Nelson, N. W. (1998). *Childhood language disorders in context: Infancy through adolescence*. Needham Heights, MA: Allyn & Bacon.

Nieto, S. (1994). Lessons from students on creating a chance to dream. *Harvard Educational Review*, 64(4), 392–426.

Nippold, M. A. (1991). Evaluating and enhancing idiom comprehension in language-disordered students. *Language, Speech, and Hearing Services in Schools*, *22*, 100–106.

Norris, J. A. (1994). From frog to prince: Using written language as a context for language learning. In K. G. Butler (Ed.), *Best practices II: The classroom as an intervention context*. Gaithersburg, MD: Aspen.

Norris, J. A. (1997). Functional language intervention in the classroom: Avoiding the tutoring trap. *Topics in Language Disorders*, *17*(2), 49–68.

Norris, J. A., & Damico, J. S. (1990). Whole language in theory and practice: Implications for language intervention. *Language, Speech, and Hearing Services in Schools, 21*, 212–220.

Norris, J. A., & Hoffman, P. R. (1990). Language intervention within naturalistic environments. *Language, Speech, and Hearing Services in Schools, 21*, 72–84.

Owens, R. E. (1999). *Language disorders: A functional approach to assessment and intervention* (3rd ed.). Needham Heights, MA: Allyn & Bacon.

Palincsar, A. S. (1986). The role of dialogue in providing scaffolded instruction. *Educational Psychologist, 21*, 73–98.

Palincsar, A. S. (1987). Reciprocal teaching: Can students' discussions boost comprehension? *Instructor*, 96(5), 56–60.

Paul, R. (1995). *Language disorders from infancy through adolescence: Assessment and intervention.* St. Louis: Mosby.

Perl, S. (1994). Teaching and practice: Composing texts, composing lives. *Harvard Educational Review*, 64(4), 427–449.

Polloway, E. A., & Patton, J. R. (1993). *Strategies for teaching learners with special needs* (5th ed.). Columbus, OH: Merrill.

Poplin, M. A. (1988). Holistic/constructivist principles of the teaching/learning process: Implications for the field of learning disabilities. *Journal of Learning Disabilities, 21*, 389–400.

Prater, M. A., Joy, R., Chilman, B., Temple, J., & Miller, S. R. (1991). Self-monitoring of on-task behavior by adolescents with learning disabilities. *Learning Disabilities Quarterly, 14*, 164–177.

Quill, M. I. (1995). Innovative educational program for communicative enhancement in students with autism. *Journal of Childhood Communication Disorders*, 8, 223–224.

Reid, D. K. (1989). The role of cooperative learning in comprehensive instruction. *Journal of Reading, Writing, and Learning Disabilities—International*, 4, 229–242.

Reid, D. K. (1996). Narrative knowing: Basis for a school–university partnership. *Learning Disabilities Quarterly, 19*, 138–152.

Reid, D. K. (1998). Scaffolding: A broader view. *Journal of Learning Disabilities, 31*(4), 386–396.

Reid, D. K., & Fahey, K. R. (1997a). *The UNC/Dos Rios Partnership on Language Diversity: Part I—The Collaborative Process* [Video documentary]. Greeley: Academic Technology Services, University of Northern Colorado.

Reid, D. K., & Fahey, K. R. (1997b). *The UNC/Dos Rios Partnership on Language Diversity: Part II—Case Studies* [Video documentary]. Greeley: Academic Technology Services, University of Northern Colorado.

Reid, D. K., & Leamon, M. M. (1996). The cognitive curriculum. In D. K. Reid, W. P. Hresko, & H. L. Swanson (Eds.), *Cognitive approaches to learning disabilities* (3rd ed., pp. 401–432). Austin, TX: PRO-ED.

Routman, R. (1991). *Invitations: Changing as teachers and learners K–12*. Portsmouth, NH: Heinemann Educational Books.

Russell, N. K. (1993). Educational considerations in traumatic brain injury: The role of the speech–language pathologist. *Language, Speech, and Hearing Services in Schools, 24*, 67–75.

Schneider, P., & Watkins, R. V. (1996). Applying Vygotskian developmental theory to language intervention. *Language, Speech, and Hearing Services in Schools, 27*, 157–170.

Seifert, H., & Schwarz, I. (1991). Treatment effectiveness of large group basic concept instruction with Head Start students. *Language, Speech, and Hearing Services in Schools, 22*, 60–64.

Sewell, A. (1982). *Black beauty*. New York: Messner.

Shachar, H., & Sharan, S. (1994). Talking, relating, and achieving: Effects of cooperative learning and whole-class instruction. *Cognition and Instruction, 12*(4), 313–353.

Simon, C. (Ed.). (1991). *Communication skills and classroom success: Assessment and therapy methodologies for language and learning disabled students*. Eau Claire, WI: Thinking Publications.

Spector, C. C. (1992). Remediating humor comprehension deficits in language-impaired students. *Language, Speech, and Hearing Services in Schools, 23*, 20–27.

Swanson, H. L. (1993). Executive processing in learning-disabled readers. *Intelligence, 17*, 117–149.

Swanson, H. L. (1996). Information processing: An introduction. In D. K. Reid, W. P. Hresko, & H. L. Swanson (Eds.), *Cognitive approaches to learning disabilities* (3rd ed., pp. 251–283). Austin, TX: PRO-ED.

Szekeres, S. F., & Meserve, N. F. (1994). Collaborative intervention in schools after traumatic brain injury. *Topics in Language Disorders, 15*(1), 21–36.

Torgesen, J. (1982). The learning disabled child as an inactive learner: Educational implications. *Topics in Learning and Learning Disabilities, 2*, 45–53.

Turner, J. C. (1995, July, August, September). The influence of classroom contexts on young children's motivation for literacy. *Reading Research Quarterly, 30*, 410–441.

van Kleek, A. (1990). Emergent literacy: Learning about print before learning to read. *Topics in Language Disorders, 10*, 25–45.

Vygotsky, L. S. (1978). *Mind in society*. Cambridge, MA: Harvard University Press.

Wallach, G. P. (1989). Current research as a map for language intervention in the school years. *Seminars in Speech and Language, 10*(3), 205–217.

Wansart, W. A. (1990). Developing metacognition through collaborative problem solving in a writing process classroom. *Journal of Learning Disabilities, 23*, 164–170.

Wansart, W. A. (1995). Teaching as a way of knowing. *Remedial and Special Education, 16*, 323–340.

Weaver, C. (1993). Understanding and educating students with attention deficit hyperactivity disorder: Toward a system theory and whole language perspective. *American Journal of Speech–Language Pathology, 2*(2), 79–89.

Westby, C. E. (1990). The role of the speech–language pathologist in whole language. *Language, Speech, and Hearing Services in Schools, 21*, 228–237.

Westby, C. E., & Cutler, S. K. (1994). Language and ADHD: Understanding the bases and treatment of self-regulatory deficits. *Topics in Language Disorders, 14*(4), 58–76.

Westby, C. E., StevensDominguez, M., & Oetter, P. (1996). A performance/competence model of observational assessment. *Language, Speech, and Hearing Services in Schools, 27*, 144–156.

Wilcox, M. J., Kouri, T. A., & Caswell, S. B. (1991). Early language intervention: A comparison of classroom and individual treatment. *American Journal of Speech–Language Pathology, 1*, 49–62.

Wisconsin Department of Public Instruction. (1989). *Strategic reading in the content areas* (Bulletin No. 9310). Madison: Publication Sales, Wisconsin Department of Public Instruction.

Wong, B. Y. L. (1993). Pursuing an elusive goal: Molding strategic teachers and learners. *Journal of Learning Disabilities, 26*, 354–357.

Wong, B. Y. L., & Jones, W. (1982). Increasing metacomprehension in learning disabled and normally achieving students through self-questioning training. *Learning Disabilities Quarterly, 5*, 228–240.

Classroom-Based Interventions for Speech Problems

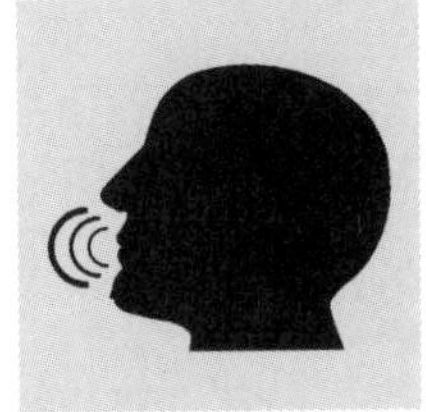

Chapter 11

Kathleen R. Fahey

Children who have speech problems, including those related to hearing and vision, face challenges in classrooms regarding learning and social interactions. The nature and characteristics of seven of these problems, defined and described in Chapter 8, include hearing impairment and deafness, visual impairment and blindness, motor speech disorders, phonological and articulation disorders, fluency and prosody disorders, and voice disorders. In this chapter, these problems are considered from the perspective of how teachers, speech–language pathologists (SLPs), and other specialists provide classroom-based interventions.

The rationale for collaborative, classroom-based intervention for language and learning problems is discussed in Chapter 9. The focus on individual strengths as well as weaknesses, the realization that language is embedded in situational contexts, and the recognition that human systems are integrated and part of the whole person are important underpinnings of the framework for classroom-based interventions for hearing, vision, and speech problems. With this framework in mind, this chapter emphasizes assessment and intervention strategies within classroom contexts.

Classroom-Based Assessments

In the early elementary grades teachers and SLPs assess the progress of individual students on a daily basis. When particular children appear to be developmentally delayed, teachers and specialists attempt to determine the causes of such delays. Initially, assessment might involve observation of the student during activities throughout the school day. For example, if a student appears to have trouble listening to teacher instructions in the classroom, observation might reveal that the background noise is interfering with hearing the more distant single voice of the teacher. When the student is involved in face-to-face communication or is listening to others in small groups, the problem may not be as evident. Because hearing in this case is a possible problem, referral to the school district's audiologist for hearing testing is the prudent course of action.

With regard to speech problems, students in early grades may evidence articulation, fluency, or voice problems that have not been formally evaluated. Observation of the characteristics of the problems and their influence on academic and social development leads to referral for testing by the SLP. The classroom is one of the most important environments for the SLP to observe the specific nature and severity of the problem, and its influence on academic and social development.

Assessment strategies within classroom contexts include checklists, criterion-referenced tests, naturalistic assessment, and dynamic assessment. These, along with assessment and planning strategies (journaling and focus teams), are described in Chapter 10. The following example illustrates how a checklist, naturalistic assessment, and dynamic assessment strategies can be used to assess a student who stutters.

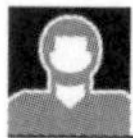

Raul

A sixth grader named Raul is finding it more and more difficult to participate verbally in classroom dialogue. The teacher notices that he avoids raising his hand during discussion, even when he undoubtedly knows the answers to questions. When Raul does speak, he looks down at his desk, becomes highly dysfluent, becomes flushed in the face, and answers in nonelaborative statements. The teacher and SLP observe Raul so that decisions can be made about his eligibility for speech intervention.

They observe Raul across several days within the month during different times, academic subjects, and participatory activities. A checklist is used to document the characteristics of the dysfluencies (e.g., part-word repetitions, silent blocks, prolongations), their frequency of occurrence, and the strategies Raul uses to cope with them. This information provides the team with a description of the problem and an estimate of its severity. However, to gain insight into the situations where his stuttering varies, and its impact on his social and academic growth, the adults must observe Raul in naturalistic contexts. Small group interactions in the classroom and lunchroom, at the playground or more formal sporting events, and even in the home are important to observe. These contexts are especially important for observing social, functional communication. The teacher and SLP can use journaling to note the setting, the type of interactions occurring (e.g., conversation, discussion of an event in a story), the perceived comfort level of Raul during interactions, the type and amount of stuttering, and so on. Journaling can help them observe interactions, compare interactions across situations, and reflect on the variables that influence Raul's fluency.

This process can specifically inform any other team members about potential intervention goals and methods to achieve them. Once such goals and methods are determined, dynamic assessment is a valuable avenue for determining the amount and type of support needed for successful interactions. In this case, Raul could use self-talk to review fluency-enhancing strategies prior to speaking. The teacher or SLP and even Raul's parents could continue to use checklists and naturalistic observation, conferring with Raul periodically about his use of the strategies and determining when or whether additional support is necessary. Or perhaps Raul could learn to use these assessments to evaluate his own progress.

Strategies for Teaching and Learning

The teaching and learning strategies described in Chapter 10 for students with language and learning problems are also appropriate for students with hearing, vision, and speech problems. Recall that the strategies such as dialogue, cooperative learning, verbal mediation, scaffolding, reciprocal teaching, and self-monitoring involve students in *interaction* with self, peers, and teachers. Thus, they provide numerous opportunities for students to engage in conversation with others, solve problems, benefit from prompts and models of more complex language structures, receive support for their own expansions, and evaluate learning from individual perspectives. Students who have sensory or speaking limitations are prime candidates for interactional strategies. Such students require frequent opportunities to engage in meaningful communications within contextually based situations. The remainder of this chapter focuses on teaching practices in the classroom that support students with hearing, vision, and speech (i.e., phonology and articulation, fluency, and voice) problems.

Hearing Impairment and Deafness

Hearing loss can be mild to profound and of a temporary (conductive) or permanent (sensorineural) nature. The types and degrees of hearing loss are explained in Chapter 8. It is important that educational planning teams know and understand how hearing loss affects each student because the levels and types of support will vary in accordance with each student's hearing profile (audiogram). For some students accommodations may be sufficient, whereas for others accommodations and modifications become necessary.

Hearing impairments affect students' verbal language development and in turn their development of literacy, academic success, and social interactions (Brackett, 1997; Brackett & Maxon, 1986; Davis, Elfenbein, Schum, & Bentier, 1986). Most students receive their education in regular classroom settings, which provide many opportunities for learning, including hands-on practice, use of technology, self-paced instruction, and peer-to-peer instruction (Brackett, 1997). Although teachers regard their experiences with students with hearing impairments as positive, they report that they lack preparation to deal with such students and are provided little support and information regarding the impact of hearing impairment on development and learning, the use of hearing aids or auditory systems, ideas for adapting curricula or materials, and modifications of teaching techniques (Luckner, 1991). It is important, then, that SLPs, audiologists, and teachers of individuals with hearing impairments provide in-service training and classroom consultation to general education teachers to help them become better equipped to support students with hearing impairments in general education classrooms.

The assessment and intervention team must develop specific objectives for students within the classroom. Accommodations and modifications must be clearly delineated and the levels of support from the team members must be determined. Shared responsibility for the educational success of each student requires that all team members learn about the impact of hearing impairment and the techniques that lessen its impact for students. Therefore, it is vital that the educational audiologist or teacher of individuals with hearing impairments be an active member of the team. This professional can have a significant impact on the education of students with hearing loss through engaging in assessment and intervention activities with students, their family, members of the classroom, and the support team.

When a student has fluctuating hearing loss due to recurrent middle ear fluid and infection (see Chapter 8 for a description of otitis media), the audiologist should perform periodic hearing testing. When a loss is detected, parents must be informed so that medical management can occur. In addition, the classroom teacher and SLP should be informed about the amount of loss and its implications for classroom learning. Recommendations for classroom accommodations that help to maintain student participation include short-term preferential seating, frequent monitoring of student comprehension, and reminders to students to keep parents and teachers informed about their hearing status.

When a sensorineural hearing loss is present, the audiologist provides the team with interpretations of how the loss is likely to affect communication, educational programming, and psychosocial development in the classroom. He or she collaborates with the teacher of the hearing impaired, SLP, and general education teacher to make recommendations regarding interventions, accommodations, and modifications in classrooms. Audiologists also provide group and individual counseling to students who are deaf and hearing impaired regarding hearing loss, hearing aids, FM systems (defined later), and other concerns. In some cases the school counselor may become involved in short- or long-term personal and social concerns of students (Grunblatt & Daar, 1994). In particular, middle and high school students may have difficulty adjusting to the use of hearing aids or FM systems due to the social implications of wearing such devices (Maxon, Brackett, & van den Berg, 1991).

The audiologist also determines and then monitors the proper fit and functioning of hearing aids and personal or classroom listening devices, and analyzes classroom noise levels and acoustics so that the listening environment is optimal. Noise levels in public schools average 60 decibels (dB), with a range from 53 to 74 dB (Maxon & Brackett, 1978). The relationship between the background noise and a new signal, such as a teacher's voice, is called the signal-to-noise ratio (S/N). A student using a hearing aid requires +15 to +30 dB S/N to recognize the new signal. One can imagine how difficult it is for students using hearing aids to focus on what is being said by a teacher or peer when environmental noise is amplified.

The S/N can be improved significantly in classrooms through the use of FM systems. Individual students wear receivers that amplify the voice of the teacher, who speaks into a microphone. An alternative to individual FM systems is having the entire classroom wired for amplification of the teacher's voice. There is evidence that amplification benefits students with hearing impairments, fluctuating or minimal hearing loss, learning problems, phonological and language disorders, and auditory processing problems (American Speech-Language-Hearing Association, 1996; Blake, Field, Foster, Platt, & Wertz, 1991; Flexer, Millin, & Brown, 1990; Stach, Loiselle, & Jerger, 1987). If an FM system is being considered for a student, the audiologist should demonstrate the appropriate device and the settings that are most appropriate for the level of hearing loss or other problem, demonstrate its use, and work with the student and teacher to determine the situations when the device will be used in the classroom. The audiologist also provides checks of amplification devices, troubleshoots problems, and arranges for repairs when needed. He or she provides direct instruction to students and parents about the care and maintenance of hearing aids and teaches students to recognize problems so that parents and teachers can be informed (Lipscomb, Von Almen, & Blair, 1992).

When an amplification device is under repair, the audiologist should confer with the teacher and SLP to increase instructional support for the student. The student may require an increase in visual information and written language; more direct face-to-face communication; a peer who can model tasks and provide demonstration when necessary; and increased teacher, SLP, and self-monitoring.

Oral communication can be developed in students even when the hearing loss is severe and especially when hearing aids are provided early (Paterson, 1994). Sign language is often learned in conjunction with oral language, and deaf students may communicate exclusively in sign language. When sign is the primary mode of communication, and the student is in the general education classroom, a full-time interpreter acts as mediator between the student and others. This communication strategy is highly effective in instructional settings, but it has limitations in social situations. Students who sign tend to miss out on comments other students make to each other during tasks and casual conversation (i.e., the underground talk) that occurs naturally in classroom settings. Interactions outside of the classroom can be limited when the interpreter is not present to act as a mediator. The reduced social interactions faced by students who are deaf or severely hearing impaired can impact their self-confidence around peers and their development of social interaction competencies (Antia & Kreimeyer, 1997). Thus, teachers and intervention specialists should encourage frequent social interactions between students with hearing impairments and their classmates. Guided intervention to increase social skills can include such interactions as greetings, sharing materials, assisting peers with tasks, conversing, complimenting others, responding appropriately to emotions of others, and even refusing requests and arguing effectively (Antia & Kreimeyer, 1997).

Another important mode of communication for students with hearing loss or deafness is written language. Literacy acquisition should be a primary goal and receive maximum emphasis in the elementary through high school curricula. Direct literacy instruction should begin as early as possible because phonological awareness and metalinguistic awareness are important for reading and writing. Written, tactile (touch), and kinesthetic (movement) cues can heighten such awareness for students with hearing impairments. Students need explicit teaching of unstressed grammatical forms, such as plurals and past tense, as well as connector words, including articles, prepositions, and conjunctions (Nelson, 1998; Paul, 1995). In addition, instruction in oral and written discourse is an important consideration in providing students with strong interaction skills for educational, social, and employment opportunities (Kretschmer, 1997).

Students are expected to listen throughout the school day to a variety of types of information presented at varying loudness levels and with varying degrees of background noise and competing messages. However, students are rarely taught how to listen or what to listen to. Truesdale (1990) suggested that teachers and other team members use "whole-body" activities to teach students the art of listening. The emphasis on explicit instruction in listening behaviors is to make students aware of the active nature of listening. Classroom activities include discussion of listening behaviors, observation of others, listing do's and don'ts, determining interferences to listening, role-playing listening situations, and writing about listening. These activities are appropriate for all students regardless of their level of hearing ability; thus, they can easily be incorporated into general classroom instruction. For older students, listening tips can be presented as a handout in content-area classrooms, with verbal reminders provided as new information is being learned.

The school environment is an important setting for the prevention of hearing loss through education. School-age children participate in many leisure activities that expose them to high levels of noise and put them at risk for noise-induced hearing loss. Noise levels accompanying motor vehicles, firearms, fireworks, amplified music, lawn mowers, and power tools are responsible for the increasing incidence of hearing loss, especially in boys above age 10 (Chermak, Curtis, & Seikel, 1996). Parents, teachers, and specialists have a role in prevention through education about the dangers of loud noises, the effects that loud noises have on the hearing mechanism, and the benefits of wearing hearing protection (earplugs or ear cuffs). Such information can be easily incorporated into the health and science curricula. The audiologist, teacher of the hearing impaired, or SLP can provide students with information about the structures and functions of the outer, middle, and inner ear and discuss with students the activities that put them at risk for damaging their hearing. A problem-solving approach with peers can be effective in promoting prevention.

Chermak et al. (1996) used a collaborative model to include speech and hearing professionals, general education teachers, students, and their families in a hearing conservation project for fourth-grade students. Teachers were provided materials to conduct in-class activities. Students assumed instructional roles through reciprocal teaching and peer education techniques, and pamphlets were sent home to involve parents in the project. Marked changes occurred in the hearing conservation practices of the fourth graders.

In summary, students with hearing impairment or deafness have several challenges within the educational setting. The educational team must work collaboratively to understand assessment data so that the educational and social implications of each student's loss are clearly defined. They must determine the appropriate classroom accommodations and modifications to provide maximum opportunities for full participation. Team members and the student, if possible, must monitor student progress and be alert to changes in hearing status due to otitis media or nonfunctional hearing aids or FM systems. Oral communication or sign language should be encouraged in both academic and social settings, and literacy acquisition should be the primary goal in each grade and throughout the educational curriculum. Students should be taught effective listening practices in classrooms and small group settings. Finally, professionals working in educational settings have an obligation to provide information about the damaging effects of loud noise and to work with students to prevent hearing loss through educational efforts.

A decision tree for supporting students with hearing impairment and deafness is provided in Figure 11.1. Team members, the student, and parents should

1. Does the student have a fluctuating or permanent hearing loss? → YES
   - a. Discuss concern with the student and parents. Make referral to audiologist and other intervention specialist as appropriate.
   - b. Audiologist determines nature and extent of loss through audiological testing. Teachers may complete behavioral checklists about hearing and listening in the classroom.
2. Does the student have fluctuating hearing loss due to middle ear fluid? → YES
   - a. Inform parents and recommend medical management.
   - b. Provide accommodations:
     - Preferential seating
     - Frequent monitoring of student comprehension
     - Check hearing status daily
3. Does the student qualify for special education as hearing impaired or deaf?

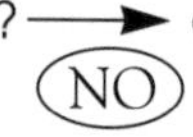

→ NO
   - a. Teach hearing loss prevention to all students.
   - b. Collaborate with teachers of students with hearing impairments to enhance oral and written language.
   - c. Collaborate with the interpreter to mediate instructional and social interactions.
   - d. Teach social skills.

→ YES

Students may use hearing aids and other amplification devices.
- Collaborate with audiologist to monitor proper fit and functioning.
- Refer students for counseling regarding amplification issues.
- Increase support to students when devices are under repair.
- Work with the speech–language pathologist to incorporate language needs into the classroom.

Figure 11.1. Decision tree for language intervention in classrooms for students with hearing problems.

carefully determine the types and amounts of support necessary for successful classroom participation. As students participate more in such decisions, their input about comfort level and degree of personal benefit is important for team members to consider. The success of the plan is contingent upon the collaboration of the team, the student, and family members.

Visual Impairment and Blindness

The early cognitive, social, and linguistic problems that can result from severe visual impairment or blindness were discussed in Chapter 8. Limited or absent visual information regarding objects, actions, and people relationships restrict these areas of growth at least during the first few years. In particular, infants with visual impairments do not relate to objects or people in the same way that sighted infants do. They miss the benefit of gestures, facial expressions, color, size, shape, and action that inform others about the world. Despite the lack of visual information, students with visual impairment do advance in all areas of development, especially when families and educators provide appropriate support. However, teachers and SLPs should be watchful because such students may have weaker foundations in language than their sighted peers (Paul, 1995).

Language skills should be carefully monitored during classroom instruction and activities. Because the visual and experiential basis for word meanings and concepts may be deficient, teachers and SLPs should assess word knowledge and relationships as new information is learned (Ratner & Harris, 1994). Preteaching of vocabulary may be necessary, especially when new vocabulary is accompanied by visual information for sighted students. For example, the word *topography* is easily explained by showing students a topographical map and having students measure differences in height. It is much harder to explain height differences in the landscape when the map is not visualized or the demonstration of height differences is not seen. Thus, students may require other types of experiences, such as the use of tactile and kinesthetic cues, to understand height differences in the landscape. For instance, they can feel and compare height differences of classmates or experience changes in the landscape by climbing ramps with various gradients.

Syntactic structures involving description (adjectives), reference (pronouns), and space, time, or direction (prepositions) can be difficult for students with visual impairment or blindness. These students may confuse words that convey these concepts or have difficulty understanding sentences containing these forms (Paul, 1995; Ratner & Harris, 1994). Cause–effect relationships among events and situations also may be difficult to understand. Teachers and the SLP can determine whether an individual student is experiencing difficulty and explore ways to minimize these difficulties. They can teach the forms and then help the student apply his or her knowledge within the classroom environment.

Students who are visually impaired or blind are at a disadvantage with regard to social interaction with peers in and outside the classroom. Because they do not see how others use gestures, facial expressions, body proxemics, and so on, they appear to be socially underdeveloped. For instance, the distance speakers maintain from each other is often defined implicitly by culture. Sighted people observe this social physical distance and adjust their bodies to maintain it when speaking with others. Those with visual impairment need verbal direction and explanation regarding how to establish and maintain social distance. They can judge distance through offering to shake the hand of someone or judge it based on the volume of the other person's voice. Variations in social distance depending on the situation and the communication partner can be taught through discussion and role playing.

Students who are visually impaired or blind must depend on listening skills and auditory memory in classroom learning situations. This requires sustained effort in the use of these cognitive processes. Thus, students may require frequent breaks from the demands of listening and remembering. They may also need assistance in transferring what is heard into long-term memory through highly redundant instruction with many examples. Strategies that require students to retell information, monitor comprehension, and engage in dialogue with others are useful for integrating new information with existing knowledge.

Literacy acquisition and development is a primary goal throughout the school years. For students with visual impairment or blindness, alternative systems such as Braille or computer scanning devices provide the learner with access to written language. The special education teacher not only teaches the use of such systems to the child and family members but facilitates their use within the classroom. Because reading and writing are critical to academic success, the student requires maximum opportunity to read and write. Teachers must be accommodating and welcome the input of the specialist who can provide strategies for monitoring student learning. The SLP and the special education teacher can work together with the student and general education teacher to determine appropriate language interventions that can be provided through written language instruction.

In summary, students who are visually impaired or blind need accommodations in classrooms to maximize their ability to participate with their peers. The potential cognitive, linguistic, and social challenges they experience can be minimized through careful planning and early intervention techniques.

Students may need support in language and learning strategies, literacy development, and social interactions. The decision tree in Figure 11.2 is a guide for professionals who provide interventions within classroom settings.

Severe Speech and Physical Impairments

Students who have motor limitations involving the structures of the speech mechanism (i.e., jaw, lips, tongue, hard and soft palate), the vocal mechanism (i.e., larynx, vocal cords), or the respiratory system (i.e., lungs, muscles of respiration) have moderate to profound difficulties with the production of speech. Such problems can result from neurological conditions, such as cerebral palsy, or from structural injuries that interfere with normal functioning of systems. (Refer to Chapter 8 for a review of such problems.) Students who have difficulty with speech production are at a distinct disadvantage in classrooms. Reduced or absent verbal communication limits cognitive, linguistic, and social development.

Students acquire language through hearing it in natural contexts and by participating in socially reinforcing interactions with family members and others. When speech development is hampered by structural and functional problems, interactions from the child are limited to visual, gestural, and vocal attempts. The restricted ability to practice language verbally and use it for communication results in reduced development of expressive language structures, including phonology, morphology, syntax, semantics, metalinguistics, and pragmatics. Thus, language knowledge and its use for academic and social interactions are often impoverished when students arrive at school. It is important that students receive intervention for language delays from the SLP within the classroom and in small group settings outside the classroom when appropriate. Teaching and learning practices that engage the student in dialogue with peers and promote self-monitoring (see Chapter 10) are particularly necessary for students with severe speech and physical impairments (SSPI).

Alternative and augmentative communication (AAC) systems provide students with SSPI access to interactions with their family members, support team, and peers. It is vital that such systems are provided early and modified as students increase cognitive, linguistic, and social abilities. Low-technology systems, such as picture boards of objects, actions, and attributes, provide the student opportunities to request, comment, refuse, describe, and express feelings or states. High-technology systems expand the student's ability to use functional communication through voice output capabilities and written language. It is important that parents, teachers, and specialists work together to make sure that students participate often with peers in small groups. An aide or

1. Does the student have visual impairment or blindness? ↓ YES
   a. Discuss concerns with the student and parents. Advise parents to seek evaluation of sight (e.g., ophthalmologist, optometrist).
   b. Vision specialist determines nature and extent of vision loss. Teachers may complete behavioral checklist about vision in the classroom.
2. Does the student qualify for special education as being visually impaired or blind?

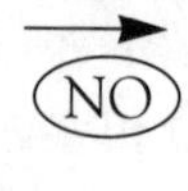

Support the student through regular teaching and learning strategies. Observe the student for other difficulties (e.g., hearing, language).

↓ YES

   a. Teach language skills checking for comprehension during classroom activities.
      - Collaborate with the SLP to increase word knowledge and word relationships.
      - Teach the syntactic uses of adjectives, pronouns, and prepositions for space and direction.
      - Collaborate with the SLP and special education teacher to teach social rules and interactional events (i.e., pragmatics).
   b. Teach strategies that enhance cognitive processing, such as self-monitoring of comprehension, dialogue with peers, and short- to long-term memory transfer.
   c. Collaborate with special education teacher to teach reading and writing through Braille or computer scanning systems.

Figure 11.2. Decision tree for language intervention in classrooms for students with visual problems.

peer should be attentive to the student and encourage frequent and meaningful participation.

Literacy instruction is a critical goal for students with SSPI. Koppenhaver and Yoder (1993) found that only five studies in the literature pertain to classroom literacy for this population. Studies suggest that students with SSPI receive *less* literacy instruction when compared to nonimpaired peers, and they are often passive and noninteractive with peers during classroom instruction. These findings parallel others showing that students in special education often receive less intensive instruction in reading and writing. Many variables help to explain the difficulty teachers and specialists have in providing successful literacy instruction. Koppenhaver and Yoder stated that "the poor quality of literacy instruction provided to children with SSPI can be traced to many different and overlapping sources, including the lack of teacher training programs, contextual complications introduced by assistive technology and the absence of a specific curriculum, the difficulties in communication that AAC users and speaking partners encounter across contexts, and the absence of valid and reliable literacy assessments to monitor student progress" (p. 9).

In a survey of 22 highly literate adults with SSPI, Koppenhaver, Evans, and Yoder (1991) found that all were regularly read to as children, they engaged in reading for pleasure and for completing classroom assignments, and they participated in many activities that promoted reading acquisition. It is interesting to note, however, that activities were not provided for their development of writing (Koppenhaver & Yoder, 1993). Writing instruction is an important area that team members must include in the educational plan. Students who have physical challenges can select letters and words from communication boards or computer keyboards to write or they can access letters and words through scanning and selection computer devices. Several suggestions for promoting development of speaking, reading, and writing in students with SSPI are provided in Table 11.1 (Foley, 1993; Koppenhaver & Yoder, 1993).

In summary, it is important that students with SSPI have opportunities to interact with classroom peers both during classroom activities and in other school, community, and home environments. Peers should understand that respect for others is required during interactions and that verbal or physical actions that demean or harm the student with SSPI will not be tolerated. Educationists should work with students in classrooms to understand the special needs of students with SSPI and encourage their support and participation in the academic and social interactions of the classroom. When physical challenges restrict the student's mobility and dexterity, modifications may be necessary in the physical arrangement of classrooms and the materials the student uses during classroom activities. Accessibility to equipment and materials and removal of barriers that limit participation are the responsibility of the intervention team. Some questions and decisions that teachers and specialists should explore for students with SSPI and their families are provided in

Table 11.1
Ideas To Promote Language Instruction for Students with Severe Speech and Physical Impairments

1. Examine how time gets used and the amount of wait time (for readying equipment, repair of devices, between activities) by children with severe speech and physical impairments (SSPI) in classrooms. Minimize delays in instruction through preplanning.
   - Preplan time needed to prepare equipment and materials, and accomplish this preparation prior to the start of the school day or period.
   - Encourage peer assistance with preparations by accepting volunteers and providing specific planning and organizational tasks (e.g., turning on computer, clearing the work area, moving chairs so that area is wheelchair accessible, gathering appropriate materials).
   - Load software programs or find the appropriate pages in texts.
2. Provide independent literacy activities whenever guided instruction is not occurring.
   - Independent listening or reading of taped books
   - Spelling and other metalinguistic activities
   - Computer-based or other commercial word puzzles and literacy games
   - Interactions with others through group problem-solving activities
   - Practice activities for mathematics or other content areas
3. Seek greater balance across instructional activities and the use of materials.
   - Plan activities that balance listening, speaking, reading, and writing.
   - Emphasize language activities that use meaningful contexts such as stories, children's narratives, and discussions about real-life events.
4. Increase student opportunities to have control over their own learning.
   - Allow student choices in oral and written activities.
   - Encourage students to construct meaningful oral and written texts.
   - Allow the use of oral and written language to serve many communicative purposes.
   - Provide students with the means for choosing activities, asking for assistance, and terminating activities.
   - Allow opportunities for students to interact with each other about language activities.

(*continues*)

Table 11.1 *Continued.*

5. Use resources to expand teacher knowledge and skill in teaching students with SSPI.
   - Attend continuing education seminars in working with students who have SSPI.
   - Read and discuss techniques for teaching students with SSPI.
   - Consult with manufacturer representatives of augmentative or alternative communication devices about their use.
   - Access the Internet for the ISAAC CONFER bulletin board posted by the International Society for Augmentative and Alternative Communication.
6. Teach specific literacy skills in language-based classroom programs.
   - Increase phonological awareness through sound segmentation and manipulation activities.
   - Increase automaticity of word recognition through software programs with speech output devices.
   - Increase comprehension and use of complex syntactic structures through sentence breakdown and sentence combination practice and grammatical judgment tasks.
   - Increase comprehension of narrative and expository texts through software programs that provide speech output for reading aloud and playback.

Figure 11.3. Team participation should always include the student and family members as well as strategies that can be used effectively in the classroom and home.

Phonological and Articulation Disorders

The ability to acquire and use speech sounds of one or more languages requires intact cognitive, physical, and linguistic systems. Delays in the acquisition of the sound system can result in intelligibility problems, limitations in phonological awareness, delays in reading and writing, and underdeveloped social competence. Traditionally, students with weak phonological and articulation abilities left their classrooms to receive speech therapy singly or in small groups. In some cases, especially when target sounds are being learned and practiced, these sessions can be appropriate and productive. However, when

1. Does the student have severe structural or functional speech and language problems?

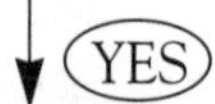

   a. Discuss concerns with student and parents. Make referral to speech–language pathologist, physical therapist, occupational therapist, and other intervention specialists as appropriate (e.g., regarding visual, hearing, cognitive, behavioral problems).
   b. Use a collaborative model to assess speech, language, and learning (and other areas when appropriate) through classroom-based tools.

2. Does the student qualify for special education due to speech and language impairments?

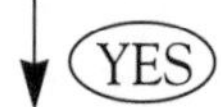

   a. For nonspeaking students, collaborate with the SLP and physical and occupational therapists to explore augmentative or alternative communication devices that will increase language learning and participation in individual and classroom interactions.
   b. Collaborate with intervention specialists to teach reading and writing using augmentative or alternative technology when appropriate.
   c. For students who speak with some degree of impairment, increase student opportunity to participate verbally in small supportive groups.

3. Does the student have temporary difficulties with speech and language (e.g., due to reconstructive surgery, temporary tracheotomy)?

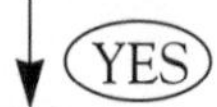

   a. Create opportunities for participation through writing or other modes of communication.
   b. Consult with the SLP to monitor speech improvement.

Figure 11.3. Decision tree for language intervention in classrooms for students with severe speech and physical impairments.

the student begins to transfer newly learned sounds, or when high exposure to sounds and their manipulations is the primary goal, intervention should be provided in the classroom.

Masterson (1993) advocated the provision of phonological intervention in classroom settings. She cited many advantages, including "increased relevance of linguistic targets; additional opportunities to learn the social dynamics of group settings, including turn-taking conventions and listening skills; and cost effectiveness" (p. 5). Further, she pointed out that classroom interventions allow teachers to become familiar with and participate in the language goals and procedures for specific students. Classroom intervention for phonological delays in the early grades can be incorporated in activities that enhance phonological awareness and metalinguistic awareness, such as rhyming, alliteration, and word and sentence games. Particular goals for individual students can be infused into these strategies. For example, a student who uses the simplification strategy called cluster reduction (e.g., *nake–snake*, *tee–tree*) may spend more time in guided practice of rhymes or alliterations containing clusters (e.g, *tree*, *tray*, *try*, *true*). Repeated storybook readings (Hoffman, 1997) provide opportunities for the scaffolding of students' utterances to assist them in producing more complex phonology. In addition, techniques such as providing a cloze ("The little boy was very __ "), forced choice ("Is this a shell or a sell?"), preparatory set ("What happened to the tiger?"), or relational terms ("Because of . . .," "So then . . .") exercise assist students in practicing difficult or new forms.

Masterson (1993) discussed several methods appropriate for collaborative, classroom-based phonological intervention. Some of the methods require that the SLP participate in direct, explicit instruction of students, whereas other methods involve collaborative, indirect involvement. The team is responsible for determining the nature of the problem and for selecting specific goals and the most appropriate methods of intervention for each student. Some variables to consider in planning interventions include the age of the student, related language and literacy goals, and the degree of phonological problems.

Some students have pronunciation difficulties, but they understand and have fully developed phonological systems. They do not have problems in phonological awareness, metalinguistic development, or delays in reading and writing acquisition. Due to structural irregularities such as severe dental or occlusal problems, cleft lip and palate, facial malformation, or slight motor weakness or incoordination, speech sounds are distorted or substituted. The most common errors for school-age children include lisping on one or several sounds (i.e., /s, z, ʃ, tʃ, dʒ, ʒ, θ/) and distortion or substitution of the glides and liquids (i.e., /r, l, j, w/). These errors can make intelligibility difficult for some children or simply make the speaker sound immature. As students enter middle and high school, sound errors become quite noticeable as they sound incongruous next to the more mature syntactic and semantic structures being produced.

Speech therapy for articulation problems consists of having the student identify the faulty pronunciation, learn new motor behaviors that result in correct pronunciation of the sound(s), practice the sound(s) in words and utterances, and generalize the correct pronunciation to conversational levels. Individualized and small group instruction is an effective way for students to receive this type of intervention. However, teachers can help assess the progress of each student so that appropriate generalization opportunities can be provided in the classroom. For example, a student working on correct production of /s/ and /z/ can practice these sounds when asking a question, reading aloud, or participating in group activities with other students. Depending on the group, it may be appropriate for the student to seek evaluation from peers or the student can self-evaluate and receive feedback from the teacher, SLP, or parents later in the day. Teachers can also provide subtle reminders to students to focus on integrating newly learned sounds into speaking activities. For instance, a cue such as the index finger to the lips could remind a student to use a correct "th" sound.

In summary, delays in the acquisition of the sound system can result in problems involving speaking, metalinguistic development, reading and writing, and social interactions. Assessment and intervention strategies for phonological delay and articulation problems are relevant and advantageous within general education classrooms. They not only involve general and special education teachers and SLPs in collaborative practices, but also allow students to work on their speaking within functional environments. The team considers several factors for each student, including the nature and severity of the problem, age, and related goals (e.g., reading and writing, social competence), and then determines when and how classroom interventions occur. Figure 11.4 provides decisions about classroom-based intervention for speech problems, including articulation or phonological problems, as well as voice and fluency problems.

Fluency Problems

Many preschool-age children experience periods of dysfluent speech. Most decrease and gradually eliminate stuttering without intervention. However, some children persist in stuttering into elementary school. Although early

1. Does the student demonstrate characteristics of stuttering, voice, or articulation and phonological problems?

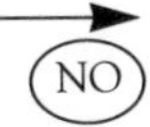

   a. Document characteristics of the problem.
   b. Discuss concerns with students and parents and make referral to speech–language pathologist (SLP).
   c. Use a collaborative model to assess speech through classroom-based tools and norm-referenced tests.

2. Does the student qualify for special education as speech–language impaired?

NO →
   a. Consult with SLP to determine techniques for monitoring fluency, voice, and articulation or phonology.
   b. Support student through dialogue, scaffolding, and development of self-monitoring.
   c. Teach student prevention techniques for voice problems.

YES ↓

Fluency

Collaborate with SLP to determine specific ways to reduce environmental demands.

a. SLP provides teachers and parents with information about the nature of stuttering and factors associated with stuttering.
b. SLP helps teachers and parents identify and modify situations that increase stuttering.
c. SLP helps teachers and parents to discuss feelings and attitudes about stuttering and to modify these so that comfortable interactions occur.

Voice

Collaborate with the SLP to provide a vocal hygiene prevention program to all students.

a. Students learn about the behaviors that can cause voice problems.
b. Students identify behaviors that they observe in themselves and others.
c. Students discuss prevention and use self-monitoring to eliminate behaviors.
d. Assist students receiving voice therapy to transfer techniques to the classroom and outside of the classroom.

Articulation/Phonology

Collaborate with SLP to provide rich experiences in language and literacy.

a. Confer with students when breakdowns in communication occur. Show students that mispronunciations change meaning.
b. Provide phonological awareness training in early grades in classroom-based activities.
c. Implement the Cycles approach (Hodson & Paden, 1983) or provide meaningful language context for hearing and producing target sounds.

(*continues*)

Figure 11.4. Decision tree for language intervention in classrooms for students with speech production problems.

Fluency	Voice	Articulation/Phonology
SLP provides specific strategies to teachers and parents to decrease time pressures, language complexity, and difficult interactions. a. Students may work directly with SLP to learn to modify stuttering behaviors or incorporate fluency enhancement strategies. b. Older students may work with SLP to learn cognitive and self-instructional strategies that enhance self-concept. c. Help students transfer fluency, cognitive, and self-instructional strategies into classroom. d. Provide repeated storybook readings using scaffolding to focus student on complex or difficult phonology. e. Teach students to self-monitor correct articulation, use cues to help students remember to use strategies, and provide information about student progress to SLP.		

Figure 11.4. *Continued.*

intervention for these children increases the likelihood that they will become more fluent (Meyers & Woodford, 1992; Ramig, 1993), a small number of students continue to stutter throughout high school and into adulthood. Although students who stutter are no more shy, nervous, or insecure than fluent peers, negative stereotypes can influence how parents, teachers, and peers relate to students who stutter (Lass et al., 1992). This particularly obvious speech problem leads to negative reactions and attitudes by others, which can cause the student who stutters to develop deep feelings of inadequacy, helplessness, embarrassment, fear, and a sense of failure (Berkowitz, Cook, & Haughey, 1994; Daly, Simon, & Burnett-Stolnack, 1995; Fosnot, 1995). Because stuttering occurs within speaking interactions and with people and situations that may help or hinder fluent speaking, it is important that interventions also occur during interactions (Gottswald & Starkweather, 1995). This is the most compelling argument for classroom-based interventions for stuttering.

Indeed, the focus of intervention for stuttering in public schools has shifted to classroom-based approaches in recent years. Gottswald and Starkweather (1995) mapped out two specific components for preschoolers. The first is to reduce the environmental demands that increase stuttering through education of parents and teachers. This goal involves the participation of the SLP, the general or special education teacher, and the parents. The SLP can provide information to the teachers and parents about stuttering and the factors associated with increases and decreases in dysfluent speech. This education process, with those who closely interact with the student, allows them the opportunity to obtain accurate information and identify situations and factors in the environment that influence the student's stuttering. The ability to identify such situations and factors allows parents and teachers to modify or capitalize on them. Because parents and teachers naturally react to stuttering, the team should also discuss feelings and attitudes such as anxiety, guilt, fear, and anger (Zebrowski & Schum, 1993). Desensitization experiences through books, videotapes, and discussion can help teachers and parents discuss feelings and attitudes openly. Once teachers and parents identify emotions, they then can learn to reduce them and replace them with positive, comfortable interactions.

The second component in an intervention plan for preschoolers is to strengthen the student's capacity for fluency. The SPL, teacher(s), and parents identify factors that result in high fluency demands (e.g., time pressures, language complexity, stressful interactions). The goal of intervention within this component is to reduce the environmental demands so that the student is given opportunities to speak at the highest level of fluency possible. Gottswald and Starkweather (1995) provided specific strategies of how these factors can be reduced for increased fluency (see Table 11.2). For example, adults can eliminate interruptions during the student's speaking turn so that the student does not feel pres-

Table 11.2
Reducing Fluency Demands for Preschool Children

Factor	Strategy
Time	Use a slow rate of speech by adding pauses and slowing oral movements.
	Reduce the rate of turn-taking in conversations by inserting a 2-second pause before responding to the student.
	Eliminate interruptions.
	Allow sufficient time to converse with the student and eliminate distractions and activity that may increase communicative pressure.
	Establish periods of quiet time to reduce stress and anxiety. Encourage nontalking activities during quiet time.
Linguistic Complexity	Identify the types of language demands placed on the student that increase stuttering.
	Lessen language demands through scaffolding explanations or phrasing questions that require less output from the student.
Social Interactions	Provide opportunities for interactions and presentations in small groups rather than large groups.
	Focus on the content of the student's message rather than on the stuttering behaviors, and compliment the student's language, voice, and self-expression abilities.
	Provide relaxed opportunities for interactions with others.
	Increase predictability by structuring the student's activities and by using routines. Prepare the student when changes in routine are expected.
	Respond to the student's feelings with openness and help the student express feelings through modeling.

Note. Adapted from "Fluency Intervention for Preschoolers and Their Families in the Public Schools," by S. R. Gottswald and C. W. Starkweather, 1995, *Language, Speech, and Hearing Services in Schools, 26,* pp. 117–126.

sured and can communicate her ideas completely. Some clinicians also provide intervention to parents who demonstrate communicative and interpersonal stress during interactions with their children (Rustin & Cook, 1995).

These two components enable the SLP, teacher(s), and parents to work together to modify the environment so that the preschooler experiences increased fluency. These techniques also can be used for older students; however, in elementary school and beyond, the intervention typically includes the student directly.

Daly et al. (1995) recommended two phases of treatment for adolescent students. The first phase consists of speech treatment that focuses on modifying stuttering behaviors and using fluency enhancement strategies. The second phase consists of strategies to change the student's self-concepts from negative mental attitudes, feelings, and beliefs into positive thinking about themselves as communicators. The second phase is accomplished through teaching cognitive and self-instructional strategies, which include relaxation, mental imagery, affirmation training, and positive self-talk. The tenets underlying intervention for older students who stutter are summarized in Table 11.3.

To summarize, the SLP should collaborate with general and special education teachers to reduce stereotypic reactions and attitudes about stuttering, modify factors that contribute to high fluency demands, and encourage the use of fluency and cognitive strategies in academic and social activities within the classroom. In addition, teachers and parents should be alert to teasing and bullying from others and enforce strict policies against verbal or physical abuse of students who stutter. Refer to Figure 11.4 for decisions about classroom-based interventions for speech production problems, including fluency (as well as phonology and articulation and voice).

Voice Problems

Students in elementary, middle, and high schools participate in many activities that lead to potentially damaging consequences on their voices. Cheering, yelling during sporting events or concerts, imitating voices of cartoon or film

Table 11.3
Tenets of Treatment for Adolescents Who Stutter

- Teachers, parents and, speech–language pathologists (SLPs) must demonstrate belief and confidence in the student's capacity to change.
- Concrete and realistic goals must be understood and agreed upon by the student.
- Treatment sessions must be frequent (2 to 3 times weekly) to facilitate progress and to develop a trusting relationship.
- A combination of cognitive, self-instructional, and speech treatment strategies results in a successful outcome.
- The teacher and the SLP must engage in many roles to listen, support, challenge, and provide guidance to the students.

Note. Adapted from "Helping Adolescents Who Stutter Focus on Fluency," by D. A. Daly, C. A. Simon, and M. Burnett-Stolnack, 1995, *Language, Speech, and Hearing Services in Schools, 26,* pp. 162–168.

characters, talking through the night during sleepovers, and smoking are examples of abusive practices that can cause voice disorders. Because these abusive behaviors are changeable, voice disorders caused from abuse can be prevented.

Prevention of voice disorders in students begins with education (Andrews, 1991; McNamara & Perry, 1994; Pindzola, 1993). The topic of prevention can be included in the health curriculum, and basic anatomy and functioning of the larynx can be included in science when the human body is being discussed. Knowledge about the characteristics and purpose of the larynx alerts students to its important biological and vocal functions. Information about the proper care and use of the larynx during speaking, during respiratory ailments, and for intentionally changing pitch, loudness, and quality can reduce the chance that abuse will occur due to lack of knowledge about good vocal hygiene. Students should engage in dialogue about the types of vocal behaviors that can be abusive and the situations where such behaviors are likely to occur. The heightened awareness of behaviors and situations can lead to self-identification and reflection about vocal abusive practices. A discussion that encourages students to problem solve about ways to eliminate vocal abuse helps all students hear the variety of solutions to everyday situations and construct plans to implement them in their own lives. Students can role-play to make the situations and solutions directly applicable to their age, experiences, and environments.

Pindzola (1993) provided specific suggestions of commercial and homemade materials that can be used in vocal hygiene programs for young children. Suggestions are plentiful for working with adolescent students as well (Aaron & Madison, 1991; Andrews & Summers, 1991; Burk & Brenner, 1991; Conroy, 1989; Nichols, Middleton, & Brand, 1990).

Students who have been diagnosed with voice disorders from vocal abuse or from other conditions (see Chapter 8) and are receiving voice therapy from the SLP, need support from teachers, parents, and peers to effectively transfer appropriate use of vocal techniques into the classroom. The team can encourage the student to use self-talk, self-monitoring, and other metacognitive strategies that help the student plan, execute, and evaluate vocal productions according to the learned techniques. For example, a student may learn the purpose and procedures of "easy onset" of voice during speech therapy sessions. After considerable practice in the use of this technique, the student can try it during some classroom activities. The SLP, teachers, and parents can determine which activities provide practice opportunities and self-monitoring both in school and at home. For instance, a small group discussion about a film might be selected, allowing time for each student to express opinions and ideas. The student might use self-talk to review the principles of the technique. During speaking, the student can judge the effectiveness of the technique in reducing laryngeal tension and producing a better vocal quality. The student then might use a checklist or comment sheet to record observations that can be shared later with the SLP, parents, and teacher(s).

In summary, vocal abuse by students can lead to voice disorders. Therefore, prevention of vocal abuse is the responsibility of educationists and parents through education about abusive practices and their effects on the vocal folds. Students with voice disorders can receive intervention in the general education classroom. Team members can encourage students to use metacognitive strategies to eliminate vocal abuse and to practice good vocal hygiene and specific techniques determined by the team. Refer to Figure 11.4 for intervention decisions about speaking problems, including voice problems (as well as phonology and articulation and fluency).

Summary

Teachers, SLPs, and parents are seeking more opportunities to collaborate in assessing, planning, and implementing interventions within classroom contexts. Although norm-referenced testing and pull-out therapy are appropriate for some students, classroom-based services have the added benefit that they inform professionals, parents, and the students themselves about the impact of communication problems on academic and social functioning. This information has direct application on designing, implementing, and evaluating educational programming for students.

Interventions for hearing, vision, and speech problems depend on the characteristics of the problem, the severity in terms of functional communication and learning, and the effect of previous intervention decisions on the present ones. Intervention teams must be knowledgeable about these factors as they make decisions about classroom interventions.

Literacy instruction is a critical area of intervention for students with sensory losses and speech production problems. Instruction in reading and writing not only teaches students about the structures and functions of language, but opens up an important avenue for learning and communicating.

Educationists have a special role in the prevention of hearing, vision, and speech problems. Opportunities for education about abusive practices that risk intact hearing, vision, and speech should be provided in the health and science curriculum. Further, students with such problems should have the right and freedom to be educated in a comfortable and healthy environment that does not tolerate verbal or physical abuse from others.

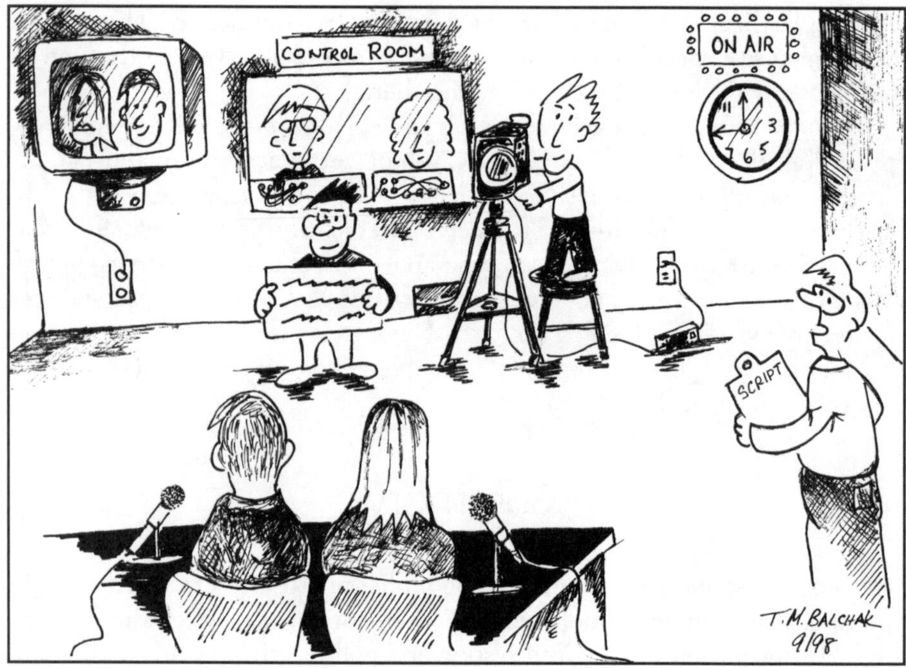

Students who have sensory or speaking limitations are prime candidates for use of interactional strategies. Such students require frequent opportunities to engage in dialogue, cooperative learning, verbal mediation, scaffolding, reciprocal teaching, and self-monitoring.

References

Aaron, V., & Madison, C. (1991). A vocal hygiene program for high school cheer leaders. *Language, Speech, and Hearing Services in Schools, 22*, 287–290.

American Speech-Language-Hearing Association Task Force on Central Auditory Processing Consensus Development. (1996). Central auditory processing: Current status of research and implications for clinical practice. *American Journal of Audiology, 5*(2), 41–54.

Andrews, M. L. (1991). The treatment of adolescents with voice disorders: Some clinical perspectives—An introduction. *Language, Speech, and Hearing Services in Schools, 22*, 156–157.

Andrews, M. L., & Summers, A. C. (1991). The awareness phase of voice therapy: Providing a knowledge base for the adolescent. *Language, Speech, and Hearing Services in Schools, 22*, 158–162.

Antia, S. D., & Kreimeyer, K. H. (1997). The generalization and maintenance of the peer social behaviors of young children who are deaf or hard of hearing. *Language, Speech, and Hearing Services in Schools, 28*(1), 59–69.

Berkowitz, M., Cook, H., & Haughey, M. J. (1994). A non-traditional fluency program developed for the public school setting. *Language, Speech, and Hearing Services in Schools, 25*, 94–99.

Blake, R., Field, B., Foster, C., Platt, F., & Wertz, P. (1991). Effects of FM auditory trainers on attending behaviors of learning-disabled children. *Language, Speech, and Hearing Services in the Schools, 22*, 111–114.

Brackett, D. (1997). Intervention for children with hearing impairments in general education settings. *Language, Speech, and Hearing Services in Schools, 28*, 355–361.

Brackett, D., & Maxon, A. B. (1986). Service delivery alternatives for the mainstreamed hearing impaired child. *Language, Speech, and Hearing Services in Schools, 17*, 115–125.

Burk, K. W., & Brenner, L. E. (1991). Reducing vocal abuse: "I've got to be me." *Language, Speech, and Hearing Services in Schools, 22*, 173–178.

Chermak, G. D., Curtis, L., & Seikel, J. A. (1996). The effectiveness of an interactive hearing conservation program for elementary school children. *Language, Speech, and Hearing Services in Schools, 27*, 29–39.

Conroy, K. (1989). *How your voice works: A voice modification program*. Chatsworth, CA: Opportunities for Learning.

Daly, D. A., Simon, C. A., & Burnett-Stolnack, M. (1995). Helping adolescents who stutter focus on fluency. *Language, Speech, and Hearing Services in Schools, 26*, 162–168.

Davis, J., Elfenbein, J., Schum, R., & Bentier, R. (1986). Effects of mild and moderate hearing impairments on language, educational, and psychosocial behavior of children. *Journal of Speech and Hearing Disorders, 51*, 53–62.

Flexer, C., Millin, J., & Brown, L. (1990). Children with developmental disabilities: The effects of sound field amplification in word identification. *Language, Speech, and Hearing Services in Schools, 21*, 177–182.

Foley, B. E. (1993). The development of literacy in individuals with severe congenital speech and motor impairments. *Topics in Language Disorders, 13*(2), 16–32.

Fosnot, S. M. (1995). Some contemporary approaches in treating fluency disorders in preschool, school-age, and adolescent children. *Language, Speech, and Hearing Services in Schools, 26*, 115–116.

Gottswald, S. R., & Starkweather, C. W. (1995). Fluency intervention for preschoolers and their families in the public schools. *Language, Speech, and Hearing Services in Schools, 26*, 117–126.

Grunblatt, H., & Daar, L. (1994). A support program: Audiological counseling. *Language, Speech, and Hearing Services in Schools, 25*, 112–114.

Hodson, B., & Paden, E. (1983). *Targeting intelligible speech: A phonological approach to remediation*. San Diego: College-Hill.

Hoffman, P. R. (1997). Phonological intervention within storybook reading. *Topics in Language Disorders, 17*(2), 69–88.

Koppenhaver, D. A., Evans, D. A., & Yoder, D. E. (1991). Childhood reading and writing experiences of literate adults with severe speech and motor impairments. *Augmentative and Alternative Communication, 7*, 20–33.

Koppenhaver, D. A., & Yoder, D. E. (1993). Classroom literacy instruction for children with severe speech and physical impairments (SSPI): What is and what might be. *Topics in Language Disorders, 13*(2), 1–15.

Kretschmer, R. R., Jr. (1997). Issues in the development of school and interpersonal discourse for children who have hearing loss. *Language, Speech, and Hearing Services in Schools, 28*, 374–383.

Lass, N. J., Ruscello, D. M., Schmitt, J. F., Pannbacker, M. D., Orlando, M. B., Dean, K. A., Ruziska, J. C., & Bradshaw, K. H. (1992). Teachers' perceptions of stutterers. *Language, Speech, and Hearing Services in Schools, 23*, 78–81.

Lipscomb, M., Von Almen, P., & Blair, J. C. (1992). Students as active participants in hearing aid maintenance. *Language, Speech, and Hearing Services in Schools, 23*, 208–213.

Luckner, J. L. (1991). Mainstreaming hearing-impaired students: Perceptions of regular educators. *Language, Speech, and Hearing Services in Schools, 22*, 302–307.

Masterson, J. J. (1993). Classroom-based phonological intervention. *American Journal of Speech-Language Pathology, 2*(1), 5–9.

Maxon, A. B., & Brackett, D. (1978). *The mainstreamed hearing-impaired child: Data and descriptions*. Short course presented at American Speech-Language-Hearing Association Convention, San Francisco.

Maxon, A. B., Brackett, D., & van den Berg, S. A. (1991). Classroom amplification use: A national long-term study. *Language, Speech, and Hearing Services in Schools, 22*, 242–253.

McNamara, A. P., & Perry, C. K. (1994). Vocal abuse prevention practices: A national survey of school-based speech–language pathologists. *Language, Speech, and Hearing Services in Schools, 25*, 105–111.

Meyers, S. C., & Woodford, L. L. (1992). *The fluency development system for young children*. Buffalo, NY: United Educational Services.

Nelson, N. W. (1998). *Childhood language disorders in context: Infancy through adolescence*. Needham Heights, MA: Allyn & Bacon.

Nichols, G., Middleton, G., & Brand, M. (1990). *Be a smooth talker*. Bellingham, WA: Voice Tapes.

Paterson, M. M. (1994). Articulation and phonological disorders in hearing-impaired school-aged children with severe and profound sensorineural losses. In J. E. Bernthal & N. W. Bankson (Eds.), *Child phonology: Characteristics, assessment, and interventions with special populations* (pp. 199–226). New York: Thieme Medical.

Paul, R. (1995). *Language disorders from infancy through adolescence: Assessment and intervention*. St. Louis: Mosby.

Pindzola, R. H. (1993). Materials for use in vocal hygiene programs for children. *Language, Speech, and Hearing Services in Schools, 24*, 174–176.

Ramig, P. R. (1993). High reported spontaneous stuttering recovery rates: Fact or fiction? *Language, Speech, and Hearing Services in Schools, 24*, 156–160.

Ratner, V., & Harris L. (1994). *Understanding language disorders: The impact on learning*. Eau Claire, WI: Thinking Publications.

Rustin, L., & Cook, F. (1995). Parental involvement in the treatment of stuttering. *Language, Speech, and Hearing Services in Schools, 26*, 127–137.

Stach, B. A., Loiselle, L. H., & Jerger, J. F. (1987, November). *FM systems use by children with central auditory processing disorders*. Paper presented at the annual convention of the American Speech-Language-Hearing Association, New Orleans.

Truesdale, S. P. (1990). Whole-body listening: Developing active auditory skills. *Language, Speech, and Hearing Services in Schools, 21*, 183–184.

Zebrowski, P. M., & Schum, R. L. (1993). Counseling parents of children who stutter. *American Journal of Speech-Language Pathology, 2*(2), 65–73.

Classroom-Based Interventions for Written Language

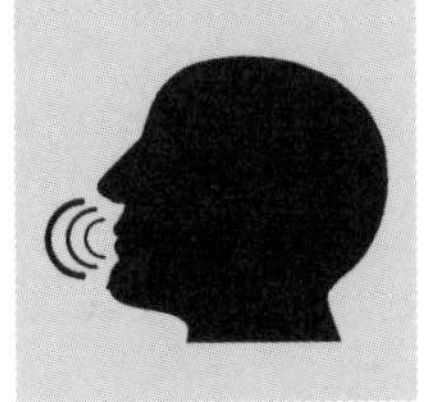

Chapter 12

Ginny Helwick and Kathleen R. Fahey

The acquisition of oral and written language is a complex process involving cognitive, linguistic, and social development that begins in infancy and continues throughout adulthood. The interactions that children engage in with families and other caregivers provide the situational contexts for listening and speaking, as well as recognizing and interacting with print. As children enter preschool and kindergarten, their well-developed oral language systems and developing knowledge of written language allow full participation in school and community activities.

Children who have underdeveloped oral language systems or language(s) other than Standard American English (SAE) are at a disadvantage with regard to the acquisition of written language. In children's native language these systems develop simultaneously from about age 2 or 3. When the native language is delayed or different from SAE, the relationships between oral language and print become less developed and result in delays in reading and writing. To some degree, the old notions of "readiness" may also cause adults to limit exposure to written language experiences in favor of oral language experiences. The purpose of this chapter is to discuss ways that general and special education teachers and speech–language pathologists (SLPs) can collaborate to provide assessments and interventions for written language development of students who exhibit any of these difficulties.

For students with language problems, classroom situations requiring listening, speaking, reading, and writing can be daunting. It is important that the intervention team carefully consider students' strengths and coping strategies, the situations that tax their capabilities, and ways in which each student can participate and learn successfully. Accommodations and modifications in the general education classroom can create a positive and facilitative atmosphere for students with problems.

Ginny Helwick has taught both general and special education at the elementary level for 32 years. She is currently a special education teacher at Meeker Elementary School and a doctoral student in the Division of Special Education at the University of Northern Colorado, both in Greeley, Colorado.

Classroom environments that promote learning from an integrated language perspective (Pappas, Kiefer, & Levstik, 1995) use listening, speaking, reading, and writing throughout the curriculum so that students use these modes of language in authentic situations with peers and teachers. Reading and writing then are tools of learning, not ends in and of themselves. Students whose language is not commensurate with the level of language being used during school activities must be supported by teachers and other students until language knowledge and use are strengthened. In particular, instruction in reading and writing is critical for students who have oral language problems. It helps them to gain information about the language systems and provides an additional avenue for expression of their ideas. Exposure to print should be started during the preschool years if possible, but certainly by kindergarten.

The presence of language and learning problems should not be regarded as a justification for limiting literacy experiences. In the past, fewer opportunities were provided for students with special needs to engage in authentic reading and writing experiences because it was presumed that oral language abilities were not sufficiently well developed for such experiences (Koppenhaver, Coleman, Kalman, & Yoder, 1991). Reading programs tended to consist of skill-based (phonics) drills without connections to meaning. Recent research in emergent literacy, however, has revealed that children with cognitive, physical, or communication problems benefit from connected reading and authentic writing instruction (Butler, 1979; Koppenhaver et al., 1991; van Kleeck, 1990). Such instruction not only enhances reading and writing but influences communication abilities. Koppenhaver and colleagues proposed several suggestions for the home and school that can increase the development of reading and writing (see Table 12.1).

In addition, specific teaching and learning strategies—dialogue, cooperative learning, verbal mediation, scaffolding, reciprocal teaching, and self-monitoring (see Chapters 10 and 11)—that invite interactions among students and between students and their teachers and parents about what is being learned, how it is learned, why it is being learned, and to what extent it was learned, help students with language difficulties. These strategies engage the students in active thinking and reasoning with the support of others in natural language contexts.

The Multifaceted Nature of Reading and Writing

Acquisition of reading and writing is dependent on many different abilities acquired through reading and writing practice, explicit instruction, exposure to different types and difficulty levels of literature, and an organized curricular plan.

Table 12.1
Suggestions for Parents and Practitioners To Increase Literacy for Children with Developmental Disabilities

Parents

Include children in daily routines involving print:

- Open and respond to mail.
- Use recipes to make and bake favorite foods.
- Create shopping lists by having children name items and watch or attempt spellings.
- Model and encourage children to read signs and labels at home, in stores, and while traveling in the car.
- Watch educational children's television shows and reinforce reading and writing activities.
- Model opportunities for functional and recreational uses of print (e.g., newspaper, letter writing, television guides).
- Think aloud and explain the usefulness of print during daily activities.
- Read stories aloud and relate the events and characters to the experiences of the children.

Practitioners

Incorporate reading and writing experiences into classroom routines and curricula:

- Use thematic experiences to introduce, explain, and practice new concepts (e.g., stories, drama, art, dance, cooking).
- Provide frequent interactions with nondisabled peers and encourage modeling of language (e.g., asking and answering questions, commenting, creating and retelling stories).
- Use supportive materials such as pictures, manipulatives, and storybooks to increase interactions during instruction.
- Use rereading as a vehicle for establishing new understandings and for integration of concepts and ideas.
- Read aloud from several types of literature to provide exposure to different discourses.
- Create opportunities for independent access to print-related materials and provide guidance in the use of materials.

Note. Adapted from "The Implications of Emergent Literacy Research for Children with Developmental Disabilities," by D. A. Koppenhaver, P. P. Coleman, S. L. Kalman, and D. E. Yoder, 1991, *American Journal of Speech–Language Pathology: A Journal of Clinical Practice, 1*(1), pp. 38–48. Copyright 1991 by American Speech-Language-Hearing Association. Adapted with permission.

Instruction must be continuous and progress assessed regularly (Cunningham & Allington, 1994). The question is not "Which approach should be taught?" but rather "How can teachers integrate reading and writing instruction so that all student needs receive emphasis?" No single approach is best for all students. For students who find reading and writing difficult, there is no quick fix (Allington & Walmsley, 1995; Cunningham & Allington, 1994).

Classroom-Based Assessments

"Kid watching" in classrooms provides teachers with opportunities to observe students and to assess their competencies and needs (Goodman, 1979). Although formal, norm-referenced tests can be used to determine reading and writing levels, it is often more useful for teachers and SLPs to analyze each student's problems during specific, functional activities in the classroom. After analysis, activities can be designed with the students that help each one become more proficient at reading and writing. Thus, observation strategies such as checklists, criterion-referenced tests, naturalistic assessments, and dynamic assessments (see Chapter 10) are superior to norm-referenced tests for teachers who provide an integrated language curriculum.

An example may help to clarify how these assessment strategies are relevant for reading and writing instruction in classrooms. Let us consider an eighth-grade student who struggles in these areas.

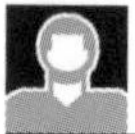

John

John is a 13-year-old who is eager to learn and is well liked by his peers. He participates in a variety of extracurricular activities. In the early elementary grades his academic progress was average; however, his oral language abilities were below average and his reading and writing development was slow. He showed great frustration and avoidance of tasks involving print. During fourth grade, his progress in school began a noticeable decline, and he is currently having great difficulty in middle school. His poor reading and writing interfere with accurate completion of classroom assignments.

Checklists

One way for teachers and specialists to observe specific factors in John's poor progress is to create a checklist that contains the essential reading and writing abilities needed within the eighth-grade classroom. Checklists are most helpful when they are constructed by the teacher, special educator, or SLP who is knowledgeable about what the students are expected to do. The professional should analyze classroom tasks so that the checklist reflects the complex array of activities required, such as in a checklist for classroom interactions (Nelson, 1998). Figure 10.1 in Chapter 10, which shows how various aspects of language are embedded in functional communication (Norris, 1997), can help to stimulate thinking about what should be included in a checklist. Once established, such a checklist can serve, perhaps with some modifications, other students as well. Collaboration could also enable the team to integrate language into all aspects of the curriculum, including fine arts, technical courses, and mathematics.

In John's case, the teacher, SLP, and John himself might observe several different classroom activities involving reading and writing. The checklist could be completed as items are noted during the performance of activities. For example, if students are asked to read a section in social studies and respond to written questions, the observers could note how long it takes John to read, whether he uses any visible strategies to keep his place or guide his own reading, and whether he reads the questions first and then reads the section to answer the questions. Any oral language interactions could also be noted. Once the answers to the questions are written, an analysis of John's comprehension of what he read could occur and observations made about spelling, grammatical structure, organization, and writing mechanics.

Criterion-Referenced Assessment

Teachers and SLPs can also observe John by testing his knowledge of reading and writing of eighth-grade (or lower or higher) material. This criterion-referenced method provides a fairly quick way to assess skills in a large group or of a specific individual (Nelson, 1998; Paul, 1995). A spelling test of words that students are expected to write accurately could be given through dictation. Tests of reading speed and comprehension could be devised (or selected from published materials) from narrative and expository texts. A miscue analysis could be accomplished as John reads aloud. The value of this kind of testing lies in its focus on specific curricular areas. It yields information that could inform instruction in classroom activities, such as teaching comprehension strategies as John reads content-area texts (Miller & Paul, 1995). Criterion-referenced testing is limited in perspective in that it assumes that the items observed comprise the act of reading and writing, and that students of a particular age or grade have or should have a "level" of competence.

Naturalistic Assessment

Another type of assessment approach that views the student's reading and writing abilities within social and academic situations is naturalistic assessment. Teachers, specialists, and SLPs work together to determine the many situations routinely encountered by students to read and write. Observation may take place in several situations, such as small learning groups, the classroom, pull-out special education classes, the library, after-school club meetings, and the home (Lund & Duchan, 1993). To assess John's ability to participate in publishing the school paper, where members' roles and responsibilities can be observed, the observer must watch him perform a designated task. The observer might use a note-taking strategy such as journaling to document impressions. The goal of this type of assessment is to determine what types and amount of support are needed for successful learning and participation within various situations (Silliman & Wilkinson, 1991).

Dynamic Assessment

Once interventions are in place, dynamic assessment strategies help teachers and specialists determine whether they are effective. If John is using specific decoding strategies during reading, he, the teacher, and the SLP must evaluate whether the strategies are helping him decode print more easily and accurately. If the strategies are not being used or do not appear effective, team members search for more productive strategies. An advantage of this assessment strategy is that it encourages interaction among the student, teachers, and SLP and fosters self-evaluation as an important learning component. It also provides opportunities to try many different strategies and adopt those that benefit the student. Notice that the assessment strategies outlined for John are easily accomplished within the daily activities of classrooms and, therefore, do not require the student to be absent from a class to engage in evaluation sessions with specialists.

Teaching Cognitive Strategies for Reading and Writing

Readers and writers who approach literacy from a strategic perspective actively and purposefully take charge. They set purposes for reading and writing, identify and use appropriate strategies, integrate new and existing information, demonstrate confidence and positive self-concept, and use self-monitoring techniques (Routman, 1991). These strategies afford the student control over mental operations that allow for deliberate reflection on and manipulations of written language (Clay, 1991; Tunmer & Cole, 1991). Thus, students can monitor whether the words and sentences make sense, whether they know the vocabulary, and whether they have read or written the text accurately.

Three strategies students use for effective reading and writing are searching, self-monitoring, and self-questioning. Schwartz (1997) defined *searching strategies* as those that enable readers "to gather cues for an initial attempt to read a text, make multiple tries at different words, and self-correct some errors" (p. 42). The cues include print (graphophonemic), grammatical structure (syntactic), and meaning (semantic). When teachers teach word recognition, they focus on searching strategies that make the cues explicit to students. Students who have limited ability or experience to employ searching strategies benefit from teacher and peer modeling, dialogue about how cues help, and practice using such cues during authentic, contextual reading and writing activities.

The second strategy, *self-monitoring,* requires students to assess and evaluate their learning attempts (see also Chapter 10). Teachers guide their students to use cues during reading and writing and then ask them to judge their effectiveness. Confident readers and writers can typically express how they approach tasks and what they do when they encounter difficulty. Many poor readers do not engage in self-monitoring, because they lack both awareness of the cues and strategies to assess and evaluate learning. Self-monitoring strategies, however, can be taught and applied to classroom activities (Davey, 1985; Schwartz, 1997). Teacher and peer modeling, dialogue about strategies, teacher use of verbal mediation, and scaffolding are some ways that help students develop self-monitoring strategies.

A particular self-monitoring strategy that encourages independence is *self-questioning*. In this strategy, the student hears common questions asked by other readers and writers as they evaluate their work and practices asking questions that provoke analysis of what was learned. For example, a student who is reading about water pollution can ask several questions prior to reading based upon background knowledge and the title of the story or text, or after reading to check comprehension. Some general questions prior to reading might focus on what the reader expects to find out about water pollution, such as causes, prevention, cost to taxpayers, and environmental consequences. Questions after reading might focus on whether expected information was presented, what additional issues were addressed, what the author's purpose was in writing the passage (e.g., information, call to action), and what information the student wishes to know that was not presented. Small group discussions are helpful because students may have different questions that all students benefit from hearing. Students who have difficulty generating questions benefit from cooperative learning or reciprocal teaching environments in which other students talk about learning processes and the information being learned.

Students who have moderate to severe reading and writing problems may require specific, intense, and explicit instruction in searching, self-monitoring, and self-questioning strategies. Instruction can be provided within minilessons in the classroom and then applied during subsequent reading and writing experiences. For example, during a context-embedded phonics minilesson about long vowel patterns, the students might collectively identify words from the text with long vowel sounds. The teacher, specialist, SLP, or other student shows the cues that represent the pattern and then models a questioning strategy. For example, "What pattern do I see in the words *cane, rate, bake, bone*, and *fire* that tells me the vowel is long?" Some children may need verbal direction (e.g., "Remember to ask yourself questions") or visual cues (e.g., pointing to questions printed on the board), which can be reduced or eliminated as students become more proficient and independent in the use of these strategies.

In summary, reading and writing development begins during the preschool years as the oral language system continues to develop. Because students who have oral language problems are at risk for delays in the development of written language, early experiences with reading and writing are critical, and intensive instruction that invites interactions with other students, parents, teachers, and SLPs is warranted in many cases.

Students who have reading and writing difficulties must be observed during classroom activities so that teachers and SLPs understand the nature of the problems and how the problems interfere with classroom learning. Classroom-based assessments (e.g., checklists, criterion-referenced tests, dynamic assessment) provide opportunities for such observation, which leads to interventions that support student learning.

Three cognitive strategies students use for effective reading and writing are searching, self-monitoring, and self-questioning, which allow students to discover and use cues to evaluate learning and to analyze what was learned. Students with language problems may require specific, intense, and explicit instruction in cognitive strategies.

Teaching Literacy

The remainder of this chapter focuses on teaching and learning strategies for reading and then writing. The development of these modes of language involves integration of several abilities that develop simultaneously as students learn to read and write. Although the various abilities are discussed separately for reading (i.e., phonological awareness, decoding and fluency, and comprehension) and writing (i.e., process, structure, and form), teachers, specialists, and SLPs should teach these together in the service of comprehension and expression.

Most students acquire reading and writing through a balanced language arts program that includes equal proportions (20%) of five components: (1) the teacher reading literature with student discussion, (2) phonics and word study, (3) shared reading experiences, (4) independent reading, and (5) writing (Daniels, Zemelman, & Bizar, 1998; International Reading Association & National Council of Teachers of English, 1996). It is important to realize, however, that students with dyslexia (see Chapter 4) need more intense instruction in phonics and word study.

Teaching Reading

In her 1990 summary of the existing reading and reading education research for the U.S. Congress, Adams concluded that instruction that leads to phonemic segmentation and phonological coding is crucial to learning to read and is especially important for students with significant reading delays (i.e., those labeled as having learning or reading disorders or dyslexia). What was new about her conclusion was that such instruction is best carried out in *context*, that is, that texts should be carefully coordinated with the content and schedule of phonics lessons. Furthermore, she concluded that reading is an *interactive* process; it proceeds neither from the top down (i.e., from meaning to syntax) nor from the bottom up (i.e., from distinctive features to letters, to letter strings, to words). Instead, reading is a process in which readers must derive information from all of those knowledge sources *simultaneously*. Two instructional implications that emerge from this understanding are (1) that the integrity of the reading process needs to be maintained during instruction—that the only way to learn to read is to practice reading text—and (2) that reading instruction needs to be broadly based for all students, including those labeled as having dyslexia (see also Wise, 1991).

Consequently, the bottom–up, multisensory and phonics interventions so often advocated in special education may be useful when intensive phonological coding or phonemic awareness instruction is warranted (i.e., for students with severe delays). Among such multisensory and phonics systems (there are too many to mention here—the reader should check the research connected with whatever one is recommended locally) are the *Lindamood Phoneme*

Sequencing Program for Reading, Spelling, and Speech (LiPS) (Lindamood & Lindamood, 1998), probably the best researched and most beneficial of these systems, as well as the old special education standbys, the Fernald (1943) VAKT (i.e., visual, auditory, kinesthetic, and tactile) and the neurological-impress method (Heckelman, 1969), which have not been strongly supported by research evidence (Bartel, 1995). These systems, particularly the LiPS Program, often prove quite important to the progress of students with severe reading impairments, but they should not constitute the entire reading program. Although they address one aspect of the reading process, they are not reading. Teachers and SLPs should begin with text in which there are numerous examples of the skills to be developed, then shift focus to instruction with specific target skills, and end each lesson with those skills being reembedded into text. When it is necessary to use isolated, bottom–up instruction, it should be accompanied by additional, holistic instruction with a strong emphasis on authentic writing and invented spelling (Allington & Cunningham, 1996). Never should multisensory or phonics instruction be the students' *only* reading instruction. Such single approaches often contribute to the cumulative delays in the development of vocabulary, syntax, and knowledge acquisition that were identified by Stanovich (1986).

Facilitating Phonological Awareness and Other Metalinguistic Abilities

The importance of metalinguistic development as it relates to reading and writing was discussed in Chapter 4. Students benefit from learning and talking about how particular forms and functions of language work (Paul, 1995). Phonological awareness includes knowledge about words within sentences, syllables within words, sounds within words, rhyme, sound–letter correspondence, and so forth. These understandings emerge during the preschool years and continue to develop through early elementary school as students engage in reading and writing. Students who have highly developed oral language and who experience literacy-rich environments at home begin school with strong backgrounds and abilities in phonological awareness. Those who have delayed or different oral language development and little or no experience with literacy need high exposure and explicit teaching of phonemic awareness and segmenting. Phonological awareness is highly associated with early reading and writing development, especially as it relates to word recognition (decoding) and spelling (encoding). Therefore, it is an important ingredient to include in literacy instruction (Ball, 1997; Blachman, 1989; Catts, 1991; Clay, 1991; Cunningham & Allington, 1994; Liberman & Liberman, 1990; Snowling, 1995; Stanovich, 1986; Tunmer & Cole, 1991).

Because students enter school with varying degrees of understanding of the phonological structure of oral and written language, teachers, parents, and SLPs must determine the extent to which experiences and explicit teaching should receive focus in classrooms. In the early elementary grades, it is prudent to provide some instruction for all students. An early emphasis on awareness of syllables, rhymes, alliteration, sound–letter relationships, spelling patterns, invented reading and spelling, and so on, provide opportunities for students to gain phonological awareness and other metalinguistic information (e.g., grammatical structures, homonyms, silent letters). Adams (1990) stressed that phonological awareness involves developing knowledge of print: "Children must induce that print symbolizes language and that print holds information" (p. 60).

Activities that promote student awareness and knowledge of print at home and in the classroom include grocery lists, newspapers and books, letters and other mail, notes from parents and teachers, and labels on food or other items. These everyday uses of written language teach students how words look (e.g., word length and configuration) and the identity of letters in uppercase and lowercase forms, as well as provide opportunities to practice printing letters and writing whole words. Some ideas for teachers to help emergent readers to develop phonological awareness are included in Table 12.2 (Frost & Emery, 1996; Jenkins & Bowen, 1994). Instructional strategies should stress integration of language, metacognitive thinking, and practice for increasing students' ability to use phonological information automatically.

For students with language and learning problems, phonological awareness is often delayed. Such students require increased instruction and intense practice within *meaningful* language contexts so that they continue to develop in this area and consequently improve their success in reading and writing. Note, however, that phonological awareness is a part of oral and written language; therefore, students should have experiences in using their knowledge in authentic speaking, reading, and writing situations.

Ball (1997) described phonological awareness tasks as existing on a continuum of linguistic complexity. Simple tasks require shallow processing of phonological information, such as in sound play involving rhyme and alliteration. More complexity is required when students categorize or produce words according to their initial sounds and make rhymes by substituting the initial sound for another sound while retaining the rest of the syllable. For example, the word *fish* can be changed to *dish, wish,* and *swish.* Tasks involving rhymes are useful because they facilitate the ability to segment spoken and written language (Adams, 1990). Further complexity is inherent in tasks requiring segmentation of syllables and individual sounds in words. The alphabetic principle known as sound–symbol relationships requires segmentation of words into

Table 12.2
Interventions for Increasing Phonological Awareness

Integrated Instruction

- Reveal reading and spelling as companion processes by encouraging students to spell the words they can read.
- Provide regular practice with contextually meaningful materials.
- Introduce vocabulary and story components and encourage story retelling.

Promote Metacognitive Strategies

- Discuss the goals and purposes of each activity.
- Increase awareness of the similarities, differences, and patterns of speech sounds and symbols in words.
- Use modeling, verbal review, and relational language to increase metacognitive abilities.
- Use positive, explicit, and corrective feedback to increase students' understanding of errors during reading or writing.

Increase Phonemic Awareness and Its Relationship to Phonics

- Use rhymes, alliteration, or stories with predictable and repetitive sequences of words and phrases.
- Point out predictable sound and spelling patterns in words.
- Use flannel board stories to introduce sound–symbol relationships and orientation concepts such as top, bottom, left, and right.
- Encourage pretend reading of books.
- Discover segmentation and blending of syllables in words through tapping and counting games.
- Make rhymes or use key words to manipulate sounds within words.
- Read connected text, moving finger from word to word.
- Provide instruction in the alphabet principle through segmenting and blending activities.
- Use visual and manipulative materials to make phonemes concrete during segmenting and blending activities (e.g., add, delete, substitute, rearrange).
- Provide regular exposure and practice of words in connected and meaningful materials to increase word recognition and reading fluency.

sounds and the association of sounds to letters. The highest complexity of phonological awareness requires conscious analysis and manipulation of sounds within words. The ability to substitute, omit, add, and rearrange sounds is important for the development of spelling. For instance, the word *brink* can be changed to *ink* by deleting the first sound. The word *sunset* without *sun* is *set*. *Door* plus *knob* is *doorknob*. These progressively new insights about oral and written language are strengthened during guided and incidental literacy experiences within the home and classroom environments.

Explicit teaching of phonological awareness for students with language and learning problems should be structured so that linguistic complexity and context relevancy are kept in mind. Because students gain information about words gradually as they encounter them during a variety of tasks and complexity levels, it is likely that some students will become aware of an aspect of word segmentation or manipulation before another more complex aspect. Thus, instruction between levels of complexity should be fluid, allowing students to gain experience in a variety of phonological tasks. The levels of complexity are valuable for determining progress in phonological awareness and for making adjustments in the instruction, so that students are successful and continue to build competence in this area.

Decoding and Fluency

Students who have strong phonological awareness abilities learn to read from a natural progression of abilities they already possess. They sound out words, recognize whole-word sound and letter patterns, predict words from the semantic and syntactic context, and read for meaning. As students gain knowledge and experience in decoding words, they read larger units such as phrases and sentences quickly and automatically (Allington, 1983). As speed, fluency, and the ability to self-monitor develop, students increase the amount of reading and adopt silent reading in place of oral reading. They use all available cues necessary for fluent reading by engaging in reading for enjoyment, during functional daily living, and in learning new information. For these students, reading is both enjoyable and rewarding (Routman, 1991). Good readers become even better by reading. Clay (1991) described reading as a self-extending system, where good readers become better as a result of their own efforts, while poor readers fall further behind. She contended that good readers develop a "forward thrust" that enables them to develop, control, and use aspects of this self-extending system. Behavioral signs that teachers, parents, and SLPs can observe in students regarding the development of inner control include (a) facility with the oral language system in speaking, manipulating, and constructing meaning; (b) gaining concepts about print;

(c) attending to visual information contained in sentences, words, syllables, and letters; and (d) hearing sounds in oral language sequences.

"Decoding is the process of extracting sufficient information from printed word units so that the word's location in the mental lexicon and its associated meaning are activated. Stated in less technical terms, it is the process of recognizing printed words" (Tunmer & Cole, 1991, p. 388). Although word recognition is a necessary part of reading, the ability to recognize words is only one part of the reading process. Although single words are seen in the environment, such as on written labels or street signs, written words are typically in the context of sentences. In that the main purpose of reading is to comprehend what is written, individual words must be related to each other for the sentence to make sense. Thus, readers use word recognition strategies along with syntactic and semantic information to assist in decoding written sentences. Other cues such as sight word knowledge, the visual configuration of words, and knowledge about topics also help the reader. Thus, students make use of their knowledge of oral language to gain cues about written language. They read sentences with anticipation as they predict what came before and what is likely to come after words. It is not uncommon for students to substitute words based on their expectations from surrounding grammatical and semantic structures. As long as substitutions do not change the meaning of the sentence and disrupt comprehension, readers keep reading.

Students with language problems (e.g., poor phonological awareness, delayed knowledge and use of grammatical structures, semantic network and retrieval problems) find it difficult to use the phonological, syntactic, and semantic cues to recognize words during reading. Decoding is often very slow and unsuccessful much of the time, hampered by poor use of phonological information, poor prediction of the types of words being decoded (e.g., noun, adjective, verb), and limited vocabulary knowledge. Therefore, interventions for students with language problems must include strategies to help them recognize and use cues, many opportunities to practice reading and writing, and support and guidance as they learn to read and write.

Strategies for Early Elementary Students

Many decoding strategies are available for parents, teachers, SLPs, and students to choose from. Some students, especially those who have language or learning problems, require intensive exposure through first modeling and verbal mediation (often of strategies used by classmates), then explicit teaching of a variety of strategies, practice in their use, and, when applied, evaluation of their usefulness (Cunningham & Allington, 1994). This sequence of instruction is useful for teaching a variety of strategies, so that teachers, SLPs, and students discover which provide the greatest access to word recognition and under what circumstances. Notice that students who struggle with reading do not require *different* approaches than other students. Rather, they need explicit and intensive support and practice in authentic and meaningful activities, along with ongoing evaluation and adjustment toward the strategies they find most beneficial (see also Chapter 4 on the development of written language).

At the beginning of Table 12.3, some goals for teaching decoding and fluency strategies are listed. These goals serve as a reminder that reading encompasses much more than word recognition and speed. Although these two aspects are important and necessary, readers need to be able to monitor their reading so that the meaning is received and understood and so as to select appropriate strategies for accurate and efficient reading. To monitor comprehension and to select and use appropriate strategies, students need instruction in the decoding strategies as well as in metacognitive strategies that enable them to think about reading.

Young students benefit from seeing contextual print and hearing what it says from others (e.g., parents, teachers, SLPs, peers). As they develop word recognition from exposure to it, they begin to read more fluently with the model. Strategies such as *shared reading* provide students the opportunity to experience reading in an ongoing and meaningful manner (Cunningham & Allington, 1994; Rhodes & Dudley-Marling, 1996; Routman, 1991). Other similar techniques include *choral reading* (reading simultaneously) and *echo reading* (reading after the model). The first stories that early elementary teachers, parents, SLPs, and students might share are ones that are highly predictable; that is, they contain highly redundant yet interesting information, predictable sentence patterns, words used with high frequency, and pictures. Some stories that contain rhyming, alliteration, repeated expressions, and so forth, also provide opportunities for phonological awareness building and teaching word recognition patterns and rules.

As students attempt to read independently, they need assistance in decoding unknown words. Early elementary students are at different levels in this process, and some have strategies already in use, whereas others do not have such strategies or the strategies are not effective with them. It does not take long for teachers and SLPs to identify what strategies are in place and which need further development or alternatives. Thus, teachers, SLPs, and students must think about strategies that help the student decode. Metacognitive strategies seek to teach students to ask questions. During decoding, students ask whether words make sense in the context of the phrase or sentence given previous information. This question facilitates student thinking about semantic cues. If the word does not make sense, the student must then employ some specific decoding strategies. If it does make sense, the student can keep reading.

Table 12.3
Decoding and Fluency Strategies for Oral and Silent Reading

Goals

- Read for meaning
- Increase automaticity in letter and word recognition
- Relate word recognition to meaning
- Self-monitor oral and silent reading
- Select appropriate decoding strategies
- Repair miscues
- Monitor and adjust rate

Strategies

Use Predictable Contexts

- Assisted reading
- Shared reading
- Repeated reading (radio, choral, or echo reading; reader's theater)
- Sustained silent reading
- Recording and reading books
- Reading together or to younger children
- Reading different genres

Increase Metacognitive Strategies

- Think alouds
- Self-questioning (Does it make sense? sound right? look right?)
- Group questioning
- Discussion
- Peer assistance in selection and use of strategies

Promote Decoding Strategies

- Sound it out
- Stretch out the syllable
- Make meaningful substitutions
- Find smaller words or syllables within words
- Reread the sentence
- Use context cues

(*continues*)

Table 12.3 *Continued.*

Allow Practice Strategies

- Repeated reading
- Cloze procedures
- Phonemic awareness activities
- Phonemic analysis and synthesis activities

Encourage Rate and Fluency Strategies

- Read phrases as meaningful units
- Use context to predict grammar and meaning
- Adjust speed depending on purpose for reading
- Practice reading at independent levels with variations in speed
- Practice reading aloud, then silently
- Practice rate flexibility techniques

Students should also ask whether the word sounds right, that is, think about the word in relation to the syntactic characteristics of the surrounding words. In English, nouns precede and follow verbs but adjectives only precede nouns. Finally, students ask whether words look right. This question alerts the students to focus on the letters making up words and directs their attention to prefixes, suffixes, and word configurations.

When students encounter words they do not know, several decoding strategies can be used. A *sounding-out strategy* is common, yet some students have difficulty retrieving sound–symbol relationships, whereas others have difficulty synthesizing the parts into a combined whole. Other strategies that rely on knowledge of phonics include *stretching the word* so that syllables receive emphasis, *trying word substitutions* or best guesses based on how the word looks, and *breaking words into smaller known words*. Strategies that focus more on deriving meaning from surrounding context include *rereading the sentence to predict words*, *using syntactic and semantic cues*, and *isolating parts of sentences to direct student focus*.

In addition to the goals discussed previously, Table 12.3 provides strategies for the development of fluency. "Fluent reading is characterized by a rapid and smooth processing of text and an apparently effortless construction of meaning" (Rhodes & Dudley-Marling, 1996, p. 154). Reading fluency is facilitated when students broaden their focus from individual word recognition to the construction of meaning, take advantage of their knowledge of the interrelated language systems, and take risks (Rhodes & Dudley-Marling, 1996). Fluency develops simultaneously with word recognition as students gain knowledge and experience. Further, the level of fluency is dependent on the type of material students are reading. For example, first-time reading of new information is often read at a slower rate and errors in decoding occur due to unfamiliarity. Through experience, however, subsequent readings become more rapid and smooth. Proficient readers develop an awareness of how they and others read fluently during oral and silent reading. Less proficient readers do not develop this awareness. They need more explicit teaching of what proficient readers do when they read. For example, Rhodes and Dudley-Marling (1996) suggested that students watch more proficient readers and note particular behaviors, interview others about reading, and directly discuss with teachers and others their beliefs and attitudes about reading.

Many of the strategies already mentioned facilitate the development of reading fluency. For early elementary students and students with severe reading problems, techniques should be used that provide opportunities for students to participate at a higher level of functioning through modeling and scaffolding (Pearson & Gallagher, 1983). Support is gradually decreased as students are able to take more of the responsibility for reading. *Assisted and repeated reading techniques* are useful because they provide the student with a proficient model and support during reading, as well as plentiful opportunities to practice reading for fluency (Rhodes & Dudley-Marling, 1996). Students are invited to hear others read and then to read along with others as they gradually assume more responsibility for recognizing words and using their knowledge of context and language systems to predict words within sentences. Assisted reading opportunities can be provided that do not require the teacher–student, direct instruction format. Several alternatives, discussed by Rhodes and Dudley-Marling, include unison reading within pairs or small groups of students, prerecorded tapes with headphones for student practice, captioned videos, parent participation, and teacher aide assistance. As students develop fluency at one level, practice should occur at that level so that they experience reading in an easy and almost effortless manner. Students can experiment with reading faster and slower or using visual aids to keep place or encourage faster reading. Some readers read faster during silent reading because they do not have to pronounce each word aloud as when reading orally. Thus, oral reading can be followed by silent reading so that students experience reading when pronunciation is eliminated as a factor. Some activities that use repeated reading to promote fluency and comprehension include radio reading (students read to an audience to convey meaning), readers theater (scripts of plays), choral reading (interpretive reading of text), recording books (self-evaluation and assisted reading for younger children), reading to younger children, reading different formats of the same text, and sustained silent reading (scheduled periods of silent reading each day) (Rhodes & Dudley-Marling, 1996).

Strategies for Older Elementary and Middle School Students

By the fourth grade most students read with high accuracy and fluency. Thus, teachers expect reading assignments to be completed correctly and independently. Some students, however, are not independent readers during later elementary school and middle school. They require continued support during reading tasks in classrooms. Classrooms that provide integrated language experiences are excellent environments for instruction and support in written language development. General education teachers, special educators, and SLPs collaborate to provide instruction and support for individual students who have written language needs.

For older students, assessment of the nature of the problem must include information about past assessment, instruction, and remediation techniques. It is not helpful to students when they are assessed repeatedly only to find similar results, or when they receive the same instruction that has proven to be unsuccessful. Often the student has insightful understandings about his or her own difficulties. Teachers and SLPs should discuss with their students what successes and difficulties they have. Once the strengths and weaknesses are identified, joint decisions can be made regarding the nature and extent of instruction. Some students will need instruction and practice in metacognitive strategies, using graphophonemic, syntactic, and semantic cues during reading, and strategies for recognition and repair of miscues. Others will need focused instruction in particular reading strategies. Teachers, parents, SLPs, and other specialists must work collaboratively to construct a plan that provides such instruction within and throughout the student's curriculum.

For older students with moderate to severe reading problems, all of the techniques previously mentioned can be modified for appropriate use, taking age, interests, and reading level into consideration. Although all may not be appropriate as classroom activities, parents, teacher aides, and student assistants can help individual students in small groups or during individual practice time at school, during focused pull-out intervention sessions if necessary, and in the home.

Consider John, the 13-year-old eighth-grade student described earlier in the section on assessment. Because John has not developed independent reading accuracy and fluency, his comprehension of reading is also poor. In addition, his delayed oral language skills most likely have resulted in reduced metacognitive strategies and use of linguistic cues during reading. Poor reading ability reduces this student's access to information enjoyed by other students.

For John, poor reading is a barrier to academic success. John's intervention team has the challenge of determining how reading can be improved within a curriculum that focuses on content-area knowledge. In the past, this student would have been removed from his eighth-grade classroom for part of the day to receive focused instruction in reading. This approach to reading instruction often lacks integration and changes substantially the curriculum other students are receiving within the classroom. Contextual instruction and practice may help students learn new strategies during reading, but these strategies need practical application so that students become more successful reading within their classrooms.

Teachers with an integrated approach use supportive strategies to enhance reading during classroom activities. For instance, a peer assistant might be engaged to support John during silent reading. When an unknown word is encountered, John must use a think-aloud strategy (modeled previously by the teacher, parent, or peer) to select from several decoding strategies (e.g., reread, substitute a word that makes sense, break the word into syllables), which can be provided in a notebook with examples. The assistant can then respond to each decoding attempt by confirming that the strategy resulted in correct decoding or by instructing the student to try another strategy.

John can also keep a journal of difficult words that can be practiced for increased automatic recognition. Not every miscued word should be recorded in the journal; rather the student determines which words are likely to be encountered again.

Another strategy to help John gain access to the information is for small groups to read the text silently and then discuss what was read. Although John may continue to have difficulty reading, he benefits from the discussion about the text's content. As John rereads the text, he can think about the information previously discussed. Discussion prior to reading is also helpful for all students because they activate background knowledge and use prediction to anticipate what the text contains. Key vocabulary can be introduced orally and on the board or in a handout so that students recognize and understand new words.

Older students who want to improve their rate should be taught rate flexibility techniques (Mullen, 1987). Rate flexibility involves consciously recognizing and adjusting reading speed depending on the reading situations. Table 12.3 also includes some options for helping students determine an appropriate reading rate based on student needs, materials, and situations. For example, students can deliberately read faster when the goal is to determine the main ideas of paragraphs in expository texts or the gist of a narrative story. Reading can be slowed down when details are being sought or new information is being read that requires reflection.

Comprehension

Reutzel and Cooter (1996) described reading comprehension as obtaining meaning from written material by categorizing new information and associating with prior knowledge. However, reading is not simply a transfer process where readers decode, categorize, and associate information. It is an interactive process that requires individuals to become engaged in thinking and reasoning for a variety of reasons during many different situational contexts. Therefore, reading competence must be considered within a social perspective as well as an academic one. Four ingredients—interest, mind-set, purpose, and mental schema—must be considered in helping students develop and improve comprehension of written texts.

A student's *interest* in reading is a key factor in comprehension. Each student has several interest areas, often because of previous experience. Interest is important because background knowledge and experience with topics can be used to engage the reader in reading and discussion, which sets the stage for increased motivation to read further about the topic. In addition, background knowledge helps students make sense of written materials and recognize its meaningfulness and relevance in their lives (Poplin, 1988; Rhodes & Dudley-Marling, 1996).

Choice is an important ingredient in reading development. "The additional freedom offered by choice increases the probability of accomplishment for a reader" (Hansen, 1987, p. 28). Therefore, students need access to many different books that vary in topic and level of difficulty. Students choose books as they become acquainted with materials made available in classrooms, libraries, and home; as they see others choosing books; as they read and enjoy specific topics and authors; and as they try a variety of books at varying difficulty levels (Hansen, 1987).

Choice has been shown to be important for students who have difficulty reading. Fink (1996) conducted interviews with 12 adults with dyslexia who eventually developed competence in reading through persistence in using decoding strategies, reading avidly, and reading about topics that were of passionate interest. Fink found that their reading fluency developed 3 to 4 years later (about 10 to 12 years of age) than peers and word recognition difficulties remained to some extent. In addition, as children, they relied on context to a great extent for simple word identification and comprehension, which was more reliable when a familiar topic was being read. Despite these difficulties, all of the adults had passionate interests and read very specific types of information. Their knowledge of the text structure (i.e., genre), through previous reading experiences and knowledge of the topic, enabled them to be accurate readers, writers, and professionals in specific fields. The implication for classroom teachers regarding instruction for students with reading problems was stated strongly by Fink: "Teachers should provide captivating materials based on each student's strengths, prior knowledge, skills, and interests" (p. 277). This study also has implications for leisure reading in the home. Parents should encourage their children to select materials that are interesting and motivating. For instance, a teenage girl may willingly read and enjoy a teen magazine about clothes, makeup, dating, and music rather than a novel about something that does not interest her.

The second important ingredient for reading development is the *mind-set* of the reader. Because reading is an interactive process, students must be able to focus attention and concentrate on the text. When interest is high and the student is ready to read, focused attention and concentration allow the student to decode and comprehend the text. However, when interest is low or when the student is distracted either by external factors (e.g., noise, movement, talking) or internal factors (e.g., anxiety, restlessness, negative feelings and attitudes), reading can be disjointed and unproductive. Some readers can decode text almost unconsciously as they think about something else. It is only after reading a paragraph or even an entire page that the lack of comprehension becomes evident to the reader. Proficient readers recognize this problem and refocus attention and concentration, reread the text, or stop reading altogether. Less proficient readers have difficulty self-monitoring (see Chapter 4). It may take such readers longer to recognize their own lack of attention and concentration and repair strategies are less likely to occur.

Comprehension involves thinking about what is read within the context of the *author's purpose* as well as the *reader's purpose* for engaging in the act of reading. This third ingredient allows readers to adjust their mind-set and the way in which they engage in reading. For instance, a novel that takes place in a historical context, such as Michener's (1974) *Centennial,* can certainly inform the reader about past events in the United States. Reading, then, can be directed toward obtaining historical facts. However, when given as an assignment in a high school literature class, students may engage in critical analysis of the text structure, explore the motivations of characters, and discuss literary devices the author uses. In this example, comprehension involves critical thinking and reasoning, which students demonstrate through discussion, comparison, reflection, and perhaps writing. These activities require much more than reading for basic understanding or for enjoyment of the story as setting, characters, episode, and resolution unfold.

Purposes for reading vary, just as purposes for speaking depend on situations and goals. Teachers ask students to read for many different reasons, including (a) broadening their interest about topics; (b) giving them practice reading; (c) teaching strategies for decoding or comprehension; (d) gaining new information; (e) providing background for discussion; (f) assessing reading skills; (g) accessing content knowledge; (h) engaging in reflection, analysis, comparison; and (i) extending knowledge for writing. Most students learn to recognize what type of reading the situation calls for and adjust their reading strategies accordingly. They adjust attention, concentration, effort, speed, decoding accuracy, and comprehension and memory strategies depending on what purposes they identify as important. Less proficient readers are less flexible in recognizing situational cues that alert them to purpose and they have difficulty making adjustments in how they read to suit specific situations (Rhodes & Dudley-Marling, 1996).

In addition to interest, mind-set, and purpose, students comprehend texts more fully when they have a *mental schema* about narrative and expository text structures, as well as other literary genres (e.g., poetry, letters). Students obtain experience with narratives and poetry early on through storybook reading, nursery rhymes, and songs in the home and preschool. As they listen and respond to adults and other children, they learn about the predictable nature of these genres. Such knowledge about the text structure helps them anticipate and use it when they read independently. Although some expository texts may be used by some parents and teachers during the preschool years, the predominant genre is narrative because of the high interest children have in stories.

During the elementary grades and beyond, students read textbooks or select library books around particular topics. The text structure of expository reading (see Chapter 2) is much different from that of narratives and requires students to develop a mental schema based on titles and subtitles; introductions and summaries; pictures, graphs, and charts; italicized or underlined key concepts; and other devices that help readers understand, organize, and remember information. Students must learn to focus on the text structure as a way to explore the content of the text.

Narrative and expository text structures are learned as students gain experience in their use and as the special features of each are brought to an awareness through instruction. Students who have language problems often do not show interest in text structure differences and find the structures difficult to learn. Such students need explicit teaching and many examples of structures found in reading material, so that the mental schemas for the structures become an avenue for comprehension of texts during reading.

Comprehension will, of course, be influenced by the reader's ability to decode using graphophonic, semantic, and syntactic cues, as well as to adjust speed and fluency. Decoding and fluency skills in combination with the four ingredients (interest, mind-set, purpose, schema) discussed previously require that all these components be part of the reading curriculum throughout the school years. Comprehension strategies, though, cannot be taught as separate skills according to a preset time schedule. Rather, strategies to derive meaning from text *must* be integrated into all literacy opportunities throughout each day (Hagerty, 1994). Comprehension instruction involves assisting, defining, demonstrating, modeling, describing, and explaining (Reutzel & Cooter, 1996). While teachers can assess students' ability to answer questions through writing or circling choices on worksheets, comprehension strategies are not *taught* through these practices.

Instructional methods for reading comprehension are most effective when they involve the reader in applying active strategies for deriving meaning from text. Because all students require strategies for reading comprehension, it is appropriate and desirable for teachers, SLPs, parents, and students to experiment with strategies as partners engaged in discovery. Knowing that students have different experiences and levels of success with reading, and knowing that students with language problems face challenges in the development of reading, team members must recognize that quick fixes are rare and one approach does not fit all students' needs (Allington & Walmsley, 1995). Therefore, they must be flexible and allow students plenty of time to try strategies in a variety of contexts. Students must be encouraged to evaluate the usefulness of strategies so that they can practice successful ones, abandon unsuccessful ones, and experiment with new ones.

Comprehension strategies for narrative and expository texts are listed in Table 12.4. They are divided into three main areas of active participation focusing on what the reader does prior to reading (prediction), during reading (self-monitoring), and as a follow-up to reading (reflection).

Prediction Strategies

Readers can improve comprehension of texts by engaging in strategies that foster prediction. Clay (1991) recommended that adults and peers orient students to books prior to reading by drawing attention to important ideas, discussing pictures (or other visual cues), and providing opportunities for students to hear new words that are contained in the text. In other words, readers should determine the purpose for reading text (e.g., for enjoyment, to learn about a topic, to compare information) and think about the topic or theme based on their own experiences. Teachers and SLPs guide students in using prediction when they ask them to brainstorm questions or recall knowledge about a topic. Students can generate questions that they think will be answered in the text ("From this title I think the story is about . . ."), and teachers and SLPs can use these questions as a basis for scaffolding so that the questions and discussions become focused. Team members may provide opportunities for students to preview the text by looking through it for cues about what the story or

Table 12.4
Comprehension Strategies for Narrative and Expository Texts

Prediction

Goals

- Set purpose for reading
- Preview text and vocabulary
- Activate prior knowledge
- Link prior knowledge to new information

Strategies

- Brainstorming
- Self-generated questions
- Previewing text
- Think alouds
- Prereading plan (PreP)
- Survey, question, read, recite, review
- What you know, want to know, learned
- Directed reading and thinking activity

Self-Monitoring

Goals

- Read fluently
- Self-correct
- Question
- Predict
- Reread
- Revoice and paraphrase
- Summarize content
- Self-appropriate strategies
- Use visualization
- Use metacognitive strategies

(*continues*)

Table 12.4 *Continued.*

Strategies

- Self-generated questions
- Think alouds
- Backtracking
- Margin notes and highlighting
- Writing summaries
- Interactive reading guides
- Story, event, or concept maps
- Mental imagery
- Creating analogies
- Modeling experiences
- Graphic organizers

Reflection

Goals

- Critique and evaluate
- Recognize part-to-whole and whole-to-part relationships
- Analyze information
- Apply information
- Discover new insights
- Create associations

Strategies

- Small group discussions
- Reciprocal teaching
- Question–answer relationships
- Role plays, debates, drama
- Creative writing
- Graphic organizers and semantic maps
- Story and text frames
- Written book reports
- Written reaction logs
- Written dialogue journals
- Creative art forms

chapter is about, such as by attending to titles and subtitles, pictures or graphs, the summary, and study questions. The goal of teaching prediction strategies is to increase student awareness of the cues provided by different text structures so that the cues can be used to comprehend the information during reading. Educators can choose from a variety of strategies to accomplish the goal. Notice that the strategies are metacognitive in that they focus student attention on thinking, reasoning, remembering, and organizing information.

Self-Monitoring Strategies

When students are engaged in reading, they need strategies to monitor their own comprehension of the text. Self-monitoring involves being able to keep track of one's own decoding and fluency skills, using self-correction strategies when needed. Self-monitoring also involves self-questioning during reading as information is comprehended. Students learn the value of reading information more than once and gradually gain ability to paraphrase the information and construct summaries.

Reading instruction must include strategies that enhance students' abilities to comprehend texts independently. Comprehension involves not only understanding the content of what is read, but also the ability to critique and evaluate the information. Critical reading involves categorizing new knowledge, associating it with previously learned information, and questioning its accuracy and relevance in relation to the reader's purpose.

Flexibility in the selection of strategies is also an important aspect of comprehension monitoring. When misinterpretations occur during reading, students not only must recognize the source of the problem (e.g., decoding error, ambiguous meaning, missed line of text), but must select and use appropriate strategies leading to the repair of the misinterpretation. Several strategies can be taught to readers that assist them in comprehension monitoring. Some examples included in Table 12.4 are helpful for improving reading fluency and repair, whereas others focus on the student's active participation in thinking, reasoning, and evaluating texts. Such strategies include mental imagery ("I see the scene in my head"), creating analogies ("This reminds me of ______"), thinking aloud when a problem is encountered ("This word ______ is new to me"), and modeling experiences ("How would I feel in this situation?"). The following example shows how a self-monitoring strategy can be used. In the Newbery award–winning book, *The Giver,* by Lois Lowry (1993), Jonas is receiving memory for his community. He is surprised when he sees colors, because people in his community see only black and white. The reader does not know this right away, however, so to make sense of the text at that point, the reader can use a self-questioning or a metacognitive think-aloud strategy, such as "I wonder what's so unusual about Jonas seeing a red sled? I thought when he has foggy images, it's because he sees into the beyond. Jonas thought this too. As I read on, I found out it was him being able to see color."

Reflection Strategies

Reflection strategies to facilitate comprehension are also important for students to employ after reading texts, because they engage students in activities that promote remembering what was read, relating new information to prior knowledge, applying information to personal knowledge and experience, analyzing meanings, creating associations, and evaluating the quality and usefulness of information. Techniques that promote interaction between students (e.g., small group or class discussion, reciprocal teaching) allow them to benefit from the perceptions of others as students create and respond to questions, summarize information, and reenact portions of text. Many strategies involving writing are used by students to organize information for enhancing understandings of relationships (e.g., semantic maps, graphic organizers), to assist with writing after reading (e.g., story and text frames, creative writing), and to summarize or reflect on what has been read (e.g., written book reports, written reaction logs, written dialogue journals). Finally, occasionally team members can engage students in projects that involve artistic media such as creating models, dioramas, maps, cartoons, films, brochures, photography, and drawings, or through dance, drama, role plays, and debates.

Summary

Reading and writing instruction results in successful comprehension and expression for most students when it is balanced across several components. Students who have severe reading and writing problems may benefit from intensive phonological coding and phonemic awareness training, but as skills develop they must be reembedded in authentic reading and writing activities.

Students learn to segment the language and recognize its many components during home and preschool activities. The observations that we ask students to make about language components when they enter school can vary in complexity. Therefore, educationists should analyze the difficulty of phonological coding and phonemic awareness activities and adjust expectations or scaffold when students encounter problems.

Many teaching and learning strategies are available to teachers, SLPs, and students for improving decoding and fluency during reading. Word recognition strategies focus on the identification and use of cues (e.g., phonological, semantic, syntactic) and the benefits of practice within meaningful texts. Instruction in word recognition and fluency should be context embedded and should be accompanied by instruction in employing metacognitive strategies, such as self-monitoring and self-questioning.

Teachers, specialists, SLPs, and parents assist students' comprehension of texts by (a) providing opportunities to read in areas of high interest, (b) helping them regulate mind-set, (c) clearly conveying or helping students determine purposes for reading, and (d) developing mental schemas for different types of text structures. Further, teachers help students acquire comprehension strategies that can be effectively used prior to reading, during reading, and as a follow-up to reading that involve the student in active participation with others and the development of thinking and reasoning abilities. Prediction, comprehension monitoring, and reflection strategies engage the reader in construction of meaning through thoughtful interaction with texts. The strategies should be taught and practiced during authentic reading activities in the elementary grades. In the middle and high school years, students should select strategies that maximize comprehension. Students who have language problems will likely need assistance in determining which strategies are most beneficial and support in the use of strategies during classroom, small group, and individual reading activities.

4 Teaching Writing

Most children observe writing in their home and community environments long before they begin school. They see parents making lists, paying bills, writing notes, and writing on computers; siblings completing homework assignments, writing notes to friends, and writing for enjoyment; and community workers such as bank tellers, waitpersons, ministers, and salespersons writing as a function of their jobs. These early experiences sustain the motivations of preschool-age children to pick up writing utensils such as crayons, pens, or chalk, and play with keyboards on typewriters and computers to experiment with writing. Through feedback from others and their own ability to learn from experiences, children discover that symbols convey meaning. Thus, for most children, these early activities lead to continued success with writing as more formal instruction occurs in schools (Zinsser, 1988) (see also Chapter 4).

Children who have language problems are often those who have not engaged in early writing behaviors. They may not have had the opportunity to find experimentation with writing to be enjoyable or profitable. In addition, when children have delayed oral language skills or poor visual or motor skills, adults may limit writing opportunities due to belief that such competencies are necessarily precursors to written language development. It is important, then, that parents, teachers, SLPs, and other specialists recognize the importance of early experiences with writing, so that the writing process is developed along with the interest to write.

In the previous section, four ingredients were identified as important for the development of reading: interest, mind-set, purpose, and mental schema. These ingredients are also important considerations as students begin to write. Students benefit from making choices about what they write about, and when students have personal interests and reasons for writing, the outcome is both more relevant and more useful (Zinsser, 1988). As students gain positive experiences with writing, they begin to take more risks without the fear and frustrations that are sometimes associated with writing. Additionally, through reading and writing experiences, along with teaching of different types of writing schemas, students learn to vary their writing for different purposes.

Writing is a process that develops through instruction, practice, and feedback. Because it is an interactive process, however, it cannot be taught effectively as an isolated subject comprised of discrete skills. Writers learn to write for a variety of purposes and with varying degrees of formality and structure depending on the situations and purposes they have for writing. For example, a note written by one classmate to another may be on a small scrap of paper hastily written in pencil with little attention to complete sentences, proper grammatical form, and spelling accuracy. The same student may write a well-formed paragraph summarizing a book chapter as an assignment for a science class. Indeed, at all levels, students are capable of understanding and internalizing purposes for writing. However, for some students, especially those with language problems, explicit information about the purposes and types of writing along with instruction in spelling is necessary.

Writing is one way that individuals communicate with others, but it is also a vehicle for intrapersonal thinking and reasoning. When we write our thoughts, we clarify ideas, sequence them in logical ways, and extend our own understanding of topics through reflection. In fact, writing is an emergent process that requires "percolation" as we engage in thinking, writing, reflection, and rewriting (Routman, 1991). Therefore, teachers can facilitate thinking and reasoning in students by promoting writing as a way to learn (Zinsser, 1988). Students also benefit from hearing other writers talk about the process of writing. Discussion about what writers do when they write brings students to an awareness of the process and encourages individuals to think about what they do. This metacognitive activity helps students to think about writing as communication.

Process

Writers engage in a process involving several components. Some call them prewriting, writing, and rewriting, whereas others refer to them as rehearsal, drafting, revision, editing, and publishing (Calkins, 1994). Although the components appear to be organized sequentially, proficient writers continuously revisit and revise their work in a spiral-like manner. This allows them to interact with their writing as an integrated process.

Rehearsal

Rehearsal is engaged in as writers determine their interests in topics, purposes for writing, and the intended audience. Young writers and students with language and learning problems often benefit from some discussion about these issues and even some choices to narrow their selections. For example, teachers can provide choices regarding topics, purposes, and variations of target audiences. Choices that are not selected for one assignment can be reserved for another so that students gain multiple experiences. Rehearsal also includes gathering information about the topic prior to writing. For young writers this may involve activating background knowledge and experience such as with brainstorming, asking others what they know, reading or listening to books from libraries, watching films, and so on. Older students may be expected to find multiple sources from libraries, access information from the Internet, or conduct experiments. As information is gathered, students can take notes, retell the information to others, or tape-record summaries of information. As the writer begins to write, the information, purpose, and audience must be continually kept in mind and the work must be revisited to maintain these aspects as the work develops.

Drafting and Revising

Drafting and revising occur as writers put ideas on paper. The writer must attend to many aspects of writing, including selecting the genre, conveying ideas, organizing information, constructing grammatical sentences, selecting words, and spelling words. Any one or all of these aspects can be difficult for writers, resulting in slow and inaccurate attempts. However, the very nature of these stages allows writers to revise their product and make changes in each aspect as they read and reflect on the work. Revision can and should occur numerous times so that writers continue to develop and refine writing as a communication tool.

Editing

Editing involves proofreading and correcting. The writer must stand apart from his or her text and look critically at it so that it can be refined. The writer rereads the text, looking specifically for errors in sentence structure and grammatical forms, spelling, punctuation, word choice, and conveyance of ideas. Editing is a continuous process during writing and it should be incorporated into instruction right from the beginning so that writers include it in the earliest stages of writing. Students learn through instruction and practice that correct use of language is both important and powerful (Graves, 1994).

Sharing and Publishing

The last component of writing is called sharing and publishing, which provides opportunities for writers to use it as a form of social interaction. The interaction can take many different forms, such as individual or group discussion about the topic, constructive criticism about the writing itself, interaction about how the topic can be expanded, discussion from opposing viewpoints, and so forth. Students invite others such as friends, family members, teachers, and classmates to read their work and engage in some form of interaction. Some key learning outcomes of publishing texts have been suggested in *Dancing with the Pen: The Learner as Writer* (1995):

1. Learners are interested and motivated to publish their work.
2. They consider and use design in the presentation of text.
3. They take audience into account.
4. They dialogue about the layout of texts with other students.
5. They learn about and practice various publishing media, forms, and styles.
6. They use resources and time effectively.

The sharing and publishing of writing allows students to celebrate writing and to showcase their work. Sharing places high value on writing, and emphasis placed on producing polished products motivates students to consider giving their writings as gifts.

Structure

Students learn about the stages of writing through daily experiences with reading what others have written and engaging in writing for a variety of purposes. Yet, students need instruction in these components as they extend their writing abilities. Some students, who find writing difficult, need greater amounts of instruction, guidance, and support. Teachers, specialists, and SLPs must observe students as they write to determine the amount and level of support each student needs.

Cunningham and Allington (1994) suggested several strategies for supporting students' writing development in classrooms. These are (a) shared and group writing activities, (b) writing before and after reading, (c) modeling the writing process, (d) modeling specific writing genres and forms, and (e) writing with computers. Notice how most of these strategies involve a community of learners who interact among themselves and with teachers to improve writing (Hansen, 1987). Some of the strategies also allow students time to write alone. However, interaction with others about the writing can occur whenever necessary.

Shared and group writing activities are similar to shared and group reading activities discussed earlier. In the early elementary grades, teachers may involve children in shared writing by engaging them in discussion about a topic, then recording the ideas in well-formed standard English. After reading the sentences aloud, the teacher, specialist, or SLP can ask students to provide input about expanding ideas, editing sentence length, modifying word choice, and correcting spelling and punctuation errors. Older students might listen to a movie or lecture, taking notes during the presentation. Afterward, they can compare notes and modify them to reflect all the ideas. Group writing typically involves students in pairs or small groups who construct a document together by engaging in dialogue and participating in various roles (e.g., writing, editing, sharing ideas). This cooperative learning situation results in a draft that contains the best efforts of the group. Young writers will need more guidance and support from teachers as they construct their drafts. Older students should be more independent in writing, but each student contributes to the whole and learns from peers' strengths.

Because reading and writing are connected processes, teachers and SLPs should deliberately tie them together in instruction. When students read about a topic before writing about it, they think about the topic in an organized fashion with old and new background information readily available. Reading prior to writing also activates interest and purpose for writing, as well as provides a concrete example of how the topic is presented within a specific text genre (e.g., narration, exposition, poetry). As students read, they can use techniques such as constructing graphic organizers, answering prepared questions, outlining, and creating response logs that contain thoughts, feelings, and predictions. Each of these techniques can include prepared frames that guide students to discover specific types of information. For example, if the reading lesson is about the training of astronauts, students can read to identify the types of training involved (e.g., technical training about the ship, training about how the body responds in weightless conditions, scientific training for conducting experiments). A graphic organizer in the form of a semantic web can be provided to help students categorize such information. Older students might receive an outline structure to guide them in organizing and summarizing main ideas and supporting information.

When students write before reading, they focus their attention on a topic and recall information from previous experiences with the topic. They can participate in discussion and write what they know about the topic prior to reading more about it. After reading they can add to their informational list or paragraphs. This technique is particularly useful for students who have difficulty focusing their mind-set to the topic, activating prior knowledge, or becoming motivated to read.

Proficient writers are typically keen observers who both watch and listen to others. Thus, modeling is an important avenue teachers can use to teach students about writing. A think-aloud strategy along with demonstration of writing helps students see and hear what writers think about. The dialogue and modeling during sentence construction, word selection, spelling, and editing allows students direct access to a teacher's thinking. Young writers benefit from high exposure to modeling. Modeling can be replaced gradually by cooperative learning as students notice errors and begin to offer ideas about how to correct them.

Young children love to listen to stories read aloud by family members and caregivers; thus story schemes are familiar to most children as they enter school. Poetry and songs may be familiar to students from families who read nursery rhymes aloud and listen to children's songs on tapes or videos. However, we cannot assume that all kindergarten students have been exposed to these forms, and other text structures may not be at all familiar. Therefore, different forms of writing should be modeled and taught in the early grades. For example, when stories are being read, students should focus on predictable schemes that stories contain (e.g., setting, characters, event or problem, solution, ending) and expanded schemes as stories become more complex.

When content-area books are introduced, students should be instructed in their purposes; the use of titles and subtitles; the use of visual aids such as graphs, charts, and figures; study questions presented at the beginning or end of chapters; and so forth. Other forms of texts, such as letters, poems, instructional manuals, and summaries, should be modeled and discussed. Rather than teach each genre as a separate entity using distinct instructional methods, teachers can use strategies that promote success across genres (Conrad, 1997). Familiarity with genres can be facilitated first by having students read examples so that they gain exposure to text content and structure. Discussion about the text structure can highlight the common elements within narratives and expository structures. Next, story or text frames can be used to engage students in thinking about how the elements are constructed. Such frames contain open-ended sentences that guide students in text organization based on the genre being used. Teachers can engage inexperienced writers in shared learning activities where modeling is used during completion of the frame. More experienced writers can complete frames on their own and expand their creativity in word choice, sentence structure, and use of cohesive devices.

Expository writing is often more complicated than other forms for students. This is because texts contain new and varied content with unfamiliar vocabulary within topics, and most students lack experience with the text structures (Conrad, 1997; Rhodes & Dudley-Marling, 1996). In addition, several types of expository structures are possible, including problem–solution, compare–contrast, sequence, cause–effect, and time order (see Figure 12.1). Text frames that make the structures explicit help students recognize the structures during reading, learn key words and phrases for writing, and guide them toward being able to write using the structures appropriate to each type. More experienced students can compare text structures across different expository texts. For example, as students research about astronomy, they can compare a problem–solution text with one that has a compare–contrast structure. Additionally, students can practice writing in different styles by using text frames.

Text structure (see also Chapter 2) is important for the development of writing, as is paragraph structure. Students must learn about the words and phrases that convey relationships in accord with the selected text structure. For example, in writing about volcanos using a cause–effect structure, students may include phrases such as these: "Volcanos are *(definition)*. They occur when *(explanation)*. The gases *(process)*. The results *(effects)* of volcanoes (e.g., effects on vegetation, animals, atmosphere, people, property)." The use of key words can also be effective in guiding students to structure paragraphs. For instance, in a text involving a sequence of ideas or steps, words such as *first, second, next*, and *after* may be suggested.

Students must also practice paragraph structure to include a topic sentence, elaborated ideas about the topic, and a conclusion. One way to organize paragraphs is to use occasion–position statements for topic sentences, followed by explanations, and ending with a conclusion. The occasion–position is a two-part topic sentence that introduces the reason for writing (e.g., event, problem, idea, circumstance), called the occasion, and what is going to be explained, the position statement. Several explanatory sentences follow the position, and finally a conclusion restates or summarizes the position from the topic sentence to finish the paragraph (Auman, 1993).

In a science class, students may be studying about rivers and oceans, which includes study of the water cycle. A student can begin writing a paragraph

TEXT FRAMES

Problem-Solution Text Structure

__________ had a problem because __________.
Therefore, __________.
As a result, __________.
Problem something bad; a situation that people would like to change
Action what people do to try and solve the problem
Results what happens as a result of the action; the effect or outcome of trying to solve the problem

Compare/Contrast Text Structure

Comparison

__________ and __________ are similar in several ways. Both __________ and __________ have similar __________. Also, both __________ __________.

Contrast

__________ and __________ are different in several ways. First of all, __________, while __________. Secondly, __________. In addition, while __________, __________. Finally, __________, while __________.

Sequence Text Structure

Here is how a __________ is made. First, __________. Next, __________. Then, __________. Finally, __________.

Cause and Effect Text Structure

Because of __________, __________. __________ caused __________. Finally, due to __________, __________. This explains why __________.

Time Order Text Structure

The events leading up to __________ were: First, __________. Second, __________. Third, __________. Fourth, __________. Finally, __________.

Adapted from Armbruster, Anderson & Ostertag (1989)

Figure 12.1. Expository text frames. From "Exploring Informational Text with Students," by L. L. Conrad, 1997, *Colorado Reading Council Journal, 8,* p. 7. Copyright 1997 by the Colorado Council Internation Reading Association. Reprinted with permission.

about the water cycle by using the occasion "water is everywhere" and the position "as it cycles it takes different forms": "As long as there is water everywhere, it will be cycling through different forms." The following sentences of the paragraph explain the position of the water cycle through the different forms: "First of all, water evaporates from lakes, rivers, and oceans. Next, the water vapor rises, cools, and forms clouds." The explanations continue until all of the cycle is explained. The last sentence restates the position for a conclusion: "In fact, water is continuously cycling through different forms at the same time."

A related strategy for helping students write paragraphs is the puzzle strategy. The teacher, specialist, or SLP cuts apart paragraphs into sentences and students rearrange and paste them in a logical manner. This metacognitive task heightens awareness of how key words, text structure, and the flow of ideas are conveyed through writing.

As computers become common in households and classrooms, students have greater access to their use for writing. Software programs provide several opportunities for students to develop writing skills, including word processing; organizing texts; creating professional looking reports, newsletters, and advertisements; using visual aids such as graphs, charts, and pictures; and editing for grammar and spelling errors (Cunningham & Allington, 1994).

Form

In addition to learning about the process and structure of writing, students must learn about form. Knowledge about written language form includes grammatical relationships such as subject–verb agreement, use of parts of speech in the noun and verb phrases (e.g., pronouns, articles, adjectives, prepositions, adverbs), capitalization and punctuation rules, and spelling. Formal instruction of these elements is often incorporated during the early grades as students learn to read and write. However, because students write from their own experiences using their own language abilities, teachers, specialists, and SLPs must use strategies that take advantage of authentic writing attempts in all grades.

Conferencing

A powerful strategy that encourages students, teachers, and SLPs to work in an interactive manner is conferencing; it allows for scaffolding, modeling, and dialogue. Cooperative learning lends itself to peer conferencing. Students write either individually or through shared writing and then conference with others about the content, structure, and form of the product. Regarding form, the teacher or SLP can use a questioning strategy to call attention to grammar, punctuation, and spelling. Often a simple cue such as "Does this sound right to you?" leads the student to self-correct the form. If self-correction does not occur, mini-lessons can be provided to specifically teach the concept. For example, a mini-lesson on subject–verb agreement might include discussion about singular and plural nouns with the appropriate verbs. Sample texts are helpful in providing practice in recognizing appropriate and inappropriate grammatical relationships, so that students then apply these relationships within their own writing. Conferencing is an appropriate strategy for all ages, but educationists might modify the time, place, and setting of conferences with older students.

Atwell (1990) used conferencing to evaluate student writing in her eighth-grade classroom by having students put successive drafts and finished pieces in a folder throughout each quarter. Students usually had between four and seven products that could be evaluated for growth. She then posted some questions for students to think about and spent time during grading week conferencing with each student about their accomplishments based on goals they had set for themselves, as well as developing future goals for the next quarter. Letter grades in writing were then determined according to how well each student met the goals.

Spelling

Spelling proficiency is one aspect of form that writers must develop. Spelling words in English requires several different strategies that involve thinking and reasoning abilities. Knowledge of graphophonemics (i.e., sound–symbol relationships), letter sequence and combination rules, silent letter patterns requiring visualization, syllable structure, morphological rules, the ability to analyze words by syllables and sounds, and the ability to synthesize sounds and syllables to make a word are important aspects in learning to spell. Emergent writers begin to explore spelling by experimenting with writing tools, matching some sounds with letters, and inventing spelling for words they want to write. Young children need the freedom to explore, take risks, test their ideas, and have fun with written language (Buchanan, 1989; Graves, 1994; Hagerty, 1994). As youngsters show interest, mind-set, and purpose, they need guidance and instruction in learning all the cues that spellers use: graphophonemic relationships, use of rules and conventions, visual word configurations, and derivational prefixes and suffixes. Graves (1994) noted that 46% of English words are spelled the way they sound, but 54% require visual memory because they have silent letters or require the application of specific rules. Thus, teachers, specialists, and SLPs must help students learn to use all of the available cues.

One of the best ways for students to become good spellers is through reading (Rhodes & Dudley-Marling, 1996). However, some students show adequate ability to decode during reading, but not adequate spelling of those words. The different abilities in reading and spelling occur because the processes involved in decoding print and encoding it are different. Decoding involves analyzing the printed word through recognition abilities, phonics strategies, use of context cues when available, and visual memory. Spelling, on the other hand, involves thinking about the word, accessing memory for its visual configuration, listening to the syllables and sounds, recalling silent letters or rules, and representing the word by writing letters in the correct sequence. Thus, students require explicit teaching of spelling strategies and practice in using them in writing activities.

Table 12.5 provides a summary of strategies that can be used for spelling instruction within an integrated language perspective. Some of the strategies are appropriate for classroom and small group instruction, whereas others provide individualized instruction for students having difficulty with spelling. All of the strategies can be modified in consideration of students' age and progress in spelling, as well as the instructional setting.

Students must attend to the spelling of words that occur frequently in oral and written language. When students are able to spell words that occur often in the language, they increase their ability to write sentences and paragraphs on their own. High-frequency word lists are useful for students to practice writing, preferably within sentences so that they express meaning. For example, words such as *was*, *the*, *can*, *at*, *for*, *with*, *a*, and *feel* do not convey meaning when spoken or written in isolation of other words. They take on meaning only when they are written within the context of an idea. Therefore, as students practice writing words in meaningful sentences, they also learn correct spellings.

Individual word lists can also be useful for students as they encounter spelling difficulties during writing. For instance, a student having difficulty with the application of rules such as "doubling the final consonant before adding a suffix" can enter examples of words in a journal. The teacher, specialist, or SLP can use the words to engage the student in mini-lessons about this rule and to encourage the student to use the words often during writing. Mini-lessons can occur in small groups as spelling difficulties occur.

Lessons in spelling can also occur with the entire class as part of the language arts curriculum. This practice is common in the early grades as children learn about using phonics strategies, whole word strategies, and visual cues to spell words. Although some children develop spelling easily, others need to have the cues made explicit. Educationists can model the thinking processes for spelling just as they can for reading. Thinking aloud helps students learn how others approach and solve the spelling problem. For students who continue to have

Table 12.5
Spelling Strategies

High-Frequency Words

- Make student lists from both high-frequency word lists and the student's own writing.
- Students practice using the words in meaningful contexts.

Personal Word Lists

- Teacher and student review writing for misspellings.
- Record misspellings in one column and conventional spellings in another column.
- Look for patterns of misspellings and plan mini-lesson to teach about patterns.
- Group students with similar needs for mini-lessons.
- Student keeps a record of the misspelled words and continues to work on them.

Practice of Misspelled Words

- Student attempts to write word correctly from previous knowledge.
- Teacher or peer provides feedback on what is correct and what needs to be changed.
- Student continues to use words correctly in writing.

Teacher Modeling of Think-Aloud Process

- Teacher collects words that are difficult for most to spell.
- Teacher demonstrates the thinking process associated with figuring out word spellings.

Proofreading and Dictionary Skills

- Use proofreading to identify and correct misspellings.
- Spell-check writing if using a word processor.
- Use spelling dictionary.
- Use hand-held spell-checker.

(continues)

Table 12.5 *Continued.*

Graphophonics

- Focus on predictable sound–symbol relationships encountered in reading and writing activities.
- Teach sound patterns within words that are difficult for students.
- Show students the high predictability of letter combinations in words that rhyme.
- Show students the high predictability of morphemes such as prefixes, suffixes, and common grammatical endings.
- Encourage a sounding-out strategy if this is an effective strategy.
- Discover rules through mini-lessons as children encounter the need for rules.
- Teach children to recognize when rules are applicable.
- Use knowledge about spelling to generalize to other unfamiliar words.

Dictionary Skills

- Teach students to use a spelling dictionary that is kept with their writing materials.
- Use the dictionary to focus on meaning of words.
- Use the dictionary to focus on information about pronunciation, spelling, and word derivations.
- Teach students to use alphabetizing as a strategy to find words.

Visual Memory Techniques

- Heighten awareness of the shapes of letters and words.
- Use word processing to make spelling attempts look like print.
- Show how misspellings cause confusions in meaning during reading.
- Focus on metacognitive thinking about whether words look correct.

difficulty, teachers and SLPs can encourage students to use the think-aloud strategy so that further guidance and support can be given.

Instruction in graphophonics during the early grades teaches students about the predictability of English spelling. Students learn about sound–symbol relationships, frequently occurring letter combinations, common prefixes and suffixes, and the patterns that allow rule application. The predictability and regularity of these patterns help students generalize what they know about spelling from one word to another. Coupled with awareness and knowledge of predictable visual patterns, students problem-solve during each attempt to spell words as they write.

Young writers should be taught to edit and revise their work; therefore, proofreading and dictionary use should be incorporated early in writing instruction. Some techniques for students in early grades include using first and last letter cues to look up words in a grade-appropriate dictionary; practicing alphabetizing words in functional activities (e.g., address books, library book location, yellow pages); looking up words to check spelling, pronunciation, and word derivations; and noting spelling similarity in words. When a word processor is being used, students should be encouraged to enter in their journals the correct spellings found through spell-checkers, so that they can practice these or receive instruction through mini-lessons. Older students should become more independent in using the dictionary during writing and editing, as well as using other tools such as a thesaurus to build variety in vocabulary. Older students can also proofread their own work, as well as help peers identify spelling and other mistakes.

Summary

Writing develops through many years of experience, instruction, practice, and feedback. The writer's interest, mind-set, purpose, and mental schemas are as important to writing as they are to reading. These attributes, along with experience and instruction in writing, help students use writing for thinking and communicating.

Writers must learn to engage in several components that make writing an integrated process. The process involves rehearsal, drafting and revising, editing, and sharing and publishing, and involve the writer in a spiral-like process in which content, structure, and form are visited and revisited, critiqued, analyzed, and modified. Teachers, SLPs, and students use many strategies to work on the structure (e.g., narrative or expository genres) and the form (e.g., spelling, punctuation, proofreading) of writing.

Summary

Educationists at all levels are faced with the challenge of determining the reading and writing needs of students, and with providing interesting and useful instruction in these processes. Depending on each student's background and experiences, language strengths and weaknesses, previous instructional successes or setbacks, and learning styles, the amount of support needed will vary. However, it is important for teachers and specialists to recognize that all students learn to read and write in similar ways as they gain experience and receive instruction. Students with language or learning problems may progress at a slower pace or may have particular difficulties in various aspects of reading and writing. Consequently, keen observation and the employment of strategies taught in a systematic fashion will help teachers, SLPs, and students determine the most effective strategies to suit individual needs.

Reading and writing are multifaceted processes that are interactive in nature. As such, they should be taught within an integrated framework in the classroom. Although each process has several components, the central goal should be that students read and write to accomplish many meaningful purposes.

Reading instruction should focus on three main areas that, when taught together, facilitate the students' use of all available cues in written language: phonological awareness, decoding and fluency, and comprehension. A focus on phonological awareness in the early grades provides students with a strong background in how sounds and sound patterns are used to create words and how words have similar sound attributes and configurations (e.g., rhymes, alliteration, consonants, vowels). Students learn how sounds can be manipulated to change not only the sounds of words but their meanings as well. This foundation in phonological awareness provides students with the background necessary for effectively interacting with written language.

The early grades are also important for focusing on decoding and fluency during reading. Phonological awareness becomes associated with written language as students learn about how words look. They experiment with letter–sound combinations, noting patterns in rhymes and alliterations, and encounter many words over and over again in sentences. Students learn that written sentences are similar to those in oral language. The predictable use of words then becomes an important cue as they decode sentences. As students gain experience in decoding, they increase their speed and accuracy during reading. Older students can have difficulty decoding and reading fluently. They may have poor phonological awareness or difficulty using the graphophonemic, semantic, and syntactic cues that other students use more easily. Strategies for teaching decoding and fluency in early elementary grades and for older elementary and middle school students focus on using predictable contexts, increasing use of metacognitive strategies, providing strategies for improving decoding per se, practicing using cues in reading, and using techniques to improve rate and fluency.

Students at all levels require instruction in deriving meaning from texts. Comprehension is after all the main purpose for reading. Reader interest, mind-set, purpose, and mental schemas are important for readers in gaining meaning from print, but must be supplemented with decoding and fluency instruction. The primary goal of instruction in reading comprehension is to engage the reader in the interactive process of constructing meaning. This is done prior to reading through prediction activities, during reading through self-monitoring strategies, and as a follow-up to reading through reflection. Strategies for each of these phases of reading were discussed, along with some ideas for using them with elementary and high school students.

Writing is also a process involving several components, which should be incorporated into classroom instruction along with reading, speaking, and listening activities. Students need to view themselves as writers by fostering interest, focusing mind-set, discovering purposes, and learning about the mental schemas appropriate to different purposes. Teachers, peers, and SLPs provide instruction, guidance, and support in the use of strategies that engage writers in rehearsal, drafting, editing, revising, sharing, and publishing. These strategies help writers engage in several metacognitive and interactive processes involving thinking, planning, reasoning, self-monitoring, searching, and interacting with others.

Because writing involves purpose, students need instruction in the various genres that are used to communicate ideas to readers. Reading across various genres helps students recognize the organizational structures common to them. Narratives typically contain setting, characters, problem, solution, and ending, whereas expository chapters contain an introduction, topic paragraphs with headings, and a summary. Experience and instruction involving analysis and discussion about the structures are necessary so that students can write using these organizational structures.

Finally, students must learn how to write so that ideas are conveyed through well-constructed sentences and paragraphs that contain proper grammar, punctuation, and spelling. Direct instruction in these aspects, along with attention to editing and revising writing in meaningful activities, allows students the opportunity to learn about the importance of form and gain experience in developing its use in authentic situations.

Interventions within classrooms for students with reading and writing problems require commitment and collaboration. Recall from Chapter 9 that teachers, specialists, and SLPs working together can remove barriers that prevent students from attaining their potentials. They must work with parents and each student to determine the type and extent of support needed. In the early grades, verbal instruction and demonstration accompany instruction in the language arts, with plenty of time for guided practice. Teachers, peers, and SLPs are more able to provide mini-lessons and use conferencing as a vehicle to individualize instruction. Moderate to severe reading problems in older students can present barriers to student learning; therefore, the team and the student must consider ways to maximize student learning while the reading and writing processes are being addressed. Occasionally, it may be necessary for some students to work on reading and writing outside of the classroom. However, collaboration can result in focusing such instruction on relevant activities that can improve the students' functioning in classroom reading and writing activities.

I THINK I'LL TRY THIS WORD AGAIN
HMMM?
AND when tweetle beetles bettle with paddles in a puddle, they call it a tweetle beetle....
T.M. BALCHAK 9/98

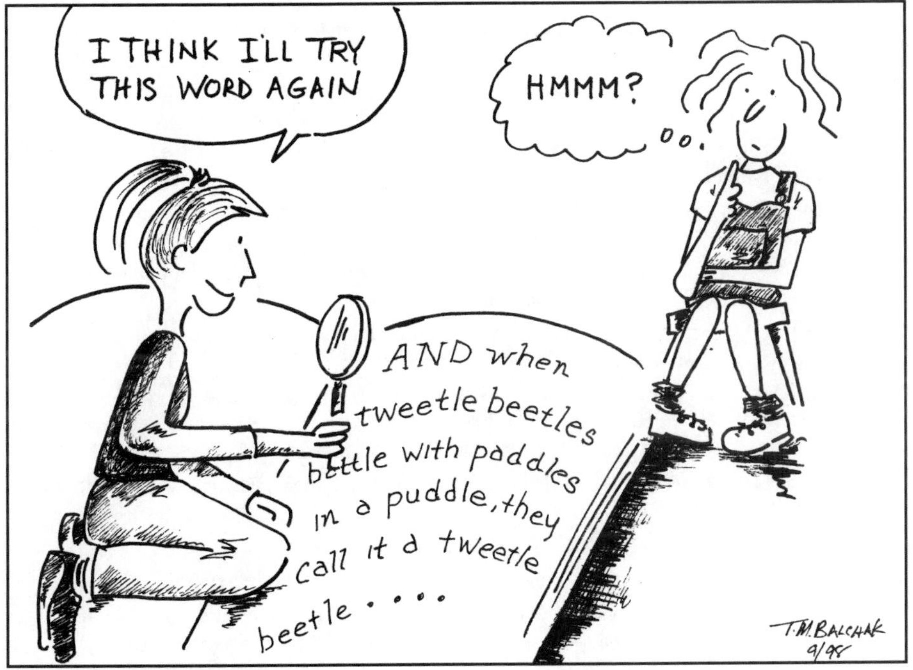

Searching, self-monitoring, and self-questioning are three powerful strategies for effective reading and writing.

References

Adams, M. J. (1990). *Beginning to read: Thinking and learning about print*. Cambridge, MA: MIT Press.

Allington, R. L. (1983). The reading instruction provided readers of different reading ability. *The Elementary School Journal, 83*, 95–107.

Allington, R. L., & Cunningham, P. M. (1996). *Schools that work: Where all children read and write*. New York: HarperCollins College Publishers.

Allington, R. L., & Walmsley, S. A. (1995). *No quick fix: Rethinking literacy programs in America's elementary schools*. New York: Teachers College Press.

Armbruster, B. B., Anderson, T. H., & Ostertag, J. (1989). Teaching text structure to improve reading and writing. *The Reading Teacher, 43*, 130–137.

Atwell, N. (Ed.). (1990). *Coming to know writing to learn in the intermediate grades*. Portsmouth, NH: Heinemann.

Auman, M. (1993). *Expository writing and content reading strategies that guarantee success for teachers and students*. Lecture in course taught at Colorado State University, Fort Collins.

Ball, E. W. (1997). Phonological awareness: Implications for whole language and emergent literacy programs. *Topics in Language Disorders, 17*(3), 14–26.

Bartel, N. (1995). Teaching students who have reading problems. In D. D. Hammill (Ed.), *Teaching students with learning and behavioral problems* (pp. 140–141). Austin, TX: PRO-ED.

Blachman, B. (1989). Phonological awareness and word recognition: Assessment and intervention. In A. Kamhi & H. Catts (Eds.), *Reading disabilities: A developmental language perspective*. Boston: College-Hill.

Buchanan, E. (1989). *Spelling for whole language classrooms*. Winnipeg, Manitoba: Whole Language Consultants.

Butler, D. (1979). *Cushla and her books*. Boston: Horn Book.

Calkins, L. M. (1994). *The art of teaching writing*. Portsmouth, NH: Heinemann.

Catts, H. W. (1991). Phonological processing deficits and reading disabilities. In A. G. Kamhi & H. W. Catts (Eds.), *Reading disabilities: A developmental language perspective* (pp. 101–132). Boston: Allyn & Bacon.

Clay, M. M. (1991). *Becoming literate: The construction of inner control*. Portsmouth, NH: Heinemann.

Conrad, L. L. (1997, Spring). Exploring informational texts with students. *Colorado Reading Council Journal, 8*, 4–11.

Crafton, L. (1994). *Challenges in holistic teaching: Answering the tough questions*. Norwood, MA: Christopher-Gordon.

Cunningham, P. M., & Allington, R. L. (1994). *Classrooms that work: They can all read and write*. New York: HarperCollins.

Dancing with the pen: The learner as writer (4th impression). (1995). Wellington, New Zealand: Learning Media.

Daniels, H., Zemelman, S., & Bizar, M. (1998, Summer). Teacher alert! Phonics fads sweep nation's schools. *Rethinking Schools*.

Davey, B. (1985, November). Helping readers think beyond print through self-questioning. *Middle School Journal*, pp. 38–41.

Fernald, G. (1943). *Remedial techniques in basic school subjects*. New York: McGraw-Hill.

Fink, R. P. (1996). Successful dyslexics: A constructivist study of passionate interest reading. *Journal of Adolescent and Adult Literacy*, 39(4), 268–280.

Frost, J. A., & Emery, M. J. (1996). Academic interventions for children with dyslexia who have phonological core deficits. *The Council for Exceptional Children*, 28(3), 80–83.

Gentry, J. R. (1982, November). An analysis of developmental spelling in GNYS AT WRK. *The Reading Teacher*, pp. 192–199.

Goodman, Y. M. (1978, June). Kid watching: An alternative to testing. *National Elementary School Principal*, 57, 41–45.

Graves, D. H. (1994). *A fresh look at writing*. Portsmouth, NH: Heinemann.

Hagerty, P. J. (1994). *Teaching spelling through writing*. Englewood, CO: Teacher Ideas Press.

Hansen, J. (1987). *When writers read*. Portsmouth, NH: Heinemann.

Heckelman, R. G. (1969). A neurological–impress method of remedial-reading instruction. *Academic Therapy*, 4, 277–282.

International Reading Association & National Council of Teachers of English. (1996). *Standards for the English language arts*. Newark, DE: International Reading Association.

Jenkins, R., & Bowen, L. (1994). Facilitating development of preliterate children's phonological abilities. *Topics in Language Disorders*, 14(2), 26–39.

Koppenhaver, D. A., Coleman, P. P., Kalman, S. L., & Yoder, D. E. (1991). The implications of emergent literacy research for children with developmental disabilities, *American Journal of Speech–Language Pathology: A Journal of Clinical Practice*, 1(1), 38–48.

Liberman, I. Y., & Liberman, A. M. (1990). Whole language vs. code emphasis: Underlying assumptions and their implications for reading instruction. *Annals of Dyslexia*, 40, 51–76.

Lindamood, P., & Lindamood, P. (1998). *The Lindamood phoneme sequencing program for reading, spelling, and speech*. Austin, TX: PRO-ED.

Lowry, L. (1993). *The giver*. Boston: Houghton Mifflin.

Lund, N., & Duchan, J. (1993). *Assessing children's language in naturalistic contexts* (3rd ed.). Englewood Cliffs, NJ: Prentice-Hall.

Michener, J. A. (1974). *Centennial*. Greenwich, CT: Fawcett.

Miller, J., & Paul, R. (1995). *The clinical assessment of language comprehension*. Baltimore: Brookes.

Mullen, J. L. (1987). *College reading and learning skills*. Englewood Cliffs, NJ: Prentice-Hall.

Nelson, N. W. (1998). *Childhood language disorders in context: Infancy through adolescence*. Needham Heights, MA: Allyn & Bacon.

Norris, J. A. (1997). Functional language intervention in the classroom: Avoiding the tutoring trap. *Topics in Language Disorders*, 17(2), 49–68.

Pappas, C. C., Kiefer, B. Z., & Levstik, L. S. (1995). *An integrated language perspective in the elementary school: Theory into action* (2nd ed.). White Plains, NY: Longman.

Paul, R. (1995). *Language disorders from infancy through adolescence: Assessment and intervention*. St. Louis: Mosby.

Pearson, P. D., & Gallagher, M. C. (1983). The instruction of reading comprehension. *Contemporary Educational Psychology*, 8, 317–344.

Poplin, M. S. (1988). The reductionist fallacy in learning disabilities: Replicating the past by reducing the present. *Journal of Learning Disabilities*, 21, 389–400.

Reutzel, D., & Cooter, R. (1996). *Teaching children to read from basals to books*. Englewood Cliffs, NJ: Prentice-Hall.

Rhodes, L. K., & Dudley-Marling, C. (1996). *Readers and writers with a difference: A holistic approach to teaching struggling readers and writers* (2nd ed.). Portsmouth, NH: Heinemann.

Routman, R. (1991). *Invitations: Changing as teachers and learners K–12*. Portsmouth, NH: Heinemann.

Schwartz, R. M. (1997). Self-monitoring in beginning reading. *The Reading Teacher, 51*(1), 40–48.

Silliman, E., & Wilkinson, L. (1991). *Communicating for learning: Classroom observation and collaboration*. Gaithersburg, MD: Aspen.

Snowling, M. J. (1995). Phonological processing and developmental dyslexia. *Journal of Research in Reading, 18*(2), 132–138.

Stanovich, K. (1986). Cognitive processes and the reading problems of learning disabled children: Evaluating the assumption of specificity. In J. Torgensen & B. Wong (Eds.), *Psychological and educational perspectives on learning disabilities* (pp. 87–131). New York: Academic Press.

Tunmer, W. E., & Cole, P. G. (1991). Learning to read: A metalinguistic act. In C. S. Simon (Ed.), *Communication skills and classroom success: Assessment and therapy methodologies for language and learning disabled students* (pp. 386–402). Eau Claire, WI: Thinking Publications.

van Kleeck, A. (1990). Emergent literacy: Learning about print before learning to read. *Topics in Language Disorders, 10*(2), 25–45.

Wise, B. W. (1991). What reading disabled children need: What is known and how to talk about it. *Learning and Individual Differences, 3*(4), 307–321.

Zinsser, W. (1988). *Writing to learn*. New York: Harper & Row.

Epilogue

D. Kim Reid

Discourse is both the content of and the context for classroom learning. Consequently, general and special education teachers as well as specialists, such as speech–language pathologists (SLPs), who work in schools must understand how it affects learning. Those students who come to school speaking developmentally appropriate Standard American English (SAE) have an academic advantage over students whose language acquisition lags behind that of their peers, whose language and culture deviate from the mainstream, or who have language learning problems. Even when the manifesting problem is not language per se (e.g., special education categories, such as mental retardation or other health impaired), language problems tend to be implicated.

Language Development

Students entering school must adjust to differences between home and school language usage. These differences typically include, but are not limited to, three forms of classroom discourse that are seldom taught explicitly—the language of curriculum, the language of control, and the language of personal identity (i.e., underground talk). Furthermore, teachers begin even in kindergarten show-and-tell sessions to shape students' language so that it conforms to the scientific concepts register, as well as SAE. Such early interventions sometimes backfire, thus confusing, embarrassing, or even silencing students who have not been introduced to this discourse at home.

The most typical form of classroom discourse is the IRE model in which the teacher directs the lesson, interacting with one student after another. Because this model requires students to answer rapidly in a few specific words and virtually eliminates interactions among students, it is not well suited to fostering growth in language. Two instructional frameworks that are more effective in many instances are teacher's revoicing and the use of instructional conversations, scripted or natural. Because teaching and learning are inherently social activities, the dialogic interactions afforded by the latter models typically get better results, especially among nonmainstream students.

Discourse Development

At least three genres of discourse develop during the school years: conversation, narrative, and exposition. Although children's immersion in conversation begins almost at the moment of birth and narrative shortly thereafter, most children acquire the bulk of their knowledge of expository language in school, often through reading and writing. The primary source of early language learning is the family and children's language experiences, which vary in almost every way that families vary. Seldom, however, do school curricula take into account the vastly different language histories that children have had prior to schooling.

Consequently, students whose conversational language does not match school expectations, for any of the reasons noted in the opening paragraph, often do poorly. As they advance through the grades, the effects can become increasingly deleterious, especially as the students encounter more and more demanding models, participate in lessons that are increasingly text based, and confront the more frequent use of figurative expressions. On the other hand, children who learned the language of schooling at home, as most middle and upper class students do, typically make the transition to school discourse easily. It is a case of the rich getting richer and the poor getting poorer, while the curriculum remains focused on the content without regard to the impact of the linguistic context.

The case of narrative development is similar. Nearly all children learn about story structures in their homes, because humans tend to use stories in day-to-day conversations. There is evidence that storytelling begins quite early, in rudimentary form at least by age 3, and develops from simple sentence strings to highly organized, interrelated units that employ literary devices, such as flashbacks. Although stories tend to predominate in preschools and elementary schools, emphasis on narration gradually wanes as the focus on exposition becomes more pronounced, beginning in the upper elementary grades and continuing throughout high school, where narratives are usually reserved for English classes. Like conversation, stories vary by culture. Who can tell a story, what emphases it should have, and what form it takes all vary. Again, however, the curriculum generally accepts only one form of story, that associated with SAE. The antidote is to accept whatever language or dialect students bring to school and to (a) immerse students in SAE (sometimes through bilingual education) and (b) help make students metacognitively and metalinguistically aware of the contrasts and similarities across those dialects and languages. Educationists must help students learn to cross linguistic boundaries at will.

Children are often introduced to exposition during the preschool years as they learn to make cookies or listen to descriptive sections of books. It becomes the dominating discourse genre in schools beginning about the fourth grade. One of the most complicated issues related to exposition is that some of the examples to which students are regularly exposed (e.g., poorly organized teacher lectures or textbooks that assume too much prior knowledge) are poorly structured. Consequently, students often must compensate for the limitations of the texts. This situation makes learning very difficult for students with language or language-related difficulties. Consequently, teachers and specialists need to pay careful attention to their own talk as well as analyze textbooks carefully, making sure that their students have the necessary background knowledge about both the content and the genre to make the transitions between what they hear or read and what they can understand.

Oral Language Development

Success in school is dependent on language competence and performance as well as the development of the language systems: phonology, suprasegmentals, morphology and syntax, semantics, metalinguistics, and pragmatics. School discourse, however, requires not only adequate acquisition within each system, but also smooth operations among them.

Children's articulation abilities develop throughout the preschool years and, by the time they enter kindergarten, are sufficiently well developed to enable them to engage in functional and intelligible communication. When children enter school, they are asked to think not only *in* language but also *about* language (i.e., metalinguistics). They relate sounds to letters of the alphabet and to combinations of these letters. The instructional emphasis shifts to phonemic awareness, which is essential to the acquisition of written language abilities. Throughout adolescence articulation and phonology continue to become refined.

Suprasegmentals begin to develop very early and by the time the infant is 6 months old, babbling has already taken on the characteristics of the child's specific linguistic environment (i.e., there are differences in the ways that Chinese and French babies, for example, babble that are linked to the language they are learning). During the elementary school years, children learn to use prosody to highlight new information and to mark grammatical structures. High school students and adults become attuned to dialects and incorporate suprasegmentals into literacy styles.

Most children say their first intelligible word at about 1 year and then augment their utterances by adding and combining morphemes. In fact, professionals determine a child's developmental age by counting morphemes to estimate the child's mean length of utterance. The larger number of morphemes, the more complex the syntax. By the time children enter school, most can produce declarative, interrogative, and imperative sentences. Still, some difficulties (e.g., with pronoun references or irregular past tense verbs) continue to exist through the early school grades. Later, augmenting syntactic complexity becomes primarily a matter of using compound and complex clause combinations to achieve longer sentences. Throughout high school and into adulthood, students continue to develop new abilities (e.g., the use of conjunctions and cohesive devices) and to refine old ones (e.g., the use of syntactic constructions to compose various discourse genres).

Semantic knowledge continues to develop throughout the life span with the acquisition of new vocabulary, new meanings for words already known, and multiple names for a single object (e.g., *sofa, couch, divan, loveseat,* etc., or calling the planet Venus both the "evening star" and the "morning star"). At first, babies convey semantic information through cries and gestures and then learn to use language. Trying to determine what an individual child knows is difficult because of differences in levels of competence and performance. We do know, however, that language growth is rapid and that even preschoolers are sufficiently sophisticated to engage in and appreciate humor. Likewise, elementary-age through high school students grow continuously in vocabulary and concept knowledge. Children generally love riddles in elementary school and more personal jokes (verbal bantering) in adolescence. As they grow, the students become more adept at both figurative language and slang. A rich source for new words and phrases in English is adolescent and young adult slang (e.g., *cool, dude, phat*). These slang terms are often adopted from other sources. *Cool,* for example, originally described jazz that was no longer hot.

For years, researchers suspected that there was some important link between oral and written language that was difficult to trace: Many students who seem to speak well exhibit difficulties with reading and writing. It was not until a few decades ago that science revealed the link to be metalinguistics. Metalinguistic knowledge does not, however, begin in school. Even very young infants have been shown to discriminate differences in speech sounds and preschoolers self-monitor the correctness of their own and others' utterances. During elementary school, students are generally taught about language (e.g., parts of speech, sentence construction) and come to recognize when language usage is inappropriate ("Did you hear how she talked to the principal?"). Among high school students metalinguistic knowledge expands to include methods for finding information and proofreading.

Because all of these systems must be acquired and then integrated into discourse structures, language is inordinately complex. In fact, children's language acquisition is so awe-inspiring that Chomsky (1976) suggested that it is not learned at all. Instead, he posited that there is an innate Language Acquisition

Device (LAD) that is specific to humans. Careful and sustained examination of interactions between parents and their children, however, revealed that, in addition to the LAD, there is a LASS, what Bruner (1978) identified as the Language Acquisition Support System. Together, they ensure that nearly all people acquire language.

Written Language Development

Literacy, however, is not acquired by everyone. The term *literacy* has been extended recently to refer to a person's ability to engage fully and effectively in his or her community. This extension recognizes that reading and writing are meaningful social and political processes. Although nearly everyone acquires oral language and there are certainly significant overlaps between oral and written language, there are also very significant differences between them. Anyone who has studied a second language as an older child or adult realizes that reading and speaking the language are very different things, as are understanding it and writing in it. The differences are physical, form, and process related, and situational and functional. Where traditional approaches to reading instruction have been either top–down (i.e., they rely primarily on semantic, syntactic, and lexical cues) or bottom–up (i.e., they rely on analysis and synthesis of phonemes in isolation), more contemporary approaches are holistic and integrated. The reason is that reading is a process that requires coordination of all cueing systems *simultaneously*. Consequently, Adams (1990) advocated teaching reading using connected texts; taking time to address strategies and abilities related to comprehending that text, including decoding; and then moving back to the connected text again. Practice reading is what promotes good reading, not isolated exercises and drills.

Furthermore, reading and writing are developmental processes. Primitive forms of reading and writing behaviors emerge with the *symbolic function* (described by Piaget, 1970)—that is, when children begin to represent activity sequences and things in words; through imitation (i.e., pretending that a broomstick is a horse), drawing, and writing; in symbolic play; and so forth. It is about that time, somewhere around the age of 2 or 2½, that students start scribbling on the walls and noticing environmental print. Thus, a child does not, as we traditionally thought, get *ready* to read and write. Reading and writing emerge gradually throughout most of the preschool years for children who are exposed to print in their environments (and continue to develop throughout the life span). The more that adults interact with children around print, especially during storybook reading, before they come to school, the more likely those children are to do well in reading and writing in school.

Language Differences

Language and culture are inextricably intertwined and, consequently, language is central to our identities. That is why schools are not neutral institutions; curriculum choices are always infused with political values (Cherryholmes, 1988). Both what is selected for inclusion and what is left out make important statements about the values of our nation. Considerable research has suggested that the closer the school environment is to the values and practices of the children's communities, the more successful the children are in school. This set of findings explains, at least in part, why students from nonmainstream groups are often overrepresented in special education classes.

Another reason is that language differences are often misunderstood as language deficiencies or even disorders. Recent laws have protected children whose native language is other than English, but there is still a problem with students of the second generation, who learn a nonstandard dialect of English at home from their parents, who are themselves just learning the English language. These students often fail to do well in school, but they are not eligible for special services or bilingual or English as a Second Language classes, and often educationists regard them as using "bad English" rather than as speaking a dialect. Many general and special education teachers as well as SLPs are from the mainstream culture and do not understand the language characteristics that members of nonmainstream groups are likely to exhibit.

Language Disorders

Although it is difficult to ascertain the causes of language delays and disorders with any assurance, a rather well-articulated classification system exists to define language difficulties. These categories include language impairments, central auditory processing disorders, attention-deficit/hyperactivity disorder, mental retardation, traumatic brain injury, pervasive developmental disorder and autism, maltreatment, and exposure to substance abuse. Although only one of these diagnostic categories focuses on language behaviors per se, all of the others include language delays or disorders as symptoms. Even though these types of categories are useful for identifying students who need services, the label seldom suggests the types of interventions that might prove useful, especially when students demonstrate mild to moderate difficulties (e.g., students who are labeled as learning disabled, mentally retarded, and emotionally disturbed). Most often, different kinds of assessments (e.g., observations, analyses of student-made products) need to be carried out to determine what the student knows and is ready to learn.

There is another group of, again, rather well-defined disorders that affect school performance. This group includes hearing impairment and deafness, visual impairment and blindness, motor speech disorders, cleft lip and palate, and speech problems (e.g., fluency and prosody, voice, and articulation and phonological problems). As with the previous group, all of these difficulties often have accompanying speech–language delays or disorders as well. In this case, however, some of the diagnoses do suggest appropriate methods of intervention (e.g., motor speech disorders, cleft lip and palate).

Language Interventions

According to the American Speech-Language-Hearing Association Ad Hoc Committee on the Roles and Responsibilities of the School-Based Speech–Language Pathologist (1999) guidelines for SLPs, the preferred approach to intervention in the late 1990s is a collaborative one. Similar statements abound in the literature of special education. There are many forms of collaboration and each is useful, even though they vary with respect to just how collaborative they are. Many times financial, situational, theoretical, or time constraints play an important role in determining how services will be delivered, and sometimes one model is better for addressing a particular kind of problem than another. Although we educationists increasingly advocate collaborative models, schools are not now organized in ways that facilitate collaborative approaches. Still, the data indicate that such models are effective and many teams throughout the country have found ways to implement various forms of collaborative activities.

The philosophy of instruction is also changing. Traditionally, interventions were carried out directly by specialists in locations removed from the general education classroom. Now students are educated in the least restricted environment (LRE), which is usually, but not always, the general education classroom. Reasons for this shift include the assumption that it is important to determine what the child is able to do (i.e., to observe how children with language delays and disorders cope and how successful they are and in what ways the students fail to meet their own needs), to teach new behaviors in the contexts in which they will be used, to teach students to become more independent learners and to self-advocate, and to alter contexts whenever possible to foster more rapid and sustained growth. Some effective, classroom-based interventions for students with language dysfunction include the teaching of learning strategies, verbal mediation, scaffolding, self-monitoring, engaging students in dialogic interactions, cooperative learning, and reciprocal teaching. Intervention strategies for students with sensory problems, motor speech disorders, cleft lip and palate, and other speech production problems are somewhat more individually specified, although many of the strategies previously listed can be useful.

Many of these same intervention strategies have proven useful for students who are having difficulties with written language. Assessments that are useful to planning interventions tend to be classroom based, rather than standardized (standardized tests are more useful to determine the student's rank order in the norming group). Some of the most important literacy strategies to be taught in the LRE are searching, self-monitoring, and self-questioning. Reciprocal teaching has been demonstrated as an effective way of teaching those behaviors to students with reading difficulties. For students who need it, phonological awareness must be addressed as well. Reading instruction must also include emphases on decoding and fluency as well as comprehension.

Interventions designed to foster writing development are process oriented: rehearsal, drafting, revising, editing, and sharing and publishing. Some activities that are useful are shared and group writing activities, modeling of the writing process and of specific genres, having students write before and after reading, using computers to write, conferencing, and attending to spelling issues.

Conclusion

This book has been an effort to elucidate the role that language plays in academic achievement and to raise issues about how language might get in the way of academic gains. It is not an attempt to be all inclusive; most general and special education teachers do not need the level of knowledge about language development, differences, and disorders that is needed by SLPs, who are hired for their expertise in this area. On the other hand, there is a good deal of knowledge about what goes on in the LRE that SLPs can benefit from as well. The data suggest that general education teachers have had some negative reactions to many of their consultation experiences, often because they thought that the suggestions were unrealistic.

In the best of all possible worlds, students, parents, and educationists would come together as equals and have sufficient time and social-interactional skills to work collaboratively not only to solve language-related problems, but also to prevent such problems from developing in the first place. We are not there yet. Still, Chapter 9 described models that have proven to be feasible and effective. We might learn from these, while keeping our eye on the ideal and moving toward it as we can. If, for one reason or another, we need to continue to work in pull-out or other segregated settings, many of the intervention strategies that have been suggested for teams can be implemented individually.

Nevertheless, the best way to honor the right to an appropriate education in the LRE for students who do not, for one reason or another, fit the general education language mold is to reconfigure the general education classroom to meet their needs—and this is the job of all educationists. The goal of meeting all students' needs requires that we educationists recognize the impact that contexts have on learning and our ability to facilitate learning by changing aspects of those contexts. Problems do not exist only within the student; they result from interactions among myriad internal and external factors. However, because discourse is both the content of and the context for classroom learning, it is probably the most important element to consider and manipulate in increasing the numbers of successes and diminishing the incidence of failure in our schools.

References

Adams, M. J. (1990). *Beginning to read.* Cambridge, MA: MIT Press.

American Speech-Language-Hearing Association Ad Hoc Committee on the Roles and Responsibilities of the School-Based Speech–Language Pathologist. (1999). *Guidelines for the roles and responsibilities of the school-based speech–language pathologist.* Rockville, MD: Author.

Bruner, J. (1978). On prelinguistic prerequisites of speech. In R. N. Campbell & P. T. Smith (Eds.), *Recent advances in the psychology of language* (pp. 242–256). New York: Plenum.

Cherryholmes, C. H. (1988). *Power and criticism: Poststructural investigations in education.* New York: Teachers College Press.

Chomsky, N. (1976). On the biological basis of language capacities. In R. W. Rieber (Ed.), *The neuropsychology of language* (pp. 1–24). New York: Plenum.

Piaget, J. (1970). *Structuralism.* New York: Basic Books.

Author Index

Subject Index

About the Authors

Kathleen R. Fahey is an associate professor in the Department of Communication Disorders within the College of Health and Human Sciences at the University of Northern Colorado, Greeley (UNC). She has also taught at Michigan State University. She is a speech–language pathologist who has 20 years of experience in the assessment and intervention of students with speech and language disorders. Her areas of particular expertise focus on school-age students who have language and learning problems and articulation and phonological problems. She currently teaches undergraduate and graduate courses in speech–language pathology and audiology, and is involved in clinical teaching in the full-time audiology and speech–language pathology clinic housed within the department. She is currently a speech–language consultant with the Colorado Department of Education, Special Education Services Unit. She has served as an elected officer in several state professional associations, most recently as president of the Colorado Speech-Language-Hearing Association.

D. Kim Reid is a professor of education at Teachers College, Columbia University, New York. She has also taught at the University of Northern Colorado, the University of Texas, and New York University. She was selected as the distinguished lecturer for the annual meeting of the Council for Learning Disabilities in 1995, distinguished scholar at the University of Northern Colorado in 1996, and Fulbright scholar to Vilnius, Lithuania, in 1998. She has taught graduate courses on language development, language problems faced by students with special needs, and language differences, and a doctoral seminar on discourse processes. She serves as associate editor of *Remedial and Special Education* and a consulting editor for the *Journal of Learning Disabilities* and the *Learning Disabilities Quarterly*. She is the author or co-author of several textbooks on learning disabilities, the *Test of Early Reading Ability–Third Edition*, and numerous articles and chapters.